Neural Development and Schizophrenia

Theory and Research

NATO ASI Series

Advanced Science Institutes Series

A series presenting the results of activities sponsored by the NATO Science Committee, which aims at the dissemination of advanced scientific and technological knowledge, with a view to strengthening links between scientific communities.

The series is published by an international board of publishers in conjunction with the NATO Scientific Affairs Division

A	**Life Sciences**	Plenum Publishing Corporation
B	**Physics**	New York and London
C	**Mathematical and Physical Sciences**	Kluwer Academic Pulishers
D	**Behavioral and Social Sciences**	Dordrecht, Boston, and London
E	**Applied Sciences**	
F	**Computer and Systems Sciences**	Springer-Verlag
G	**Ecological Sciences**	Berlin, Heidelberg, New York, London,
H	**Cell Biology**	Paris, Tokyo, Hong Kong, and Barcelona
I	**Global Environmental Change**	

Recent Volumes in this Series

Volume 268—Advances in Molecular Plant Nematology
edited by F. Lamberti, C. De Giorgi, and David McK. Bird

Volume 269—Ascomycete Systematics: Problems and Perspectives in
the Nineties
edited by David L. Hawksworth

Volume 270—Standardization of Epidemiologic Studies of Host Susceptibility
edited by Janice S. Dorman

Volume 271—Oscillatory Event-Related Brain Dynamics
edited by Christo Pantev, Thomas Elbert, and Bernd Lütkenhöner

Volume 272—Photobiology in Medicine
edited by Giulio Jori, Roy H. Pottier, Michael A. J. Rodgers, and
T. George Truscott

Volume 273—Targeting of Drugs 4: Advances in System Constructs
edited by Gregory Gregoriadis and Brenda McCormack

Volume 274—Radiofrequency Radiation Standards: Biological Effects, Dosimetry,
Epidemiology, and Public Health Policy
edited by B. Jon Klauenberg, Martino Grandolfo, and David N. Erwin

Volume 275—Neural Development and Schizophrenia: Theory and Research
edited by Sarnoff A. Mednick and J. Meggin Hollister

Series A: Life Sciences

Neural Development and Schizophrenia

Theory and Research

Edited by

Sarnoff A. Mednick and
J. Meggin Hollister

University of Southern California
Los Angeles, California

Plenum Press
New York and London
Published in cooperation with NATO Scientific Affairs Division

Proceedings of a NATO Advanced Study Institute on
Neural Development and Schizophrenia: Theory and Research,
held September 22–October 1, 1993,
in Castelvecchio Pascoli, Italy

NATO-PCO-DATA BASE

The electronic index to the NATO ASI Series provides full bibliographical references (with keywords
and/or abstracts) to more than 30,000 contributions from international scientists published in all
sections of the NATO ASI Series. Access to the NATO-PCO-DATA BASE is possible in two ways:

—via online FILE 128 (NATO-PCO-DATA BASE) hosted by ESRIN, Via Galileo Galilei, I-00044
Frascati, Italy

—via CD-ROM "NATO Science and Technology Disk" with user-friendly retrieval software in English,
French, and German (©WTV GmbH and DATAWARE Technologies, Inc. 1989). The CD-ROM also
contains the AGARD Aerospace Database.

The CD-ROM can be ordered through any member of the Board of Publishers or through
NATO-PCO, Overijse, Belgium.

Library of Congress Cataloging in Publication Data

Neural development and schizophrenia: theory and research / edited by Sarnoff A. Mednick
  and J. Meggin Hollister
      p.   cm.—(NATO ASI series. Series A, Life sciences; v. 275)
  "Proceedings of a NATO Advanced Study Institute on Neural Development and Schizophrenia:
Theory and Research, held September 22--October 1, 1993, in Castelvecchio Pascoli, Italy"—T.
p. verso.
  "Published in cooperation with NATO Scientific Affairs Division."
  Includes bibliographical references and index.
  ISBN 0-306-44996-X
  1. Schizophrenia—Physiological aspects—Congresses. 2. Schizophrenia—Etiology—Con-
gresses. 3. Developmental neurology—Congresses. I. Mednick, Sarnoff A. II. Hollister, J. Meggin.
III. North Atlantic Treaty Organization. Scientific Affairs Division. IV. NATO Advanced Study Institute on Neural Development and Schizophrenia: Theory and Research (1993: Castelvecchio
Pascoli, Italy) V. Series.
  [DNLM: 1. Schizophrenia—pathology—congresses. 2. Schizophrenia—physiopathology—congresses. 3. Schizophrenia—etiology—congresses. 4. Brain—embryology—congresses. 5. Brain—
growth & development—congresses. 6. Prenatal Exposure Delayed Effects—congresses. WM
203 N4926 1995]
RC514.N442   1995
616.89'82—dc20
DNLM/DLC   95-3584
for Library of Congress   CIP

ISBN 0-306-44996-X

PREFACE

This is the third meeting we have organized which has explored the meaning of fetal neural developmental disruption in the etiology of schizophrenia. The first was sponsored by the Schizophrenia Research Branch with the scientific cooperation of Dr. David Shore. We met in Washington; the output of the meeting was published in a book entitled, *Fetal Neural Development and Adult Schizophrenia*, Cambridge University Press, 1991. The next meeting was an Advanced Research Workshop sponsored by NATO and was held at Il Ciocco, Castelvecchio Pascoli. This meeting was reported in a NATO volume, *Developmental Neuropathology of Schizophrenia* and was edited by Mednick, Cannon, Barr and La Fosse.

The current meeting has noted several advances in the field. There are additional psychiatric illnesses which have been found to be related to maternal viral infection in the second trimester. There have been studies reported which have definitely observed a viral infection in the mothers of fetuses who later evidenced schizophrenia. More evidence has been published which has replicated the "second-trimester effect."

In the future studies will be wise to provide serological evidence of a viral infection and information on the precise viruses involved. Another important step will be to determine whether second-trimester maternal viral infection is related to a behavioral deficit in the infant. If neural development has been compromised, it might be possible to detect deficits in the infant with the proper measures. We look forward to future meetings at which these new areas might be explored.

Sarnoff A. Mednick
J. Meggin Hollister

January 1994

ACKNOWLEDGEMENTS

This volume reports the proceedings of the NATO Advanced Study Institute (ASI) on the Neural Development of Schizophrenia which was held in Il Ciocco Hotel, Castelvecchio Pascoli, Italy, from September 22 to October 1, 1993.

We would like to express our most sincere thanks to Mrs. Susan Stack without whom this meeting would never have proceeded so successfully. Susan's involvement in the meeting ranged from the proposal writing and financial planning to helping select lecturers and organizing the program. She spent countless hours in correspondence with lecturers and participants of the ASI as well as with hotel, airline and NATO staff. In sum, Susan's capacity as organizer of this NATO ASI was one of a scientist, a professional, and an administrator. We are extremely grateful to have her as an integral part of our team.

We would like to express our thanks to the lecturers who presented interesting and exciting research on the neural development of schizophrenia from a variety of disciplines and paradigms, and to the participants who provided stimulating and thought provoking questions during the discussion sections. There was general agreement that the discussion periods were unusually fruitful.

We also extend our thanks to NATO for their sponsorship. NATO must be commended for committing resources to this type of meeting that promotes multidisciplinary scientific activity.

The staff at Il Ciocco was, as always, cheerful and effective. We owe a great debt of gratitude to our friend, Mr. Bruno Giannasi, for his intelligent and patient attention to our needs. Finally, we would like to thank Judith Webb for her diligent attention to our editorial changes and for preparing the manuscript for the publishers.

Dr. Mednick's work on this volume was supported by NIMH/NIH grants K05-MH00619-RSA, MH44188, and MH46014, and Ms. Hollister's work on this volume was supported by NIH grant MH19457-03.

CONTENTS

INTRODUCTION

THE DEVELOPING BRAIN

PATHOLOGY OF THE BRAIN OF SCHIZOPHRENICS: IMPLICATIONS FOR NEURODEVELOPMENT

I. Neuroimaging Studies

A MULTIDISCIPLINARY APPROACH TO THE NEURODEVELOPMENT OF SCHIZOPHRENIA

J. Meggin Hollister, Ricardo A. Machon, and Sarnoff A. Mednick

Social Science Research Institute
University of Southern California
Los Angeles, California

INTRODUCTION

In recent years, the hypothesis that disturbances of brain development during gestation may contribute to the risk of adult schizophrenia has gained momentum. This hypothesis was, in part, given new impetus by our finding in 1988 that exposure to influenza during the second trimester of gestation increased the risk for adult schizophrenia (Mednick, Machon, Huttunen & Bonett). In this introductory chapter, we provide: a review of the evidence that supports the hypothesis of a neurodevelopmental process underlying schizophrenia, a brief introduction to the individual chapters included in this volume, and a concluding section regarding our hopes for the future of the multidisciplinary approach to understanding the neurodevelopment of schizophrenia.

Schizophrenia is a developmental process which is expressed long before the onset of psychosis. This evidence spans a variety of disciplines (and subdisciplines) that include clinical psychology, psychiatric epidemiology, and neuroanatomy. This chapter will begin with a review of the neurodevelopmental origins of schizophrenia by examining several lines of research: teratology and neurodevelopment, neuropathology, premorbid history of schizophrenia, and pre- and peri-natal factors, including obstetrical complications and maternal exposure to influenza studies.

TERATOLOGY AND NEURODEVELOPMENT

In order to provide a basis for understanding the neurodevelopmental roots of schizophrenia, we begin with two chapters which provide a historical analysis from teratology and an overall review of the neural mechanisms and processes that may be disturbed in the brains of schizophrenic patients. Chapter 2 by McClure provides a historical perspective from teratology examining the hypothesis that schizophrenia results from errors in fetal development. He reviews evidence of the various exogenous agents which can modify the embryonic development of many species of lower animals. He also reviews the role played by genetics, non-genetic maternal factors as well as the timing of the teratogen all of which can modify many aspects of teratology. He also entertains the notion whether different teratogens might produce the same or similar outcomes.

In the following chapter (3), Jones and Akbarian provide a detailed review highlighting those mechanisms of brain development that may have been disturbed in the brains of schizophrenics and which might be causally linked to the disorder. Their review is divided into three parts: Part 1 is a brief chronology of the developmental hypothesis; Part 2 outlines the principal steps in ontogenesis of the primate forebrain and reviews the morphological abnormalities, already described in brains of schizophrenics that might be linked to interference with one or more of these ontogenetic steps; Part 3 discusses the neuropathology, as related to epidemiological and other data, and the functional consequences, along with strategies aimed at further expanding the developmental hypothesis.

NEUROPATHOLOGY

Post-Mortem Studies

To date, numerous post-mortem studies of the brains of schizophrenics are consistent with the interpretation that these abnormalities originated during fetal neurodevelopment or possibly during early childhood, long before the onset of psychosis. Furthermore, these anomalies do not appear to be the result of a progressive degenerative process as is observed in Parkinson's or Huntington's Disease. The abnormalities reported in post-mortem studies indicating dysplasia include: reduced temporolimbic and thalamic structure volumes and nerve cell numbers without accompanying gliosis; cytoarchitectural anomalies in the hippocampal formation, frontal cortex, cingulate gyrus, and entorhinal cortex; and left lateralized temporal horn enlargement (Bogerts and Falkai, 1991).

Bogerts et al. (1985) compared the brains of 13 schizophrenics to 10 controls and observed a 20-30% volume reduction of the amygdala, hippocampus, and parahippocampal gyrus and a 20% volume reduction of the internal pallidum. The authors presented the hypothesis that the areas of volume reductions are those that may be selectively vulnerable to toxic substances, viruses, and perinatal hypoxia or that an inherited congenital hypoplasia may be responsible for the observed abnormalities. Falkai and Bogerts (1986) reported a reduction of hippocampal pyramidal cells without gliosis while Falkai et al (1988), using the same sample, reported a reduction of volume and cell densities in the entorhinal cortex without gliosis. Finally, Pakkenberg (1990) observed a reduction of total neuron and glial cell number in the mediodorsal thalamic nucleus and the nucleus accumbens. The above findings are considered consistent with a disorder of brain development (Bogerts and Falkai, 1991).

McLardy (1974) reported abnormal granule cell layer in the dentate gyrus of the hippocampal formation in 12 of 30 schizophrenics. The author interpreted the findings as suggestive of a developmental and not degenerative arrest. Disorientation and disarray of hippocampal pyramidal cells was reported by Scheibel and Kovelman (1981) and Kovelman and Scheibel (1984), respectively. The authors suggested that the observed abnormalities represented defective neuronal migration during embryological brain development. Benes et al. (1986) reported cytoarchitectural disturbances in the prefrontal cortex, anterior cingulate and primary motor cortex and reduction of neuronal density without gliosis. In the light of their findings, the authors argued against a progressive degeneration in the schizophrenic brain and suggested that the observed cytoarchitectural abnormalities in the cingulate gyrus might be caused by neuronal dropout early in fetal life. Jakob and Beckman (1986) reported abnormally developed temporal lobes with unusual temporal sulci and gyri in 42 of 64 schizophrenic brains as well as cytoarchitectonic abnormalities in the rostral entorhinal region of the parahippocampal gyrus. They interpreted their findings as suggestive of a disturbance of neuronal migration in the allocortex during the second trimester of pregnancy. Falkai and Bogerts (1989; 1992) also observed abnormalities in the entorhinal region that consisted of unusual location of pre-alpha cell clusters. Bogerts (1989) interprets the absence of gliosis in the hippocampus and entorhinal cortex and the altered shape of the hippocampal formation of some schizophrenics as indicative of a developmental disturbance. Furthermore, the author argues against these abnormalities being the result of pathological influences or degenerative processes occurring later in life.

Neuroimaging Studies

Neuroimaging techniques have provided a means to observe aspects of the living brains of schizophrenics. In addition, researchers are able to observe the brain structure of these individuals through the course of their illness and in some cases before the onset of psychoses. This method provides a means of ascertaining whether the observed abnormalities are progressive or whether they existed prior to the onset of psychoses. A variety of abnormalities have been observed in the brains of individuals with schizophrenia, with ventricular enlargement being the most commonly observed anomaly. Cannon (1991a) reviewed studies appearing before January of 1990 and found that 85% (24/28) reported enlargement of the third ventricle, 79% (55/72) reported enlarged lateral ventricles or ventricle-brain ratio (VBR), and 61% (19/31) reported greater cortical sulcal prominence.

Age and duration of illness have been proposed as possibly accounting for the structural abnormalities observed among schizophrenics. However, if this were true, as Cannon (1991b) noted, one would not expect the abnormalities to be present among very young subjects. The author reviewed 10 studies using teenage psychotics, first episode schizophreniform and schizophrenics within 1 to 2 years of the onset of psychosis and found ventricular enlargement in these subjects despite their younger age. Cannon (1991b) concludes that age or length of illness probably does not explain the observed findings of ventricular enlargement in schizophrenia.

Case studies by Weinberger (1988) and Woody et al. (1987) substantiate Cannon's (1991b) hypothesis. First, Weinberger studied a newly diagnosed 17 year-old schizophrenic who had had a CT scan for a sports injury 15 months prior to admission and before symptom onset. Weinberger reported abnormalities (ventriculomegaly and prominent cortical markings) in the scan taken after the psychiatric admission of the individual which were virtually identical to those from the earlier scan prior to the onset of psychosis. Second, Woody et al. (1987) described lateral, third, and fourth ventricle enlargement in a 10 year-old with recent onset of schizophrenia. The CT was done within 2 months of onset of psychosis and was confirmed with MRI. Repeat scans at 4 and 10 months after onset of symptomatology demonstrated no change in ventricular size. Breslin and Weinberger (1991) conclude that the pathology observed in the brains of schizophrenics through neuroimaging techniques is present at least at onset of psychosis and probably before.

Finally, a study which examined 15 schizophrenics on the same CT scan twice over a period of 7-9 years observed no progression of ventricular enlargement or of sulcal dilatation (Illowsky et al., 1988). Vita et al. (1988) presented similar findings in a study of 17 patients with repeat scans 2 to 5 years apart showing no significant change in the VBR over time.

In this volume we include three chapters which further explore the implications of the neuroimaging findings in schizophrenia discussed above. Chapter 4 by Eyler-Zorrilla and Cannon includes a discussion of the pattern of distribution of brain abnormalities among schizophrenics. The authors discuss the importance of using first degree relatives as controls for schizophrenics in brain imaging studies. Eyler-Zorrilla and Cannon also examine factors such as genetic risk and obstetric complications (OC's) which appear to be related to the degree of psychiatric disturbance observed among schizophrenics. They incorporate these factors into an etiological model. This model suggests that genetic risk for schizophrenia may lead to neural-developmental deficits, that by themselves lead to cortical abnormalities manifesting behaviorally as schizotypal personality disorder. However, when paired with OC's, these neuro-developmental deficits lead to structural brain abnormalities in the ventricular region and manifest as the disorder of "schizophrenia."

Rossi and Stratta in Chapter 5 discuss cerebral asymmetries observed using Computed Tomography and Magnetic Resonance Imaging among schizophrenics. The authors suggest that abnormalities in cerebral lateralization, which are developmental in origin, are related to a subgroup of schizophrenics with severe language disorder.

Chapter 6 by Bilder elaborates on three neurodevelopmental paths to schizophrenia (Bilder & Degreef, 1991). The three paths include: a defect in the early development of the medial frontolimbic cytoarchitectonic trend; a periventricular path; and a cerebral specialization path. The author concludes that the medial frontolimbic path is most likely fundamental to the development of psychosis, and that the morphologic abnormalities such as ventricular enlargement and failures in lateralization or cerebral specialization are epiphenomena contributing to the presentation and course of the disorder.

Animal Models

Animal models can be useful paradigms in our investigations of the neurodevelopmental etiology of schizophrenia. Schizophrenia research may be aided by use of these animal models because they employ <u>experimental</u> control of subjects, genetically and behaviorally---a process not feasible with human subjects. Chapters 7, 8 and 9 present plausible animal models in helping to elucidate the neuropathologic pathways in schizophrenia. Lyon and McClure (Chapter 7) propose a fetal neurodevelopmental animal model using rats. They present behavioral parallels and similarities of neuroanatomical disturbances between human schizophrenics and rats treated <u>in utero</u> with amphetamine.

Logdberg and Warfvinge (Chapter 8) present convincing arguments for using the squirrel monkey as a non-human primate model of human brain development. They review findings showing that lead and methylmercury exposure of squirrel monkeys during prenatal development produce neuropathologic changes as well as postnatal neurobehavioral disturbances. They conclude that the neuropathologic effects---including subtle disturbances in cell migration and in tissue growth and petechial white matter hemorrhages---may be pathogenetically comparable to findings reported in human cases of schizophrenia and other neuropsychiatric disorders.

In Chapter 9, de Erausquin and Hanbauer present intriguing animal data representing a model for the human susceptible period during the second trimester of fetal life. Their data support the hypothesis that if the mother is exposed to influenza (or any other similar environmental insult), increased glutamatergic stimulation of the dopaminergic neurons in the ventral tegmental area results in excessive pruning of their dendritic tree and possibly in neuronal death, thus accounting for the presence of negative symptoms in the schizophrenic patient. It is speculated that positive symptoms develop as a consequence of compensatory increases in the activity of the mesolimbic dopaminergic system.

PREMORBID HISTORY OF SCHIZOPHRENIA

Another line of evidence has examined the premorbid histories of adult schizophrenics, prior to the onset of full-blown psychosis. Pre-schizophrenics evidence abnormalities in social and motor behavior, intellectual functioning, autonomic nervous system functioning, and increases in minor physical anomalies and obstetrical complications.

Social Behavior

Many studies have found that prospective reports of school behavior distinguish children who will develop schizophrenia from those who will not (Tan et al, 1994; Schwartzman et al., 1985; Watt, 1972; Watt, 1978; Watt & Lubensky, 1976; John et al., 1982). In general, both preschizophrenic males and females were found to be emotionally unstable. Preschizophrenic males were found to be disciplinary problems for teachers, disruptive in class, highly anxious, lonely and rejected by peers. In contrast, preschizophrenic females were withdrawn, isolated and nervous. Other researchers reported children at high risk, as a group, to be less motivated, less harmonious, less emotionally stable and more verbally negative than those at low risk (Janes et al., 1983; Watt et al., 1982). Finally, poor affective control in childhood was found in other studies to predict schizophrenia in adulthood (Parnas & Jorgensen, 1989; Parnas et al., 1982a).

Motor Behavior

Disturbances in motor behavior have also been reported for children who later develop schizophrenia. Walker et al. (1994), in a study using home videos of families in which a member later developed schizophrenia, reported that the offspring who developed schizophrenia demonstrated significantly more choreoathetoid movements than their nonschizophrenic siblings. Mednick and Silverton (1988) reported other neuromotor disturbances in infants and children who later developed schizophrenia. Fish et al. (1992) have reported a neurointegrative defect, pandysmaturation, in children who are at risk for schizophrenia. Pandysmaturation is operationally defined by three criteria: 1. A transient retardation of the mean gross motor and/or visual motor developmental quotient, followed by an acceleration of the rate of development, and a return to normal levels. 2. In association with this retardation, there must be an abnormal profile of function on a single developmental examination, in which simple earlier items are failed while more difficult later-occurring items are passed. 3. The motor retardation and abnormal profile must be accompanied by a parallel retardation in growth (Fish et al., 1992).

Intellectual Functioning

Reports of poor premorbid IQ scores in schizophrenics are conflicting. Indeed, a relationship between poor premorbid intellectual functioning and schizophrenia may not exist. Moreover, the inconsistent findings may be due to the heterogeneity of schizophrenia. For instance, a subsample of schizophrenics with low premorbid IQ may exist, but due to biases in sample selection, this group of individuals may be "lost" among the larger group of schizophrenics with normal premorbid intellectual functioning. Even if such a group exists, the numbers in the subnormal group are probably small. Otherwise, more robust findings are likely to have been reported. A study by Aylward et al. (1984) found deficits in premorbid IQ, but only in males. Lane & Albee (1966) also reported a relationship between poor premorbid intellectual functioning and schizophrenia. In contrast, Mednick & Schulsinger (1965) did not observe a relationship between lower IQ and schizophrenia in a high risk sample.

Autonomic Nervous System Functioning

In other studies of high risk children, poor habituation deficits during autonomic conditioning have been observed (Mednick & Schulsinger, 1973; Prentky et al., 1981; Lykken et al., 1988). We have also reported that individuals at genetic risk for schizophrenia evidenced poor habituation of non-specific responses during a rest period before any had been diagnosed with a psychiatric illness, and subjects who became schizophrenic in adulthood also evidenced significant deficits in habituation in adolescence (Hollister et al., 1994a). We have suggested that poor habituation may be part of the constellation of heritable factors which contribute to the etiology of some types of schizophrenia (Hollister et al., 1994a).

Minor Physical Anomalies

There have been a number of studies examining the incidence of minor physical anomalies (MPA's) among individuals with schizophrenia. The advantage of measuring MPA's is that they represent evidence of disruption of fetal development due to either genetic or teratogenic factors. Two studies have reported MPA's such as dysmorphological hand development and fingertip ectodermal ridge count among schizophrenics (Bracha et al., 1991a & b). The authors suggest the anomalies are indicative of a developmental disruption occurring during the second trimester of gestation. In general, a higher incidence of MPA's is observed among schizophrenics than among the normal population (Guy et al., 1983; Gualtieri et al., 1982). In addition, Green et al. (1987;1989) report an association between higher numbers of MPA's and earlier onset of schizophrenia. Thus, MPA's provide further evidence that some type of developmental disruption is occurring during the fetal gestation of some individuals who will later develop schizophrenia.

In this volume, Jones, Murray and Rodgers report (Chapter 10) on findings which support the hypothesis that children, who as adults develop schizophrenia, show significant abnormalities in motor, cognitive and social functioning long before the onset of psychosis. The authors argue that neurological events leading to schizophrenia must occur very early since the developmental abnormalities are already observed in the first years of life. In addition, the authors speculate on the reason behind the inconsistent findings on premorbid function in schizophrenia.

PRE- AND PERINATAL FACTORS

Obstetrical Complications

The hypothesis that schizophrenia may be related to obstetrical complications (OC) is not a new one. In 1939, Barney Katz hypothesized in his dissertation at the University of Southern California that obstetrical factors are important in the etiology of schizophrenia (Dykes et al., 1991). Since that time, the literature has convincingly demonstrated the role of OC's in the etiology of schizophrenia. A specific pathologic mechanism between OC's and schizophrenia is yet to be established, however.

For a detailed and comprehensive review of the OC literature in schizophrenia, the reader should consult McNeil & Kaij (1978) or Dykes et al. (1991). None of the studies reported in these reviews have pointed to particular complications specifically associated with schizophrenia. However, Buka et al. (1993), using data from the Collaborative

Project, reported that subjects who suffered from chronic fetal hypoxia had higher rates of psychotic disorders (schizophrenia and schizophreniform), a finding that failed to reach statistical significance perhaps due to the small number of cases.

In the predecessor of this volume, Dykes et al. (1991) discussed three etiological models involving obstetrical complications as a factor. The first model suggests that certain individuals may be genetically predisposed to serious OC's which are sufficient to cause schizophrenia. The authors believe this model to be unlikely because too many infants who do not become schizophrenic later in life are born with OC's just as severe as those observed in schizophrenics. Furthermore, many individuals with schizophrenia do not experience OC's at birth (Cannon et al., 1990a & b).

The second model posits that some cases of schizophrenia are caused solely or mainly by genetic factors while other cases are caused solely or mainly by OC's (Lewis & Murray, 1987). Gottesman & Shields (1972) believe that since many identical twins are discordant for schizophrenia, some environmental factors must interact with genetic factors to increase the risk for the affected twin. However, one could argue that discordant monozygotic (MZ) twin pairs include a schizophrenic who developed the illness due to OC's (and not genetics). Although twins share the same environment in utero, they may receive differential amounts of nutrients from the mother due to placental/umbilical cord differences, as is suggested by the weight differences sometimes observed among twins.

Dykes et al. (1991) favor a third model which suggests a two-hit approach. In this model, a high risk fetus suffers a genetically predisposed (or teratogenic) disruption of fetal neural development during a critical period of gestation. The prenatal disruption or poor in utero environment may make the fetus especially susceptible to further damage from OC's. Therefore, the infant who has a strong genetic predisposition and who suffers severe OC's has a very high risk of developing schizophrenia.

Our recent finding that risk for Rhesus hemolytic disease of the fetus and newborn (Rh HDN) is related to an increased risk for developing schizophrenia (Hollister et al., 1994b) may fit the two-hit approach. Rh HDN occurs when a mother who is Rh negative develops antibodies against an Rh positive fetus, and these antibodies are transplacentally transferred to the fetus resulting in hemolysis of fetal erythrocytes. Two effects of erythrolysis (break down of erythrocytes) are hypoxia, in utero, and hyperbilirubinemia, post-partum. Both hypoxia and hyperbilirubinemia are known to damage regions of the brain implicated in the neuropathology of schizophrenia (hippocampus, hippocampus and basal ganglia, respectively).

Two hypotheses can be presented with respect to how Rh HDN fits the "Two-Hit Model" of schizophrenia and OC's. First, individuals with a genetic predisposition for schizophrenia and who suffer from Rh HDN (second hit) will be at elevated risk for schizophrenia. Alternatively, the genetic predisposition may be the genotypic combination of maternal Rh negativity/fetal Rh positivity that increases the risk for Rh HDN. And, the second-hit may be the development of Rh HDN, concomitant chronic fetal hypoxia followed by the various OC's considered secondary to Rh HDN (asphyxia, pulmonary edema and other respiratory difficulties).

Maternal Exposure to Influenza During the Second Trimester

In 1988, we first reported a relationship between viral influenza exposure during the second trimester of fetal neural development and an increased risk for adult schizophrenia (Mednick et al, 1988). Since that report, the majority of studies have replicated our basic findings (See chapters 12 & 13 for a complete review). The relationship between influenza exposure in utero and later development of schizophrenia provides additional evidence that this illness is probably of neurodevelopmental origin.

In Chapter 12, Machon and Mednick review studies finding a relationship between influenza exposure and increased risk for schizophrenia, and they present findings from their recent study that reports a relationship between second trimester influenza infection and increased risk for adult schizophrenia (Mednick et al., 1994). In addition, the authors of Chapter 4 discuss the hypothesis that the observed influenza-schizophrenia relationship might be mediated by pregnancy and birth complications or genetic vulnerability. And, they report preliminary findings implicating a relationship between influenza and the affective psychoses.

In Chapter 13, McGrath, Castle, and Murray test the strength of the influenza/schizophrenia relationship by systematically reviewing the literature and assessing how well the studies hold up in consistency, strength of association, specificity, temporality, biological gradient, coherence, and plausibility. The authors conclude that the hypothesis that prenatal influenza causes schizophrenia is far from proven, but that it has sufficient credibility to justify further scientific inquiry.

Finally, in Chapter 14, Laing, Knight, Wright, and Irving present a very comprehensive chapter that poses an interesting hypothesis that maternal infection with influenza may produce (in the mothers who are genetically susceptible) anti-brain autoantibodies which disrupt the development of the fetal brain resulting in schizophrenia later in life. The authors discuss in detail animal studies which demonstrate the teratogenic effects of maternally administered anti-brain antibodies on the developing fetus. A review of the traditional autoimmune hypothesis of schizophrenia is provided as well as detailed information on other immunological factors.

CONCLUSION

We have presented an overview of research in a variety of disciplines which support the proposition that schizophrenia results from aberrant neurodevelopmental processes. It is our contention that to unravel this complex disorder, schizophrenia, much can be gained by employing a multidisciplinary approach which meaningfully integrates the contributions of each discipline. Moreover, the diagnosis of schizophrenia undoubtedly includes a number of clinically differentiated subgroups, and it is important to keep this in awareness when evaluating and conducting research. Included in this volume is a chapter by Tienari and Wynne (Chapter 11) which is intended to remind readers of the heterogeneity of schizophrenia and to stimulate ideas for future neurodevelopmental research in schizophrenia. Tienari and Wynne present a scholarly discussion on the diagnostic and conceptual issues related to subtypes in schizophrenia. They provide a detailed historical overview of the field that has endeavored to study issues such as: differentiating "true" schizophrenia from schizophrenia-like disorders, acute vs. chronic features, classical subtyping, standardized diagnoses, the psychotic vs. non-psychotic subdivisions; the paranoid vs. non-paranoid, affective vs. non-affective, and familial vs. sporadic distinctions; and the issue of positive vs. negative symptoms.

REFERENCES

Aylward, E., Walker, E., Bettes, B. (1984). Intelligence in schizophrenia. *Schizophrenia Bulletin*, 10:430-459.
Benes, F.M., Davidson, B., & Bird, E.D. (1986). Quantitative cytoarchitectural studies of the cerebral cortex of schizophrenics. *Arch Gen Psychiatry* 44:608-616.
Bilder, R.M. & Degreef, G. (1991). Morphologic markers of neurodevelopmental paths to schizophrenia. In S.A. Mednick, T.D. Cannon, C.E. Barr, and J.M. LaFosse, (eds.), *Developmental Neuropathology of Schizophrenia*. New York: Plenum Press.

Bogerts, B. (1989). Limbic and paralimbic pathology in schizophrenia: Interaction with age and stress related factors. In S.C. Schulz & C.A. Tamminga (eds.), *Schizophrenia: Scientific Progress*. Oxford: Oxford University Press Pp. 216-226.

Bogerts, B. and Falkai, P. (1991). Clinical and neurodevelopmental aspects of brain pathology in schizophrenia. In S.A. Mednick, T.D. Cannon, C.E. Barr, and J.M. LaFosse (eds.), *Developmental Neuropathology of Schizophrenia*. New York: Plenum Press, pp. 93-120.

Bogerts, B., Meertz, E. & Schonfeld-Bausch, R. (1985). Basal ganglia and limbic system pathology in schizophrenia. *Archives of General Psychiatry*, 42, 784-91.

Bracha, H.S., Torrey, E.F., & Bigelow, L.B. (1991a). Prenatal maldevelopment of the palm/thumb in schizophrenia: A monozygotic twins study. *Schizophrenia Research* 4:274.

Bracha, H.S., Torrey E.F., Karson, C.N., & Bigelow, L.B. (1991b). A twin study of prenatal injury markers in psychosis: Timing the insult. *Schizophrenia Research* 4:250.

Breslin, N.A. & Weinberger, D.R. (1991). Neurodevelopmental implications of findings from brain imaging studies of schizophrenia. In S.A. Mednick, T.D. Cannon, C.E. Barr, & M. Lyon (eds.), *Fetal Neural Development and Adult Schizophrenia*. Cambridge: Cambridge University Press. Pps. 199-215.

Buka, S.L., Tsuang, M.T., Lipsitt, L.P. (1993). Pregnancy/delivery complications and psychiatric diagnosis: A prospective study. *Arch. Gen. Psychiatry*, 50, 151-156.

Cannon, T.D. (1991a). Sources and correlates of structural brain abnormalities in schizophrenia. In S.A. Mednick, T.D. Cannon, C.E. Barr, & M. Lyon (eds.), *Fetal Neural Development and Adult Schizophrenia*. Cambridge: Cambridge University Press. Pps. 174-198.

Cannon, T.D. (1991b). The possible neurodevelopmental significance of structural imaging findings in schizophrenia. In S.A. Mednick, T.D. Cannon, C.E. Barr, and J.M. LaFosse, (eds.), *Developmental Neuropathology of Schizophrenia*. New York: Plenum Press.

Cannon, T.D., Mednick, S.A., Parnas, J. (1990a). Two pathways to schizophrenia in children at risk. In L. Robins & M. Rutter (eds.), *Straight and Devious Pathways from Childhood to Adulthood*. Cambridge: Cambridge University Press, pp. 328-350.

Cannon, T.D., Mednick, S.A., Parnas, J. (1990b). Antecedents of predominantly negative and predominantly positive symptom schizophrenia in a high risk population. *Archives of General Psychiatry*, 47:622-632.

Dykes, K.L., Mednick, S.A., Cannon, T.D., Barr, C.E. (1991). Obstetrical events and adult schizophrenia. In S.A. Mednick, T.D. Cannon, C.E. Barr, and J.M. LaFosse (eds.), *Developmental Neuropathology of Schizophrenia*. New York: Plenum Press, pp. 121-140.

Falkai, P. & Bogerts, B. (1986). Cell loss in the hippocampus of schizophrenics. *Eur Arch Psychiatr Neurol Sci* 236: 154-161.

Falkai, P. and Bogerts, B. (1989). Morphometric evidence for developmental disturbance in brains of some schizophrenics. *Schizophrenia Research*. 2(1-2):99.

Falkai, P. and Bogerts, B. (1992). Neurodevelopmental abnormalities in schizophrenia. *Clinical Neuropharmacology*. 15 (suppl 1, part A) 498A-499A.

Falkai, P., Bogerts, B., & Rozumek, M. (1988). Cell loss and volume reduction in the entorhinal cortex of schizophrenics. *Biol Psychiatry* 24:515-521.

Fish, B., Marcus, J., Hans, S.L., Auerbach, J.G., Perdue, S. (1992). Infants at risk for schizophrenia: Sequelae of a genetic neurointegrative defect. A review and replication analysis of pandysmaturation in the Jerusalem Infant Development Study. *Arch. Gen. Psychiatry*, 49:221-235.

Gottesman, I.I. & Shields, J. (1972). *Schizophrenia and Genetics: A Twin Study Vantage Point*. New York: Academic Press.

Green, M.F., Satz, P., Soper, H.V., Kharabi, F. (1987). Relationship between physical anomalies and age at onset of schizophrenia. *American Journal of Psychiatry*, 144(5), 666-667.

Green, M.F., Satz, P., Gaier, D.J., Ganzell, S., Kharabi, F. (1989). Minor physical anomalies in schizophrenia. *Schizophrenia Bulletin*, 15(1), 91-99.

Gualtieri, C.T., Adams, A., Shen, C.D. Loiselle, D. (1982). Minor physical anomalies in alcoholic and schizophrenic adults and hyperactive and autistic children. *American Journal of Psychiatry*, 139(5), 640-643.

Guy, J.D., Majorski, L.V., Wallace, C.J., Guy, M.P. (1983). The incidence of minor physical anomalies in adult male schizophrenics. *Schizophrenia Bulletin*, 9(4), 571-582.

Hollister, J.M., Mednick, S.A., Brennan, P., Cannon, T.D. (1994a). Impaired autonomic nervous system habituation in those at genetic risk for schizophrenia. *Arch. Gen. Psychiatry*, 51:552-558.

Hollister, J.M., Laing, P., Mednick, S.A. (1994b). Rhesus hemolytic disease as a risk-factor for the development of schizophrenia in male adults. *Arch. Gen. Psychiatry*, submitted.

Illowsky, B.P., Juliano, D.M., Bigelow, L.B., Weinberger, D.R. (1988). Stability of CT scan findings in schizophrenia: Results of an eight year follow-up study. *J. of Neurology, Neurosurgery, and Psychiatry*, 51:209-213.

Jakob, J. & Beckmann, H. (1986). Prenatal developmental disturbances in the limbic allocortex in schizophrenic. *J Neural Transmiss* 65:303-326.

Janes, C.L., Weeks, D.G., Worland, J. (1983). School behavior in adolescent children of parents with mental disorder. *J. Ner. Men. Dis.*, 171:234-240.

John, R.S., Mednick, S.A., Schulsinger, F. (1982). Teacher reports as a predictor of schizophrenia and borderline schizophrenia: A Bayesian decision analysis. *J. Abn. Psychol.*, 91:399-413.

Katz, B. (1939). The Etiology of the Deteriorating Psychoses of Adolescence and Early Adult Life. Unpublished doctoral dissertation, University of Southern California.

Kovelman, J.A. & Scheibel, A.B. (1984). A neurohistological correlate of schizophrenia. *Biol. Psychiatry* 19:1601-1621.

Lane, E.A. & Albee, G.W. (1966). Comparative birth weights of schizophrenics and their siblings. *Journal of Psychology*, 64:227-231.

Lewis, S.W. & Murray, R.M. (1987). Obstetric complications, neurodevelopmental deviance, and risk of schizophrenia. *Journal of Psychiatric Research*, 21:413-421.

Lykken, D.T., Iacono, W.G., Haroian, K., McGue, M., Bouchard, Jr. (1988). Habituation of the skin conductance response to strong stimuli: A twin study. *Psychophysiology* 25:4-15.

McLardy, T. (1974). Hippocampal zinc and structural deficits in brains from chronic alcoholics and some schizophrenics. *J. Orthomol. Psychiatry* 4:32-36.

McNeil, T.F., Kaij, L. (1978). Obstetric factors in the development of schizophrenia: Complications in the births of preschizophrenics and in reproduction by schizophrenic parents. In L.C. Wynne, R.L. Cromwell & S. Matthysse (eds.), *The Nature of Schizophrenia: New Approaches to Research and Treatment*. New York: John Wiley and Sons.

Mednick, S.A., Machon, R.A., Huttunen, M.O., Bonnet, D. (1988). Adult schizophrenia following prenatal exposure to an influenza epidemic. *Arch. Gen. Psychiatry*, 45:189-192.

Mednick, S.A., Machon, R.A., Huttunen, M.O. (1994). Prenatal influenza infections and adult schizophrenia. *Schizophrenia Bulletin*, in Press.

Mednick, S.A. & Schulsinger, F. (1965). A longitudinal study of children with a high risk for schizophrenia: A preliminary report. In S. Vandenberg (ed.), *Methods and Goals in Human Behavior Genetics*. New York: Academic Press, pp. 255-296.

Mednick, S.A., & Schulsinger, F. (1973). Studies of children at high-risk for schizophrenia. In S.R. Dean (ed.), *Schizophrenia: The First Ten Dean Award Lectures*. New York: MSS Information Corporation.

Mednick, S.A., & Silverton, L. (1988). High-risk studies of the etiology of schizophrenia. In M. Tsuang (ed.), *Handbook of Schizophrenia Volume 3: Nosology, Epidemiology and Genetics*. The Netherlands: Elsevier Science Publishers, pps. 543-562.

Pakkenberg, B. (1990). Pronounced reduction of total neuron numbers in mediodorsal thalmic nucleus and nucleus accumbens of schizophrenics. *Arch Gen Psychiatry* 47:1023-1028.

Parnas, J. & Jorgensen, A. (1989). Pre-morbid psychopathology in schizophrenia spectrum. *Br. J. Psychiatry*, 155:623-627.

Parnas, J., Schulsinger, F., Schulsinger, H., Mednick, S.A. (1982a). Behavioral precursors of schizophrenia spectrum: A prospective study. *Arch. Gen. Psychiatry*, 39:658-664.

Parnas, J., Schulsinger, F., Teasdale, T.W., Schulsinger, H., Feldman, P.M., Mednick, S.A. (1982b). Perinatal complications and clinical outcome within the schizophrenia spectrum. *British Journal of Psychiatry*, 140:416-420.

Prentky, R.A., Salzman, L.F., Klein, R.H. (1981). Habituation and conditioning of skin conductance responses in children at high-risk. *Schizophrenia Bulletin* 7:281-291.

Scheibel, A.B. & Kovelman, J.A. (1981). Disorientation of the hippocampal pyramidal cells and its processes in the schizophrenic patient. *Biol. Psychiatry* 16:101-102.

Schwartzman, A.E., Ledingham, J.E., Serbin, L.A. (1985). Identification of children at risk for adult schizophrenia: A longitudinal study. *International Review of Applied Psychology* 34:363-380.

Tan, S.S., John, R.S., Mednick, S.A. (1994). Teacher reports as a predictor of schizophrenia: A Bayesian Analysis. *Schizophrenia Research*. Submitted.

Vita, A., Sacchetti, E., Valvassori, G., Cazzullo, C.L. (1988). Brain morphology in schizophrenia: A 2- to 5-year CT scan follow-up study. *Acta Psychiatrica Scandinavica* 78:618-621.

Walker, E., Savoie, T., Davis, D. (1994). Neuromotor precursors of schizophrenia. *Schizophrenia Bulletin*, in press.

Watt, N.F. (1972). Longitudinal changes in the social behavior of children hospitalized for schizophrenia as adults. *J. Ner. Men. Dis.* 155:42-54.

Watt, N.F. (1978). Patterns of childhood social development in adult schizophrenics. *Arch Gen Psychiatry.* 35:160-165.

Watt, N.F., Grubb, T.W., Erlenmeyer-Kimling, L. (1982). Social, emotional and intellectual behavior at school among children at high risk for schizophrenia. *J. Con. Clin. Psychol.* 50:171-181.

Watt, N.F. & Lubensky, A.W. (1976). Childhood roots of schizophrenia. *J. Con. Clin. Psychol.* 44:363-375.

Weinberger, D.R. (1988). Premorbid neuropathology in schizophrenia. *Lancet* 2:445.

Woody, R.C., Bolyard, K., Eisenhauer, G. & Altschuler, L. (1987). CT scan and MRI findings in a child with schizophrenia. *Journal of Child Neurology* 22:105-110.

FETAL DEVELOPMENT AND SCHIZOPHRENIA: HISTORICAL OBSERVATIONS FROM TERATOLOGY

William O. McClure

Department of Biological Sciences and Department of Neurology
University of Southern California
Los Angeles, CA 90089-2520

INTRODUCTION

A great deal of current interest about schizophrenia is centered upon the fetal development hypothesis: the suggestion that some challenge to a mother produces an error in development of her fetus which eventually results in schizophrenia in the child, now grown into a young adult. This hypothesis implicitly assumes several points. (1) Because the symptoms of schizophrenia are behavioral, we assume that the organ of the fetus which is finally affected must be the brain. We should remember that the initial challenge may act on the brain only indirectly, with a primary effect at some other tissue of either the mother or fetus. (2) Modern theories of embryonic development would suggest that the challenge to the mother would change the body chemistry of the mother and/or the fetus, thereby changing the makeup of the chemical milieu in which the fetus develops. Changes could involve the presence of chemicals which were not normally present, or the absence of - or perhaps simply alterations in the concentrations of - chemicals expected to be present. Certain of the chemical alterations must modify the structure of the fetus, probably by affecting the action of chemical inducers which regulate migration and/or differentiation of cells and cell accumulations.

In addition to these assumed points, the fetal developmental hypothesis raises other questions. Is there a single challenge, or is it necessary that two or more challenges occur together? Can there exist more than one possible challenge? Could different challenges cause different but similar forms of disease? Is a genetic predisposition required in order for the environmental challenge to be effective, or does a genetic predisposition merely increase the sensitivity of the mother-fetus combination to the challenge? Finally, and most important, what is - or are -the challenges?

A significant amount of work, chronicled elsewhere in this volume, suggests that the mother's period of peak sensitivity is at the end of the second trimenon of pregnancy, in the sixth or seventh month. The agents which may act at this time to generate children who are at very high risk for schizophrenia seem to be three: radiation; severe emotional stress; and infection with influenza virus (Otake and Schull, 1984; Huttenen and Niskanen, 1978; Mednick et al., 1988). Of these, emotional stress and influenza are probably the more significant. Challenge with either agent could alter the chemistry of either mother or fetus, and could, in principle, be responsible for developmental errors leading to schizophrenia.

Developmental errors have been studied in fields other than schizophrenia for many years. Beginning with studies of the effect of chemicals upon the fertilization and embryonic development of sea urchins in the nineteenth century, we have a rich literature concerning the action of exogenous agents upon embryonic development. Many species and agents have been examined, producing many errors in development. As more sophisticated measurements could be made, ever more subtle errors could be - and were - detected. Finally, in the 1960's, errors in behavior were related to fetal exposure to deleterious exogenous agents, and the field of behavioral teratology was born.

In the history of the fields of teratology and behavioral teratology are hidden answers to many questions which face those now working with the fetal development hypothesis of schizophrenia. Questions put to the oracle of history should be worthwhile, for their answers may contain clues to make our modern search somewhat easier.

VISIONS FROM THE PAST

Studies throughout the nineteenth century had shown that exogenous chemicals could modify the embryonic development of many species of lower animals. In all these cases (cnidarians, echinoderms, amphibians, fish) fertilization and development were external to the mother, which left the developing embryo particularly susceptible to interference. A shibboleth of the early twentieth century held that mammals, with their internal fertilization and placental development, would develop embryos which were quite resistant to external challenge from the environment. Mammals also possessed another very great improvement: they were warm-blooded. As a result, the fetus could develop in an environment of essentially constant temperature. It is difficult to appreciate the significance of the difference between cold-blooded and warm-blooded development. Externally fertilized embryos develop in a milieu which may change temperature rapidly, by as much as several degrees. These changes should wreak havoc upon a system as delicately balanced as the development of a fetus: any change in temperature would distort the loom upon which the fabric of development was being woven, causing changes in the relative rates of many biochemical reactions all of which must occur in synchrony for the system to proceed to its desired end. The embryo which developed in a medium of constant temperature was considered blessed, for it would be much less susceptible to environmental challenge. Embryos developing both internally and at constant temperature would be even more stable, and were thought to be virtually immune to perturbation by environmental changes.

This view did not infer that errors in fetal development could not occur in mammals. Malformations of fetuses were well known. Because of the prejudice in the field, however, these malformations were assumed to be wholly of genetic origin. In some cases, such as Down's syndrome, a genetic origin was known to be correct. In other cases in which a genetic etiology had not been established, it was assumed that it was only a matter of time until its genetic basis would be proven. After all, if the fetus were so well protected, an error must be genetic, must it not?

This oversimplified view of mammalian embryology was rudely corrected by the observation by Fred Hale, a Texas veterinarian, of a litter of eleven piglets each of which was born without eyeballs (Hale,1933). Both parents had normal eyes, and were able in subsequent matings to produce normal offspring. The defect appeared to originate with the nutrition of the mother of the affected litter, who had been continuously subjected to a diet deficient in vitamin A beginning five months before being bred and who was maintained upon a vitamin A-deficient diet throughout most of her pregnancy. In a series of subsequent short papers Hale provided compelling evidence supporting his conclusion that the vitamin deficiency was responsible for the observed defect. Because of the strong bias extant in the field, however, it was several years before Hale's careful work was noted, replicated, and accepted.

Dietary changes were further studied by Josef Warkany and his colleagues and students. Warkany, a physician who spent most of his research career in the Department of Pediatrics at the University of Cincinnati, was a superb scientist whose work was to provide a firm basis for a new field: mammalian teratology. In a brilliant series of experiments in the 1940's, he and his students examined the effect of riboflavin deficiency upon the fetal development of rats. They first produced deficiencies by providing mothers with diets poor in riboflavin, and reliably observed skeletal malformations in the offspring. In later experiments galactoflavin, a competitive inhibitor of many actions of riboflavin, was added to the diet to produce a deficiency similar to that observed when riboflavin was removed. The use of galactoflavin provided a great advantage over the use of riboflavin-deficient diets, for galactoflavin could easily be added or removed at specific times during pregnancy. The rapid changes thus produced in the availability of riboflavin to the fetus allowed easier study of the time of pregnancy during which a fetus was more or less sensitive; to use Warkany's term, galactoflavin was a "sharp" tool in the armamentarium of the teratologist (Warkany, 1965).

Other studies, many by Warkany or his students, established that agents which were not involved in nutrition could be teratogenic. Radiation had been shown to be teratogenic as early as 1929 (Goldstein and Murphy, 1929), and drugs which were not related to nutrition were established as teratogens when trypan blue (Gillman et al., 1948) and nitrogen mustard (Haskin, 1948) were examined. The first teratogenic hormone was cortisone, which could induce cleft palate in mice (Baxter and Fraser, 1950). Rubella was shown to be teratogenic in man in 1941 (Gregg, 1941), although the relation of this viral teratology to human teratogenicity in general was not appreciated until much later. Despite these early observations, it is likely that the full extent of the sensitivity of the human fetus to chemical teratogens was not appreciated until thalidomide, a mild sedative, caused hundreds of reduction deformities of the forelimbs in the late 50's (Lenz, 1961; McBride, 1961).

A complete history of teratology may be found in several places. Particularly interesting chapters have been written by Warkany (1965) and by Kalter (1965). Good texts are also available (Wilson and Warkany, 1965; Wilson and Fraser, 1977). In the work described in these studies are answers to many questions which are important for our consideration of fetal development and schizophrenia. Some of the more relevant of these studies will be considered in the following sections. While points will be taken from several aspects of the literature, out of deference to their painstaking contributions I shall lean particularly heavily on the work of Warkany and his students.

Genetic Effects in Teratogenicity

The genetics of the parents of the individual being studied are critically involved in the effect of teratogens. One sees this effect in virtually every study which has been undertaken, surfacing in many different ways. We shall consider two of these here; others will be discussed below in the context of different issues.

Many teratogens are species-specific. Rubella seems to be quite specific for humans, and may affect no other species (Gregg, 1941). Thalidomide does affect species other than humans, but is so much more potent in humans that its teratogenicity was not observed in preclinical pharmacological trials which utilized non-human species (mouse, rat, and rabbit are relatively insensitive to thalidomide; Wilson, 1973a, 1973b, 1977). Specificity directed toward a single species is surely a genetically defined characteristic, albeit based upon the relatively large genetic differences which exist between species.

Teratogens often affect different strains of the same species in different ways. Several comparisons are described in an article by Kalter (1965), to which the reader is referred for a more careful exposition, and from which much of the following material has been gratefully taken. Mice born to mothers treated with cortisone are quite likely to suffer cleft palate (Baxter and Fraser, 1950; Fraser and Fainstat, 1951). The strain of mouse used affects the extent of the malformation, with the incidence of cleft palate (in terms of the percentage of offspring who exhibit the defect) ranging from a low value of 12% in CBA mice to a high value of 100% in A strain mice (Table 1). Clearly the genetic makeup of the parents can affect the sensitivity of the offspring to challenge with this teratogen.

Table 1. Effect of different strains of mice on the induction of cleft palate by cortisone.[1]

Strain	Cleft palate (% of offspring)
CBA	12
C57BL	19
A	100

[1] Data selected from Kalter (1965).

These two examples define two possible effects of genetics: either an appropriate genotype is *required* before a teratogen can exert its effect, as may be true in the case of rubella, or an appropriate genotype *modifies* the action of a teratogen, as in the case of cortisone. In principle, these two possible effects represent the extremes in a continuum of activity which ranges from one extreme that exhibits an absolute requirement for a specific genotype to another extreme that displays no effect of genotype at all. Consideration of genetic effects in this way is oversimplified, but does present a measure of utility. We usually approach the study of required *vs* modifying genotypes in different ways, and it is convenient to separate them in our thinking. Furthermore, the mechanisms which underlie these two effects may be quite different. We shall encounter other examples of both cases.

Time and Method of Administration

The time during pregnancy at which a teratogen is administered can have a significant effect upon the observed action. As one of many examples, Warkany found that deficiency of riboflavin in the diet of rats before and during gestation led to the formation of young with many skeletal defects: short mandibles, cleft palate, syndactyly, fused ribs and sternebrae, etc (Warkany and Nelson, 1940). All these effects could be prevented if the diet were supplemented with liver extract, which is rich in riboflavin, or with crystalline riboflavin. A critical period existed for this effect: riboflavin added to the diet on days 13 and 14 of gestation completely prevented the defects (Warkany et al., 1942; Warkany and Schraffenberger, 1943). Critical periods are common in this work, and must be expected in any teratological study.

The way in which a teratogen is used can affect both the critical period and the observed teratology. For example, the "sharper" agent, galactoflavin, generated a more complex effect than did simple dietary restriction of riboflavin. Rats born of pregnancies which were interrupted by riboflavin deficiency induced at specific times with the use of galactoflavin did show the skeletal defects which were characteristic of dietary riboflavin deficiency, but also demonstrated abnormalities of soft tissues. If a deficiency was induced on days 7 - 13 of pregnancy, the offspring exhibited primarily skeletal and cardiac anomalies, while deficiency from days 7 - 11 led primarily to soft tissue defects. The data indicated that riboflavin deficiency could affect not only the skeleton, but also soft tissues: the heart, eyes, and urogenital systems. Of particular relevance to this Symposium, riboflavin deficiency at day 7 - 11 also caused soft tissue anomalies in the cerebrum and many other regions of the brain (Kalter and Warkany, 1957). Since the soft tissue changes were observed only when galactoflavin was employed, and were not seen in cases in which dietary riboflavin deficiency was maintained throughout pregnancy, it appears that a sharp change during pregnancy may induce results which are not observed in a long term insult. Again the lesson for us is clear: specific interference with development for only a short period of time can result in significant damage in many organ systems, and the timing and method of administration of the teratogen can significantly alter the resultant action.

The very complex relationships presented here are not unusual in the field of teratology. Warkany (1965) cautions us:

> "Although one could establish a critical period at which the abnormal environment brought on the malformations, nothing unusual happened to the mother at this critical period; the external situation was the same weeks before and weeks after the day on which the deforming changes occurred. These findings can still serve as a warning to those who believe that they can ascertain and time environmental teratogenic events with the help of an embryological timetable."

With our ever increasing knowledge of the molecular aspects of embryology, coupled with ever more sensitive methods, we should gradually overcome the caution expressed in this statement. We have probably not yet, however, reached the point at which we can disregard it altogether. Particularly in cases which deal with the development of organs as complex as the brain it seems likely that Warkany's words must still be carefully considered. Many of the interesting aspects of our field, and of this Symposium, should be considered in the light of these concerns. It is quite possible that the developmental situation is much more complex than even the most pessimistic would admit.

Can the Same Changes be Caused by Different Agents?

It is important to consider the possibility that teratologic challenge by different agents, possibly employed under different conditions, could cause the same, or nearly the same, developmental abnormality. As discussed above, the same agent acting under different conditions can induce different abnormalities. Might not the converse situation also exist?

While a proof of identity is difficult, data exist which indicate that very similar if not identical changes can be induced by different agents. In a study of skeletal abnormalities produced by developmental challenges in chicks, Landauer has examined the generation of "phenocopies": teratologies which are similar in structure to one another (as well as to a genetically derived phenotype). Phenocopies can be produced by different teratogens acting under different conditions. For example, the development of the long bones of the chick embryo could be altered to generate virtually identical structures by injecting eggs with pilocarpine at 145 hr of incubation; with insulin at 122 hr; or with boric acid at 96 hr (Landauer, 1954). These three agents certainly act by very different mechanisms, as suggested by both their known pharmacology and chemistry and confirmed by experiments in which Landauer inhibited their teratogenicity using different agents. Nonetheless, when applied at an appropriate time of incubation, each generated a morphologically identical error in skeletal development.

This situation is quite relevant to the fetal development of schizophrenia, in which more than one agent may be active. Indeed, evidence exists that either influenza virus or emotional stress may, if presented at the appropriate time of pregnancy, induce the disease.

It is possible that these two agents act, almost certainly by different mechanisms, to produce similar morphological changes in the brain; these in turn could generate similar diseases, as, for example, similar forms of schizophrenia.

Laterality of Changes

In the 1930's preoccupation with the supposed invulnerability of a mammalian fetus led to the conclusion that congenital changes must be caused by genetic effects. This was felt even more strongly in cases in which bilaterally symmetrical defects were seen. One noted textbook of the period characterized the situation (F. Lenz, in Baur et al., 1931):

> "When malformations are symmetrical, there can be little doubt that they are truly hereditary. If for instance, we find the same malformation in both hands, we can conclude with the greatest probability that the trouble is hereditary. The same thing applies to malformations which exhibit a serial homology, being of the same character both in the hands and in the feet."

Even now, knowing that the fetus is actually rather vulnerable, we expect to see teratological errors expressed in a symmetrical way: both hands should be affected in syndactyly; both sides of the palate should be equally separated in cleft palate; etc. In practice, however, data which were available in the 1940's clearly established that teratologic deformities need be neither symmetric nor bilateral.

Kalter, working with Warkany on the incidence of syndactyly induced by treatment of pregnant mice with galactoflavin, has reported effects which are not symmetrical (Kalter, 1954). In experiments using genetic variation as a tool, Kalter considered the laterality of syndactyly in nine genetic crosses which employed three strains of mice (Table 2). The occurrence of syndactyly was never completely bilateral. In even the most bilateral case (A x A), 4 % of animals showed the defect in only one of the two paws. In the least bilateral case (D x B), fully 35 % of offspring exhibited unilateral anomalies.

Table 2. Syndactyly of toes induced in rats by *in utero* galactoflavin.[1]

Cross	Total number of abnormal animals	Percentage of all animals with syndactyly expressed:			
		Bilaterally	Unilaterally	Left	Right
AxA	153	96	4	3	1
BxB	48	80	20	12	8
DxD	99	76	24	18	6
AxB	81	79	21	17	4
BxA	25	76	24	24	0
AxD	80	84	16	11	5
DxA	69	78	22	16	6
BxD	19	90	10	5	5
DxB	40	65	35	25	10

[1] A, B, and D represent three inbred mouse strains. Data selected from Kalter (1954).

These studies also indicate an unexpected bias in laterality. More often than not it is the left paw that is affected, rather than the right. In eight of the nine cases this is true; in the ninth (B x D), both sides are affected equally. In none of the nine cases does the right paw show a higher incidence of syndactyly than does the left. The probability of this distribution occurring by chance is small: $p \sim 2^{-8}$, which is about 0.004. With apologies to the oracle of statistics, one can also use a t-test to compare the left vs. right percentages;

while such a comparison has theoretical shortcomings, the results (t = 3.70, 16; p < 0.01) buttress our conclusion that these differences are not due to chance. Something occurs during the action of this teratogenic insult which favors an attack on the left paw. The experimental results indicate that genetic factors can modify the magnitude of the left/right difference, but the fundamental defect appears to require the presence of challenge by the teratogen.

The consideration of laterality need not be limited to skeletal anomalies. It seems likely that changes involving other tissues might also be observed. A particularly relevant example which involves the brain has been described by Rogers (1982). In an examination of the development of laterality in several behaviors of the chick, she found that the causative agent appears to be light, which penetrates the shell and preferentially stimulates the eye which is closer to the surface of the egg. This eye is always the right one in the strain she examined. In this case the lateral development of the brain is affected by two factors: a genetic tendency to place all embyros in a given position with regard to the egg, and an environmental challenge which exploits the genetic tendency. A similar argument may be involved in the generation of other lateralized errors in development, such as those seen in schizophrenia (Bracha, 1987; Lyon and Satz, 1991).

Effect of Gender

The results of teratologic insult may be quite different in the two sexes. In a series of pioneering studies, William Thompson and his students have shown that maternal anxiety can cause behavioral changes in the offspring. These changes were presumably mediated by developmental changes in the structure of the brain, although the neuroanatomy of animals treated in this way was not examined. In their experiments, female rats were trained in a conditioned aversion paradigm in which they could avoid shock by pressing a lever.

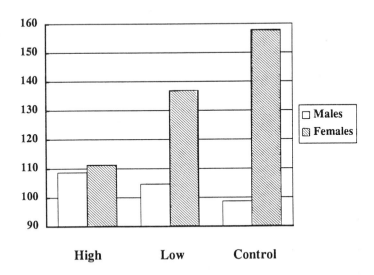

Figure 1. Effect of maternal anxiety on locomotion of the offspring. Locomotion is given in arbitrary units which are related to crossings of squares in the open field. High, high maternal anxiety; Low, low maternal anxiety; Control, mothers without added anxiety. Data replotted from Thompson and Quinby (1964).

After reaching criterion these females were mated and, during specified periods of pregnancy, were exposed to the aversive stimulus in the apparatus in which they had been trained. To provide "anxiety", the lever with which to escape was not present, and no shock was ever given. By varying the number of "anxiety" trials, conditions of high anxiety or low anxiety were established. Young born of these pregnancies showed altered amounts of running in an open field, which is in this species taken as an inverse measure of emotionality (i.e., more locomotion implies a less emotional animal). Female offspring of treated mothers ran less in an open field test of activity than did offspring of control mothers (Thompson and Quinby, 1964; Fig 2). This effect was "dose" dependent: high anxiety pups ran even less than did low anxiety animals. In contrast to females, male rats showed a small but statistically insignificant change in the opposite direction: treated male pups tended to be more active in the open field. The data document an effect which is clearly related to gender.

Genetics are again important in this effect. In a series of similar experiments in which various strains of mice were examined, Wier and DeFries (1964) have shown that the effect of maternal anxiety varies between strains. In addition to measuring the emotionality of the offspring, these workers also measured the emotionality of the parents, thereby allowing a correlation to be drawn between the parent's emotional tone and the effect of the "anxiety"-producing stimulus on their offspring. Their data allow an interpretation which is appealing, even though perhaps oversimplified: strains in which the parents were more emotional produced young which were more affected by prenatal anxiety applied to the mother. These results provide a strong signal to those considering a fetal developmental hypothesis for schizophrenia, and indicate that as mild a teratogen as anxiety - or, probably, stress - can alter the behavior of offspring in a way which is dependent upon the magnitude of the stimulus, the gender of the offspring, and the genetic composition of the mother.

Maternal Effects on Teratogenicity

A more careful examination of the genetic effect shows that the mother has an influence beyond her genetic contribution. Again using Kalter's data (Kalter, 1954), consider first the crosses of A and CBA animals. Crosses of A females and A males yield the expected 100% incidence of cleft palate; homologous crosses of CBA parents yield 12% (Table 3; cf Table 1). A cross of a mother of the A strain with a father from the CBA strain yields an intermediate sensitivity to cortisone (25%). If the reverse cross is tested, the sensitivity is again reduced (CBA female x A male; 20%). In these data the genetic effect is clearly demonstrated: crosses of two strains display a sensitivity intermediate between the two parental strains.

The mother of the more sensitive strain conveys to the cross a greater effect than does the mother of the less sensitive strain (25% vs 20%), indicating that some effect of the mother takes place. Maternal effects are well known in genetics, and may reflect either an effect from the maternal contents of the egg or/and the expanded role allowed to the mother by virtue of the contact between fetus and mother during the period of gestation.

In order properly to appreciate this phenomenon, recall that the F1 hybrids of two homozygous strains will be identically heterozygous; i.e., all animals of such a mating will be clones, as were their parents. Furthermore, the F1 hybrids from reciprocal crosses of homozygous strains will also have identical heterozygous genomes (with the exception - possibly very important - of the sex chromosomes in males). Therefore, even the relatively small but real difference between 20% and 25% is due to a non-genetic effect of the mother.

Reciprocal crosses can sometimes unearth surprising interactions between genetic inheritance and maternal effects. Consider the second set of crosses shown in Table 3, in which mice of the A strain are mated with those of the C57BL strain. C57BL parents yield offspring which are 19% susceptible to teratology with cortisone. A reciprocal cross of A mothers and C57BL fathers yields progeny with 44% susceptibility to cortisone. This pattern is similar to that seen with the A/CBA crosses: reciprocal crosses generate animals which possess sensitivity intermediate between that of the two parents. The reverse cross, however, is surprising. C57BL mothers when mated to A fathers yield offspring which are highly resistant to challenge in utero with cortisone: only 3 % of them show cleft palate. Neither of the parent strains has this level of resistance. The results of the A/C57BL cross require an interaction of genes and maternal environment which is unexpected. Despite the remarkable nature of this finding, it has been replicated both by Kalter and by others.

Table 3. Effect of *in utero* cortisone on the incidence of cleft palate in reciprocal crosses of inbred mouse strains.[1]

Cross		Cleft palate
mother	father	(% of offspring)
A	A	100
A	CBA	25
CBA	A	20
CBA	CBA	12
A	A	100
A	C57BL	44
C57BL	A	3
C57BL	C57BL	19

[1] Data selected from Kalter (1954).

These results may be extended to our consideration of schizophrenia and genetics. Dramatic effects of the genome can be seen in the sensitivity to environmental teratogens in these results with mice, and may well occur also when we consider the much more delicate challenge to fetal development which results in the brain derangements of schizophrenia. The genetic makeup of the parents can have two effects: in some cases the environmental challenge cannot act unless the genetic background allows the teratology, and an appropriate genetic composition could prevent the action. In other cases, the environmental challenge appears to cause some teratology irrespective of the genetics, but the magnitude of the effect is strongly affected by the genotype. In either case, non-genetic effects from the mother may be of significance.

Hormones as Teratogens

Hormones are excellent teratogens when employed under appropriate conditions. Many chemicals which are hormones in adult animals are known to function as inducers of embryonic development, and could easily act in an anomalous way to cause errors in development. One of the first of these to be described was cortisone, a glucocorticoid which induces skeletal anomalies in mice. Of the skeletal defects which are generated, cleft palate has probably been the most extensively studied. Induction of cleft palate by cortisone is modified by a wide variety of experimental variables: the genetic makeup of both mother and fetus; the nutritional state of the mother; maternal weight; fetal weight and gender; the time during pregnancy of the challenge; and the parity of the mother. A few of these variables have been considered above; others are also of significance, but space does not allow us to discuss them in detail. At this point it is sufficient to note the extensive studies of Warkany's students and their colleagues (Kalter, 1959; Fraser, 1977), and the great sensitivity of this system to a number of variables. A rich literature also exists in which the action of glucocorticoids upon fetal development of the brain is confirmed (Oda and Huttenlocher, 1974). There is no doubt that these results can be generalized, in principle, to other hormones acting on other tissues or organs in other species.

Viruses as Teratogens

Historically, viruses have been known to act as human teratogens since rubella was first associated causally with the formation of cataracts in the offspring of mothers infected during their first two months of pregnancy (Gregg, 1941). There is now a rich literature which discusses viruses as teratogens, and from which many lessons may be drawn. Most of these lessons are confirmations of suggestions drawn from other systems, and will not be repeated. A few new points, however, may be gleaned from the early viral literature.

Since infection with viruses usually leaves behind a marker of the presence of the virus, it is often thought that a virus acting as a teratogen should be detectable, by the usual techniques of modern biology, in either the mother, the newborn, or even in the newborn when grown into an adult. For example, rubella virus can be recovered from the cataractous lenses of infected infants for up to three years after birth (Menser et al., 1967), and has been isolated at an even later time from the brain of one child who developed a chronic progressive panencephalitis which is believed to result from infection (Weil et al., 1975).

Unfortunately, the belief that teratology caused by a virus would be easily detected is overly optimistic. At least one system has been carefully studied in which the virus leaves no detectable trace of its presence, and would not have been suspected as a causative agent were not specific experimental infections being examined. Bluetongue virus affects adult sheep with an acute and fatal illness, and is also teratogenic when present during pregnancy (Osburn et al., 1971a,b). By only a few months after birth, the presence of virions in the offspring of teratogenized mice could not be detected by any of the procedures available in the 1970's (Narayan and Johnson, 1972). Furthermore, morphological changes which were present in older affected animals demonstrated no evidence of prior infection, resembling instead non-inflammatory defects which could have been caused by simple degeneration or by errors in embryogenesis. In this case, the virus carried out its teratogenic act and then appeared to vanish from the organism. The lesson for those who study influenza and schizophrenia is, again, clear: we need not expect to see any detectable remnant of the virus in the brain of the adult schizophrenic, or even in juvenile premorbid individuals. We must not take the absence of a virus as an unequivocal indication that one was not involved.

Viral infections may also show exquisite cellular specificity. The infection produced by bluetongue virus has been followed from its early stages. The virus initially infects primordial cells of the subventricular layer of the developing telencephalon, and the developing pathology spreads from this site along pathways of migration of the affected germinal cells. Despite a rather large morphological deficit produced by the virus, the initial action seems limited to one cell type in the entire developing brain. Other germinal layers in the developing brain, such as the external granular cell layer of the cerebellum, are not involved in the action of the virus (Narayan and Johnson, 1972). There seems no reason to feel that other viruses will not be similarly selective in their sites of action.

Viruses also provide an example of a teratogen which acts indirectly. Influenza A was one of the first viruses which was recognized as teratogenic (Hamburger and Habel, 1947). Influenza virus produces a defect in development of the neural tube, with subsequent failure of closure, errors in the cervical and cephalic flexures, and collapse of the metencephalic region of the developing brain. Examination of the embryo with immunofluorescent antibody reveals that the viral antigen is present in tissues around the brain, but is not detectable in the nervous system itself. Despite extensive spread into myocardium, certain areas of the gut, and extraneural ectoderm, the virus causes no damage in these tissues (Johnson et al., 1971). An indirect role of the virus in teratogenicity was proposed, in which an initial attack upon extraneural tissues resulted in a deficit in the development of the nervous system, perhaps by restricting the availability of nutrients. While the role of influenza is discussed in detail elsewhere in this Symposium, we should remember that any teratogenic agent may act indirectly: the site of damage and the initial site of attack need not be the same. When one considers the entire system of mother and fetus, the possibilities for the site of an initial insult become very large.

CONCLUSIONS

The development of mammalian teratology in the 1940's has provided a great deal of information for those who now wish to consider schizophrenia as a disorder of fetal development. A number of specific points are established. Many different agents can be teratogenic: chemicals, including hormones and vitamins; radiation; viruses; and behavioral changes (which may act through hormones related to stress). The genetic stock of the parents is very important. Non-genetic maternal effects can modify many aspects of teratology. The timing of the environmental insult is important: the same agent can cause different teratologies when administered at different times of pregnancy. Conversely, different agents can sometimes cause morphologically identical results. Teratological challenges can induce unilateral effects. Some agents, such as viruses, show exquisite specificity, may leave no trace of their previous presence, and can act indirectly.

Our historical voices may be consulted for an answer to one key question: do the previous data support a fetal developmental etiology for schizophrenia? The answer to this crucial question is strongly affirmative: all the prior data indicate that a suitable environmental challenge could induce changes which would cause schizophrenia.

Unfortunately, the historical voices do not provide us with certain important answers. The role of genetics, for example, is not defined. In some cases the genetics of the parents modify the action of an environmental challenge, but a suitable environmental challenge may be effective regardless of the genetics of the host; in other cases an appropriate genetic makeup is required before an environmental challenge can be effective. The exact time of pregnancy at which the insult needs to occur is not easily predicted from *a priori* arguments. The specific insulting agent is not defined: any of several could be possibilities, including viruses and hormones. All of these points must yet be determined by experiment. It is at least comforting, however, to press into the scientific and medical fray surrounding schizophrenia armed with the information that the oracle of history strongly supports the fundamental tenets of the fetal development hypothesis.

ACKNOWLEDGMENTS

It is a pleasure to thank many whose time, comments, and insight I have enjoyed. Special thanks are due to John, Marlene, and Joan; to Sarnoff Mednick and Mel Lyon, who have made my work in this field so pleasant; to Harry Uylings, Larry Swanson, and others who have gracefully corrected my concepts about neuroanatomy; and to the many students whose work with me has allowed the development of the ideas in this chapter. Financial support has been generously provided by the Hedco Foundation and the NIH.

REFERENCES

Baur, E., Fischer, E., and Lenz, F., 1931, "Human Heredity", The McMillan Co., New York NY.

Baxter, H., and Fraser, F.C., 1950, Production of congenital defects in offspring of female mice treated with cortisone, *McGill Med. J.* 19:245.

Bracha, H.S., 1987, Asymmetric rotational (circling) behavior, a dopamine-related asymmetry: Preliminary findings in unmedicated and never-medicated schizophrenic patients, *Biol. Psychiatry*, 22,995.

Fraser, F.C., 1977, Interactions and multiple causes, in: "Handbook of Teratology. I. General principles and etiology", J.G. Wilson and F.C. Fraser, eds., Plenum Press, New York.

Fraser, F.C., and Fainstat, T.D., 1951, Production of congenital defects in offspring of pregnant mice treated with cortisone, *Pediatrics* 8:527.

Gillman, J., Gilbert, C., Gillman, T., and Spence, I., 1948, A preliminary report on hydrocephalus, spina bifida, and other congenital anomalies in the rat produced by trypan blue, *S. African J. Med. Sci.* 13:47.

Goldstein, L., and Murphy, D.P., 1929, Etiology of ill-health in children born after maternal pelvic irradiation. II. Defective children born after postconception pelvic irradiation, *Am. J. Roentgenol. Radium Ther. Nucl. Med.* 22:322-331.

Gregg, N., 1941, Congenital cataracts following German measles in the mother, *Trans. Ophthalmol. Soc. Aust.* 3:35.

Hale, F., 1933, Pigs born without eye balls, *Jour. Heredity* 24:105-106.

Hamburger, V., and Habel, K., 1947, Teratologic and lethal effects of influenza A and mumps viruses on early chick embryos, *Proc. Soc. Exp. Biol. Med.* 66:608.

Haskin, D., 1948, Some effects of nitrogen mustard on the development of external body form in the fetal rat, *Anat. Rec.* 102:493.

Huttunen, M.O., and Niskanen, P., 1978, Prenatal loss of father and psychiatric disorders, *Arch. Gen. Psychiatry* 35:429-431.

Johnson, K.P., Klasnja, R., and Johnson, R.T., 1971, Neural tube defects of chick embryos: An indirect result of influenza A virus infection, *J. Neuropath. Exp. Neurol.* 30:68.

Kalter, H., 1954, The inheritance of susceptibility to the teratogenic action of cortisone in mice, *Genetics*, 39, 185.

Kalter, H., 1959, Attempts to modify the frequency of cortisone-induced cleft palate in mice by vitamin, carbohydrate, and protein supplementation, *Plastic Reconst. Surg.* 24:498-504.

Kalter, H., 1965, Interplay of intrinsic and extrinsic factors, in: "Teratology: Principles and Techniques", J.G. Wilson and J.Warkany, ed., Univ. of Chicago Press, Chicago IL.

Kalter, H., and Warkany, J., 1957, Congenital malformations in inbred strains of mice induced by riboflavin-deficient, galactoflavin-containing diets, *Jour. Exp. Psych.* 136:531-565.

Landauer, W., 1954, On the chemical production of developmental abnormalities and of phenocopies in chicken embryos, *Jour. Cell. Comp. Physiol.* 43:261-305.

Lenz, W., 1961, Kindliche Missbildungen nach Medikament wahrend der Draviditat? *Deutsch. Med. Wochenschr.* 86:2555-2556.

Lyon, N. and Satz, P., 1991, Left turning (swivel) in medicated chronic schizophrenic patients, *Schiz. Res.*, 4,53.

McBride, W.G., 1961, Thalidomide and congenital abnormalities, *Lancet* 2:1358.

Mednick, S.A., Machon, R.A., Huttunen, M.O., and Bonett, D., 1988, Adult schizophrenia following prenatal exposure to an influenza epidemic, *Arch. Gen. Psychiatry* 45:189-192.

Menser, M.A., Harley, J.D., Hertzberg, R., Dorman, O.C., and Murphy, A.M., 1967, Persistence of virus in lens for three years after prenatal rubella, *Lancet* 2:387.

Narayan, O., and Johnson, R.T., 1972, Effects of viral infection on nervous system development. I. Pathogenesis of bluetongue virus infection in mice, *Am. J. Pathol.* 68:1-14.

Oda, M.A.S., and Huttenlocher, P.R.. 1974, The effect of corticosteroids on dendritic development in the rat brain, *Yale Jour. Biol. Med.* 47,155.

Osburn, B.I., Silverstein, A.M., Prendergast, R.A., Johnson, R.T. and Parshall, C.J., 1971a, Experimental viral-induced congenital encephalopathies. I. Pathology of hydranencephaly and porencephaly caused by bluetongue vaccine virus, *Lab. Invest.* 25:197.

Osburn, B.I., Johnson, R.T., Silverstein, A.M., Prendergast, R.A. and Jochim, M.J., Levy,S.E., 1971b, Experimental viral-induced congenital encephalopathies. II. The pathogenesis of bluetongue virus infections in fetal lambs, *Lab. Invest.* 25:206.

Otake, M., and Schull, W.J., 1984, *In utero* exposure to A-bomb radiation and mental retardation, a reassessment, *Br. Jour. Radiol.* 57:409-414.

Rogers, L.J., 1982, Light experience and asymmetry of brain function in chickens, *Nature* 297:223-225.

Thompson, W.R., and Quinby, S., 1964, Prenatal maternal anxiety and offspring behavior: parental activity and level of anxiety, *Jour. Gen. Psychol.* 106:359-371.

Warkany, J., 1965, Development of experimental mammalian teratology, in: "Teratology: Principles and Techniques", J.G. Wilson and J. Warkany, ed., Univ. of Chicago Press, Chicago IL.

Warkany, J., and Nelson, R.C., 1940, Appearance of skeletal abnormalities in the offspring of rats reared on a deficient diet, *Science* 92:383-384.

Warkany, J., Nelson, R.C., and Schraffenberger, E., 1942, Congenital malformations induced in rats by maternal nutritrional deficiency. II. Use of varied diets and of different strains of rats, *Am. Jour. Dis. Child.* 64:860-866.

Warkany, J., and Schraffenberger, E., 1943, Congenital malformations induced in rats by maternal nutritional deficiency. V. Effects of a purified diet lacking riboflavin, *Proc. Soc. Exp. Biol. Med.* 54:92.

Weil, M.L., Itabashi, H.H., Cremer, N.E., Oshiro, L.S., Lennette, E.H. and Carnay, L., 1975, Chronic progressive panencephalitis due to rubella virus simulating SSPE, *New Eng. J. Med.* 292:994.

Weir, M., and DeFries, J.C.. 1964, Prenatal maternal influence on behavior in mice, *J. Comp. Physiol. Psychol.* 58:412-417.

Wilson, J.G., 1973a, An animal model of human disease: Thalidomide embryopathy in primates, *Comp. Pathol. Bull.* 5:3-4.

Wilson, J.G., 1973b, "Environment and birth defects", Academic Press, New York.

Wilson, J.G., 1977, Embryotoxicity of drugs in man, in: "Handbook of Teratology. 1. General principles and etiology", J.G. Wilson and F.C. Fraser, ed., Plenum Press, New York.309.

Wilson, J.G., and Warkany, J., 1965, "Teratology: Principles and Techniques", Univ. of Chicago Press, Chicago IL.

Wilson, J.G. and Fraser, F.C., 1977, "Handbook of Teratology vol 1: General Principles and Etiology", Plenum Press. New York NY.

POTENTIAL MECHANISMS OF DEFECTIVE BRAIN DEVELOPMENT IN SCHIZOPHRENIA

E.G. Jones* and S. Akbarian

Department of Anatomy and Neurobiology
University of California, Irvine
Irvine, California

*correspondence

INTRODUCTION

Unraveling the biological basis of schizophrenia is a formidable task. At present, there is considerable interest in theories which suggest that orderly brain development is affected in this disorder and that alterations of brain organization arising from disturbed ontogenesis are causally linked to schizophrenic psychopathology. Recognition of a developmental pathophysiology in schizophrenia may be critical for further understanding the disease, and potentially important for its prevention.

Although the developmental hypothesis of schizophrenia has had some popularity for at least forty-five years (Bender, 1947), little is known about the particular developmental mechanisms, if any, that are affected in the brains of schizophrenics. Epidemiological studies have identified a number of risk factors acting during pregnancy that increase the risk of schizophrenia in offspring (Mednick and Cannon, 1991). Among these, the correlation of increased incidence with maternal influenza infection in the second trimester (Mednick et al., 1988) has received both strong and qualified support in a series of independent investigations (Kendell and Kemp, 1989; Barr et al., 1990; Crow et al., 1991; O'Callaghan et al.,1991; Sham et al., 1992). Studies of this and other risk factors suggest that schizophrenia is not solely the outcome of a deterministic process based on a faulty set of genes but also influenced by the biological environment in the prenatal and early postnatal period.

The purpose of this review is to highlight those mechanisms of brain development that may have been disturbed in the brains of schizophrenics and which might be causally linked to the disorder. The review is subdivided into three parts: Part 1 is a brief chronology of the developmental hypothesis; Part 2 outlines the principal steps in ontogenesis of the primate forebrain and reviews the morphological abnormalities, already described in brains of schizophrenics, that might be linked to interference with one or more of these ontogenetic steps; Part 3 discusses the neuropathology, as related to epidemiological and other data, and the functional consequences, along with strategies aimed at further expanding the developmental hypothesis.

The focus of the review is on the developmental pathology of the cerebral cortex, with passing comments on the basal ganglia and thalamus. Dysfunction of these forebrain regions is commonly regarded as being of primary importance in schizophrenia (Kraepelin 1919, Zec and Weinberger 1986, Crow 1990, Carlsson and Carlsson 1990, Grüsser 1991). This is not to rule out, however, involvement of midbrain and hindbrain regions in the pathophysiology of schizophrenia and morphological abnormalities in these regions have also been described (for example Bogerts et al. 1983, Karson et al. 1991, Nasrallah et al. 1991).

Chronology

The developmental hypothesis of schizophrenia came to the fore in modern times in the studies of Bender (1947), Bender and Freedman (1952), Fish (1957), O'Neal and Robins (1958) and Sobel (1961). Analyzing the postnatal psycho-motor and neuropsychological development of schizophrenics and of children genetically at risk for schizophrenia, these authors found that schizophrenics tended to show alterations in the normal pattern of psycho-motor and intellectual development during the first years of life. The implication was that brain ontogenesis is affected in schizophrenia. While these studies were mostly retrospective in nature, their principal findings have been confirmed and extended in a number of prospective studies (Fish et al., 1992) and alteration of the orderly cascade of neurological and neuropsychological development that occurs during the first year of life in a substantial proportion of schizophrenics has been referred to as a pandysmaturation syndrome (Fish et al. 1992).

In the last decade, the developmental hypothesis has been supported by neuroanatomical and epidemiological studies: Histological studies on areas of the medial temporal lobe described disturbed cortical lamination patterns in hippocampal and parahippocampal regions in schizophrenics and these patterns were interpreted as resulting from defective neuronal migration in development (Scheibel and Kovelman, 1981; Kovelman and Scheibel, 1986; Jakob and Beckmann, 1986, 1989; Arnold et al., 1991a). A significant increase in the volume of the lateral and third ventricles in schizophrenics may also reflect altered brain development since it is present in early stages of the disease and does not progress over time (reviewed in: Hyde and Weinberger 1990; Roberts and Bruton, 1990; Pfefferbaum and Zipursky, 1991). Because gliosis and other signs of neuronal degeneration are generally lacking in the forebrain in schizophrenics (Benes et al., 1986, 1991; Roberts et al., 1987; Purohit et al., 1993), the histological changes in the medial temporal lobe and the ventriculomegaly are not easily explained in terms of a neurodegenerative defect.

The neuropsychiatric assessment of at-risk infants has presented convincing, and the morphological studies suggestive evidence that brain development is compromised in schizophrenia. However, these studies cannot show whether developmental disturbances in brains of schizophrenics are directly involved in the etiology of the disease or are secondary phenomena. The answer to this particular question may lie in the results of epidemiological studies that have identified a number of risk factors such as infection with influenza virus, which act during the prenatal period and increase the incidence of schizophrenia in offspring (Mednick and Cannon, 1991; Sham et al., 1992). These studies are at present the strongest evidence for a causal relationship between disturbed brain ontogenesis and schizophrenia.

STAGES IN THE ONTOGENESIS OF THE PRIMATE CEREBRAL CORTEX

Stage 1 - Proliferative Phase

The first major step in forebrain ontogenesis is the generation of large numbers of neurons in the telencephalic ventricular epithelium. In primates, this process is largely completed during the first third of pregnancy (Rakic 1975). Substantial affections of the proliferative process should result in major architectural anomalies and smaller affections may be expected to result in at least a change in the absolute number of forebrain neurons. Major experimental disturbances, such as those engendered by the administration of cytotoxic drugs to rat fetuses (Yurkewicz et al. 1984; Jones et al. 1982) result in disastrous changes in the extent and cytoarchitecture of the cerebral cortex (Fig.1). The changes demonstrable in treated rats include loss of whole cortical areas, with altered patterns of cortical lamination and islands of ectopic neurons in the cortex that remains. These changes undoubtedly result from loss of neurons as well as from destruction of neuroglial cells along whose processes young neurons migrate to the cortex. When of modest extent, the changes in the experimental brains can resemble the cytoarchitectonic changes described in the entorhinal cortex of schizophrenic brains by Jakob and Beckmann (1986, 1989) (see below). In trying to deal with the question of reduced numbers of cortical neurons which may reflect a lesser degree of developmental cell loss in schizophrenia, it is not known if the total number of neurons in cerebral cortex, basal ganglia or thalamus are consistently altered in the disease. Absolute numbers of neurons have been determined for two forebrain regions in schizophrenics: the mediodorsal nucleus of the thalamus (Pakkenberg, 1990, 1992) and the medial temporal cortex (Falkai et al., 1988; Heckers et al., 1991a). A decrease in neurons was reported in the mediodorsal nucleus (Pakkenberg, 1990, 1992) and in the parahippocampal gyrus (Falkai et al., 1988). However, it is not clear if these reflect degeneration of neurons secondary to primary pathology elsewhere and it is not known if they have a developmentally based origin. No changes in neuronal number were found in the hippocampal formation (Heckers et al., 1991a), which is anatomically and functionally closely related to the parahippocampal cortex (Rosene and Van Hoesen, 1987) and might be expected to show changes secondary to cell loss in the latter.

Any substantial alteration in the number of forebrain neurons in schizophrenia would be expected to cause an alteration in the volume of the gray matter of the cerebral cortex, basal ganglia and thalamus. Table I shows the results of several volumetric studies that have focused upon these regions. In general, the changes described have been rather subtle and the results of different studies, apart from those on the medial temporal cortex and the mediodorsal nucleus, have often been contradictory.

Similar inconsistencies are found in the results of studies analyzing neuronal number and density in the cerebral cortex of schizophrenics. The variable results of cell counting studies performed in different regions of medial temporal cortex have been mentioned above. The largest variability between individual studies is found among those that have analyzed neuronal density in the prefrontal cortex. Decreased prefrontal neuronal density was reported in the schizophrenic samples of Colon (1970) and Benes et al. (1986, 1991), increased in those of Selemon et al. (1993) and of Daviss and Lewis (1993), and unchanged in that of Bunney et al. (1993).

The lack of profound cytoarchitectural anomalies and the inconsistent nature of the alterations in gray matter volume and neuronal density described in the forebrains of schizophrenics make it unlikely that the proliferative phase of forebrain ontogenesis is compromised in any major way in schizophrenia. Volume reduction of the medial temporal cortex and mediodorsal thalamic nucleus in schizophrenics is the most

Table 1. Gray Matter Volumes in Schizophrenia

Frontal Cortex
MRI studies

1. Suddath et al. (1990):13 twin pairs, discordant for schizophrenia, no differences in prefrontal volumes between affected and non-affected twins.

2. Jernigan et al. (1991): 42 schizophrenics, 29 controls, no significant change in prefrontal gray matter volumes.

3. Zipursky et al. (1992): 23 schizophrenics, 20 controls, schizophrenics had a significant 7% reduction of prefrontal gray matter volumes.

4. Breier et al. (1992): 44 schizophrenics, 29 controls, no significant difference in prefrontal gray matter volumes.

5. Wible et al. (1993): 14 schizophrenics, 14 controls, no significant differences in prefrontal gray matter volumes.

Cingulate cortex
MRI studies

Chou-I et al. (1993) 14 schizophrenics, 14 controls, no significant differences in cingulate cortex volume.

Temporal cortex
MRI studies

1. Suddath et al. (1989) 17 schizophrenics, 17 controls, 20% reduction of temporal gray matter volume in schizophrenics.

2. Suddath et al. (1990) 13 twin pairs discordant for schizophrenia, significant 20% reduction of temporal gray matter volume on the left side, hippocampus-amygdala complex and of parahippocampal cortex in schizophrenics. bilateral reduced 10-20% in schizophrenics.

3. Jernigan et al. (1991) 42 schizophrenics, 29 controls, 9% significant reduction in volume of hippocampus-amygdala complex and of parahippocampal cortex in schizophrenics.

4. Zipursky et al. (1992) 23 schizophrenics, 20 controls, significant 6% reduction of temporo-parietal cortex volume in schizophrenics.

5. Shenton et al. (1992) 15 schizophrenics, 15 controls, significant 19% reduction of amygdala-anterior hippocampus volume and significant 15% reduction of left superior temporal gyrus volume in schizophrenics.

Post mortem volumetry

1. Falkai et al. (1988) 13 schizophrenics, 11 controls, significant 11-34% reduction of parahippocampal cortex volume in schizophrenics.

2. Altschuler et al. (1990) 12 schizophrenics, 12 controls, parahippocampal volume significantly decreased in the schizophrenic cohort.

3. Heckers et al. (1991a): 13 schizophrenics, 13 controls, no significant differences in hippocampal volume.

Basal ganglia
MRI studies

1. Jernigan et al. (1991) 42 schizophrenics, 29 controls, 13% significant increase in volume of lenticular nucleus volume in schizophrenics.

2. Breier et al. (1992) 44 schizophrenics, 29 controls, significant 9% enlargement in volume of the left caudate nucleus in schizophrenics.

3. Swayze et al. (1992) 54 schizophrenics, 47 controls, significant differences between schizophrenics and controls only in males, but not females, 10% larger caudate nucleus volume and 9% larger putamen volume in schizophrenics.

Post mortem volumetry

1. Bogerts et al. (1985) 13 schizophrenics, 9 controls, no change in caudate nucleus or putamen volume between schizophrenics and controls.

2. Bogerts et al. (1990) 18 schizophrenics, 21 controls, no changes in caudate nucleus or putamen volumes between the two cohorts.

3. Heckers et al. (1991b) 23 schizophrenics, 23 controls, significant increase of left caudate nucleus and putamen volume in schizophrenics.

Thalamus
Post mortem volumetry

1. Pakkenberg (1990) 20 schizophrenics, 14 controls, significant, 25 - 30% reduction of medio-dorsal nucleus volume in schizophrenics.

2. Pakkenberg (1992) 12 schizophrenics, 11 controls, 25 - 30% reduction of medio - dorsal nucleus volume in schizophrenics.

consistent finding of the morphometric approaches. However, it cannot be completely excluded that proliferative activity of the portion of the neuroepithelium that produces neurons destined for these forebrain regions was compromised in schizophrenics. Yet, in the absence of major cytoarchitectonic anomalies, this seems an unlikely explanation.

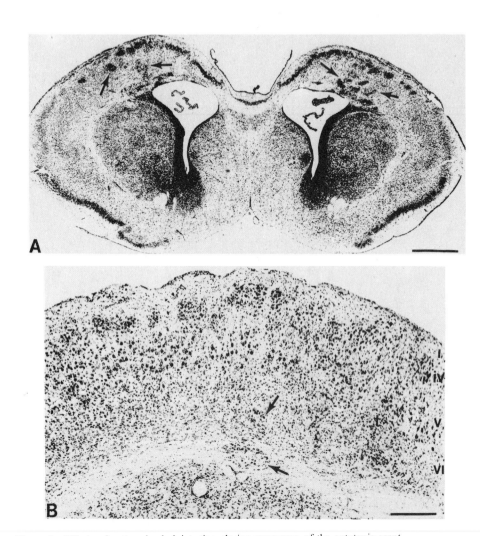

Figure 1. Effects of maternal administration during pregnancy of the cytotoxic agent, methylazoxymethanol, on cortical development in the offspring. Female rats received a single intraperitoneal dose at 14 days of gestation. The short term effect on a 19 day rat fetus is seen in A and is characterized by loss of whole cortical areas and layers and the presence of islands of cells (arrows) whose migration has been arrested. The effect on the adult cortex is seen in B and is characterized by loss of superficial cortical layers, irregular cytoarchitecture in the remaining layers and islands of ectopic cells (arrows). Yurkewicz et al., 1984. Bars: 1mm (A), 200μm (B).

32

Stage 2 - Migratory Phase

Young neurons destined for the cerebral cortex, thalamus and basal ganglia have to migrate from the ventricular neuroepithelium towards their definitive positions in these forebrain structures. During their migration, the neurons move along neuroglial fibers (Rakic, 1975, 1988), a process that, from work on cerebellar cells in vitro, is likely to be dependent upon NMDA receptors and N-type calcium channels (Komuro and Rakic, 1992, 1993). In monkey forebrain, the migratory phase is essentially limited to the second third of pregnancy (Rakic, 1972, 1974). Neuronal migration can be compromised by genetic mutations (Caviness et al. 1988) and environmental factors such as alcohol (Shetty and Phillips 1992, Miller 1993) and exposure to ionizing radiation (Rakic, 1988). These usually result in grossly abnormal cerebral gyration, such as lissencephaly and microgyria, with accompanying cytoarchitectonic malformations. In humans, a number of inherited disorders involve severe disturbances of neuronal migration: One example is the Miller Diecker form of lissencephaly, in which layers II, III and IV of the cerebral cortex are absent, the neurons originally destined for these layers having apparently settled in an abnormal position beneath the cortical plate (Richman et al., 1975; Caviness and Williams, 1979). A more frequent malformation of the human cerebral cortex, microgyria, characterized by numerous small and shallow cortical gyri, with greater than normal cell density in layers II and III, has also been explained in terms of defective neuronal migration (Richman et al., 1975; Caviness and Williams 1979). A possibly more circumscribed disturbance of neuronal migration may be found in a subpopulation of dyslexic individuals in whom parts of neocortex located in the planum temporale and adjacent regions show circumscribed micropolygyria and distortions of the normal cortical lamination pattern, characterized by neuronal ectopias in layer I and in the white matter (Galaburda et al. 1985).

At present, no conclusive evidence for a disturbance of neuronal migration has been demonstrated in brains of schizophrenics. Impaired neuronal migration has been invoked, however, to account for cytoarchitectonic anomalies described in the medial temporal cortex and hippocampal formation. These anomalies are said to include abnormal positioning and orientation of neurons in the cortex intervening between the presubiculum and the hippocampus in some (Scheibel and Kovelman, 1981; Kovelman and Scheibel, 1986; Altschuler et al., 1987; Conrad et al., 1991), but not all (Christinson et al., 1989) schizophrenic samples but the evidence upon which this interpretation is based is not clear. Cytoarchitectonic malformations of the entorhinal and insular cortex (Jakob and Beckmann, 1986, 1989; Arnold et al., 1991a) were interpreted as alterations in cell settling patterns consistent with disturbances of neuronal migration during development. In the rostral entorhinal area, these consisted of "poorly developed" lamination in the upper cortical layers and the displacement of islands of nerve cells, that are normally found in layer II, into layer III. These changes were found in approximately 50% of the schizophrenic brains examined, were more common in brains from non-paranoid schizophrenics and tended to be more prominent on the left side (Jakob and Beckmann, 1986). Associated with them were substantial reductions in cell numbers in all cortical layers, although the details of the cell counting procedures were not presented. In the insular cortex, cytoarchitectonic changes were reported in somewhat less than half of the schizophrenic brains. They consisted of reduced numbers of neurons in layers II and III, especially in the ventral insular regions adjacent to the entorhinal areas.

The cytoarchitecture of neocortical areas such as the prefrontal cortex, is within normal limits in schizophrenic brains (Benes et al., 1991; Akbarian et al., 1993a), making a migratory disturbance unlikely in this region whose function seems to be particularly compromised in schizophrenia. In the cingulate cortex of schizophrenics, an alteration in the texture of layer II, caused by the appearance of larger gaps between neuronal clusters, has been reported (Benes and Bird, 1987), but it is unlikely that this structural change reflects a disturbance of neuronal migration either. Apart from reductions in cell numbers in the mediodorsal nucleus (Pakkenberg, 1990, 1992), no significant cytoarchitectonic disturbances have been reported in thalamus or basal ganglia of schizophrenics.

Despite the lack of conclusive evidence for disturbances of neuronal migration in schizophrenia, this remains an attractive hypothesis to account for the cytoarchitectonic anomalies reported in the rostral entorhinal cortex (Jakob and Beckmann, 1986, 1989; Arnold et al., 1991a) and also for the alterations in the gyration pattern of the lateral temporal lobe, that have been described mainly in the subset of schizophrenics in which cytoarchitectonic anomalies were reported (Jakob and Beckmann, 1989). The possibility of a rather circumscribed affection of neuronal migration in the neocortex of the perisylvian region in cases of dyslexia (Galaburda et al., 1983) also suggests that this hypothesis deserves continued attention.

Stage 3 - Interactions in the Cortical Subplate

The steps involved in the establishment of the mature, highly complex pattern of connectivity of the primate forebrain are still incompletely understood. The following discussion is restricted to connection formation in the developing neocortex because few data are available on the thalamus and basal ganglia.

The formation of the complex pattern of intrinsic cortical connectivity and of the connections linking the cortex to subcortical centers occurs in a now well-understood sequence of events. In cats and primates, developing cortico-cortical and thalamocortical afferents do not grow directly into the developing cortical plate but instead, after arriving in the wall of the fetal telencephalon, rest during a waiting period lasting days or weeks in a transitional zone immediately beneath the cortical plate and referred to as the subplate (Shatz et al., 1990). The subplate is laid down subjacent to the developing cortex at the beginning of the second third of pregnancy (Marin-Padilla, 1988; Kostovic and Rakic, 1990; Shatz et al., 1990). It consists in large part of the earliest generated neurons of the cerebral cortex that initially form a primordial cortex. This is later split into the superficial marginal zone and the deeper subplate by later arriving and progressively accumulating cells of the definitive cortex. As these continue to arrive, they form the cortical plate situated between the marginal zone and the subplate. The cortical plate is the basis of the fully mature cerebral cortex.

The subplate which is particularly thick in the brains of human fetuses (Fig. 2), throughout its existence consists of early maturing neurons and a synaptic neuropil. The neurons form functional contacts with arriving thalamic afferents, with neurons in the overlying cortex and probably with one another (Marin-Padilla, 1988; Shatz et al., 1990; Friauf et al., 1990). The subplate neurons play a key role in helping establish the normal pattern of afferent connectivity in the overlying cortex and their processes which extend down into the internal capsule may guide cortical efferent axons to their targets (Shatz et al., 1990; O'Leary and Koester, 1993). The majority of subplate neurons undergo a program of physiological cell death (Chun and Shatz, 1989a). In primates, including humans, this occurs during late pregnancy and early postnatal life (Kostovic and Rakic 1990). However, substantial numbers are spared and remain throughout life as interstitial neurons of the white matter. These continue to maintain synaptic contact with the overlying cortex by means of lengthy ascending processes (Hendry et al., 1984) and are connected with the appropriate thalamic nucleus (Giguere and Goldman-Rakic, 1988).

An affection of the cortical subplate, perhaps involving altered migration patterns of subplate neurons or an alteration in their pattern of programmed cell death, may account for the distorted distribution of a subpopulation of neurons in the cerebral cortex and white matter of schizophrenics (Akbarian et al., 1993a,b). Neurons that stain for the enzyme, nicotinamide adenine dinucleotide phosphate diaphorase (NADPH-d), are normally found in a bimodal distribution, concentrated in layer II of the cortex and in the white mater immediately deep to layer VI (Fig. 3). In the prefrontal and lateral temporal areas of schizophrenics, these neurons were decreased in the cortex and in the superficial white matter (less than 2mm deep to the cortex) but increased in white matter up to 5mm deep to the cortex (Akbarian et al., 1993a,b). In

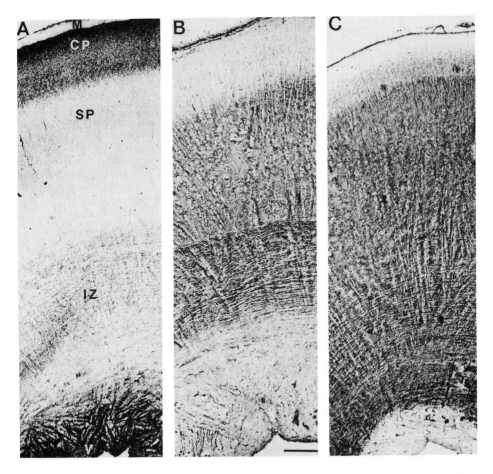

Figure 2. Adjacent sections through the wall of the cerebral hemisphere of a second trimester human fetal brain stained with thionin (A) or immunocytochemically for non-phosphorylated neurofilament proteins (B) or GAP 43 (C), showing the marginal zone (M), cortical plate (CP), subplate (SP), intermediate zone (IZ) and ventricular zone (V). Bar: 100μm.

the hippocampus and entorhinal cortex, numbers were reduced in the gray matter but the thinness of the white matter of these regions made it impossible to identify a comparable deep displacement in the white matter (Akbarian et al. 1993b). Other populations of interstitial neurons in the white matter also appear to be displaced deeply in the prefrontal cortex in brains of schizophrenics (Fig. 4). Those defined by immunoreactivity for a non-phosphorylated epitope of the 160 kDa and 200 kDa neurofilament chain and those defined by immunoreactivity for microtubule associated protein 2 (MAP2), were found to be more concentrated in deeper white matter of schizophrenics than in matched controls (Akbarian et al. 1993c).

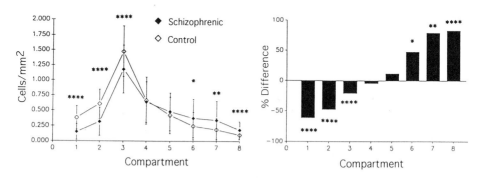

Figure 3. Left: mean density (± SD) of nicotinamide-adenine dinucleotide phosphate-diaphorase (NADPH-d)-stained neurons in prefrontal cortex and underlying white matter of a cohort of 5 schizophrenic brains (solid symbols), compared with the density in a cohort of 5 control brains (open symbols). Compartments 1 and 2 are the superficial and deep cortical layers respectively. Compartments 3-8 are successively deeper 800μm wide compartments of the white matter.

Right: Percentage difference in mean NADPH-d cell density (bars) for each compartment between the schizophrenic and control cohorts. In the schizophrenic brains, NADPH-d cells are reduced in the cortex and superficial white matter but increased in the deeper white matter. **** $p < 0.0001$; ** $p < 0.01$; * $p < 0.05$. From Akbarian et al., 1993a.

In schizophrenics, therefore, there is a change in the neuronal composition of white matter up to several millimeters beneath the prefrontal and lateral temporal cortex, and this appears to correspond to the territory of the former cortical subplate. Although a perturbation of the subplate may account for the modified distribution pattern, it is not clear if this results from an alteration in the primary migration of subplate neurons, in their pattern of programmed cell death, or from some hitherto unsuspected mechanism. The possibility that these have consequences for the organization and function of the overlying cortex is taken up below. The redistribution of NADPH-d neurons and of interstitial white matter neurons generally, does not seem to reflect an overall interference with neuronal migration to the cerebral cortex, although this originally seemed possible in view of the observations of Jakob and Beckmann on the entorhinal cortex. Subsequent investigation has revealed that the number and density of neurons in the overlying frontal cortex are not substantially altered in schizophrenics in comparison with matched controls (Bunney et al., 1993; Akbarian et al., 1993b) (Fig. 5). This leads us to focus on a primary defect in the subplate as a possible cause of the redistribution of NADPH-d and interstitial white matter neurons.

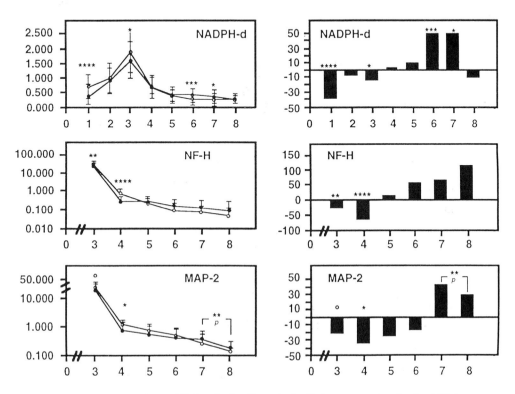

Figure 4. Left: densities of NADPH-d stained cells, and of cells immunoreactive for the 160kd neurofilament protein (NF-H) or for microtubule associated protein-2 (MAP-2) in successively deeper compartments (1-8) of the white matter beneath the prefrontal cortex in a cohort of 10 schizophrenic brains (closed symbols) and 10 controls (open symbols).

Right: Percentage differences in the densities of the three populations of cells. A similar trend is seen for the NF-H and MAP-2 cells. **** p < 0.0001; *** p < 0.001; ** p < 0.01; * p < 0.5; ° p = 0.5-0.8. Akbarian et al., 1993c.

Stage 4 - Shaping of Connectivity Patterns - The Role of Axonal Elimination

During the establishment of the normal pattern of cortical connectivity, axons grow into and out of the cerebral cortex in large numbers and to a large extent along defined trajectories. In this, they show a considerable degree of intrinsic determinism but are also guided by interactions of a molecular nature with pre-established neuroglial pathways and other structural scaffolds. Commissural, cortico-cortical and subcortical axons appear to grow out in greater numbers than those that are maintained into adulthood and the initial connectivity patterns in the early postnatal phase are to some extent less specific than those in the adult brain since many axons grow towards inappropriate targets (O'Leary and Koester, 1993). Inappropriate axon branches are later eliminated. Although most information comes from studies in rodents, there are sufficient data to indicate that comparable growth patterns occur in primates (Chalupa and Killackey, 1989; Meissirel et al., 1991; Webster et al. 1991), although the basic scheme of cortical connectivity is established prenatally (Chalupa et al. 1989, Schwartz and Goldman-Rakic 1990, 1991).

Total Neurons/Standard Strip

	Controls	Schizophrenics	p
Layer I	3.3 ± 2.1	3.4 ± 2.4	n.s.
Layer II	41.9 ± 8.4	42.8 ± 9.9	n.s.
Layer III	83.2 ± 13.2	82.4 ± 16.1	n.s.
Layer IV	37.5 ± 7.7	34.5 ± 9.2	n.s.
Layer V	42.5 ± 5.6	44.4 ± 8.5	n.s.
Layer VI	48.7 ± 7.4	50.2 ± 9.3	n.s.

Density of Small Round/Ovoid Cells

	Controls	Schizophrenics	p
Layer I	3.6 ± 2.3	3.5 ± 2.3	n.s.
Layer II	25.0 ± 6.9	24.8 ± 7.8	n.s.
Layer III	15.6 ± 6.6	17.2 ± 8.2	n.s.
Layer IV	23.8 ± 6.5	22.3 ± 7.6	n.s.
Layer V	7.8 ± 3.1	8.6 ± 4.5	n.s.
Layer VI	5.9 ± 2.6	5.9 ± 3.0	n.s.

Figure 5. Density of all thionin stained neurons (total neurons) and of the subpopulation of small round/ovoid (putatively GABAergic) cells in standard strips 250μm wide and extending through the thickness of the prefrontal cortex in a cohort of 10 schizophrenic brains and matched controls. There is no significant loss of cells in the schizophrenics, despite down regulation of GAD gene expression in the same area of cortex (cf. Fig. 8). Akbarian et al., 1993d.

Axonal elimination in primate brain most likely occurs during the first few months after birth (LaMantia and Rakic, 1990; Meissirel et al., 1991; Webster et al., 1991) during which time the final pattern of connectivity is attained and the initial overshoot of axonal connections is eliminated. Elimination of the initial large overproduction of synapses formed by the remaining axons may, however, continue for many months and even into early adulthood (Rakic et al., 1986). While the physiological and biochemical mechanisms which underlie the process of axonal elimination in the establishment of cortical connectivity are not sufficiently explored, experimental evidence in carnivores and non-human primates has demonstrated that axonal elimination in the sensory cortical areas is under the influence of sensory input from the periphery (Dehay et al. 1989, Frost and Moy 1989). Establishment, stabilization and maintenance of connections is also dependent on neurotrophic factors and ongoing neural activity. The role of neurotrophic factors in cortical development has hardly begun to be explored. However, functional nerve growth factor receptors are present in the subplate (Meinecke and Rakic, 1993) and their disappearance coincides with the period of extensive cell death in the subplate (Allendoerfer et al., 1990; Meinecke and Rakic, 1993), suggesting involvement of nerve growth factor in the early phases of axon growth and target finding. Brain Derived Neurotrophic Factor (BDNF), a neurotrophin more widely expressed in the adult brain and showing increased expression under conditions of axonal regeneration, is first expressed in the fetal monkey frontal cortex on the 121st day of gestation, when afferent connectivity is being established (Huntley et al., 1992) (Fig. 6). Delayed or perturbed expression of this neurotrophin may, therefore, have serious consequences for adequate connection formation.

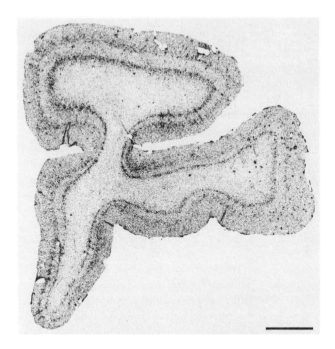

Figure 6. Autoradiogram of a section through the prefrontal cortex of a monkey fetus at 135 days of gestation, showing distribution of neurons labeled by in situ hybridization of a radioactive RNA probe complementary to the mRNA coding for brain derived neurotrophic factor. Huntley et al., 1992. Bar: 1mm.

At present, it is difficult to study cortical connectivity in the human brain, because the tracing of neuronal interconnections in post mortem tissue can only be achieved with available techniques over a few millimeters, thus excluding the examination of connections other than those intrinsic to the cortex. Therefore, it is not possible to determine directly if the specification of cortical connectivity and the process of axonal elimination have been compromised in brains of schizophrenics. A number of reported morphological abnormalities could imply a potential deficit in cortical axonal elimination in schizophrenia: Increased volume of the corpus callosum in some schizophrenic samples (Nasrallah et al., 1986; Raine et al., 1990) could indicate an incomplete elimination of transcallosal connections in some schizophrenics. The pattern of abnormalities described in the corpus callosum in schizophrenia are, however, rather variable (Casanova et al., 1990; Gunther et al., 1991). Several studies have reported a *decreased* callosal volume (Hauser et al., 1989; Rossi et al., 1989; Woodruff et al., 1993) and schizophrenics may show an increased incidence of partial callosal agenesis (Swayze et al., 1990; Degreef et al., 1992). Several authors have emphasized, that individual schizophrenic brains show an unusual variability in the volume of the corpus callosum, in comparison with those of a control cohort (Coger and Serafetinides, 1990; Gunther et al., 1991). These findings suggest that schizophrenics do not show a uniform abnormality of the corpus callosum and make it hard to predict that a defect in the normal, developmentally regulated elimination of superabundant transcallosal connections (LaMantia and Rakic, 1990) has occurred.

Disturbances of axonal elimination in the cerebral cortex of schizophrenics have also been invoked to account for a reported increase in thickness of vertical axon bundles (Benes and Bird, 1987) and increased numbers of vertical, glutamergic fibers (Benes et al., 1992a) in the cingulate cortex and for alterations in glutamergic receptor density in the prefrontal cortex of schizophrenics (Deakin et al., 1989). It is not clear if the consistently reported increase in ventricular volume results from axonal loss in the surrounding white matter.

Stage 5 - Refinement and Maturation of Functional Connections

Synaptic pruning and myelination. The formation, stabilization and maintenance of synapses in the cerebral cortex is under the influence of mechanisms that extend beyond the time window during which the basic connections are established. In the human brain, the density of cortical synapses increases during the first year of life, but later decreases progressively to reach a relatively stable number in approximately the 15th year, a further decline occurring in senescence (Huttenlocher, 1979; Huttenlocher and de Courten, 1987; Huttenlocher, 1990). Studies in frontal and occipital cortex of humans and of non-human primates have demonstrated that the elimination of overabundant synapses is a general characteristic of primate cortex, starting in early postnatal life and ending around the time of puberty (Rakic et al., 1986; Zecevic et al., 1989; Huttenlocher, 1990; Missler et al., 1993). At least in early stages, the process of synaptic pruning appears to be synchronized across the various areas of cerebral cortex, as measured by contemporaneous changes in receptor densities (Lidow et al. 1991).

A further well-known feature of the maturing primate cerebral cortex is the delayed myelination of the association areas in comparison with the primary sensory and motor areas (Flechsig, 1927). It is a general belief that increased myelination of these fiber pathways improves the functional connections between the cortical association fields and other brain structures (Weinberger, 1987; Benes, 1989). In the human brain, myelination of the association fields continues into the second decade of life, but varies considerably among individuals and potentially even extends beyond the second decade (Yakovlev and Lecours, 1967; Benes, 1989).

While there is, as yet, no convincing evidence for a disturbance of either the process of synaptic pruning or that of myelination in brains of schizophrenics, a failure in the orderly pruning of cortical synapses (Feinberg, 1982), and defects of myelination have been proposed as factors in the pathophysiology of schizophrenia (Weinberger, 1987; Benes, 1989). The main line of argument in both these theories is that the functional maturation of the prefrontal cortex, as measured by neuropsychological methods (Goldman-Rakic, 1987), occurs in the second decade of life, and thus coincides with both the terminal phases of synaptic pruning (Huttenlocher, 1990) and of myelination (Yakovlev and Lecours, 1967). This in turn coincides with the period in which the psychopathological symptoms of schizophrenia usually have their onset (Kraepelin, 1919).

Activity - dependent phenomena in cortical development. Neural activity, by which we understand the initiation and propagation of action potentials and the genesis of membrane conductance and polarization changes, is one of the most powerful factors in setting up precise patterns of connectivity during brain development (Shatz, 1990) and in the stabilization and maintenance of synaptic connections thereafter (Jones 1990). Thalamocortical axons on first entering the subplate are capable of conducting action potentials and of generating excitatory postsynaptic potentials in subplate cells (Friauf et al., 1990). These may represent signals whereby subplate influences are conveyed to the overlying cortical plate, influences which may represent signals by means of which the axons, when later invading the cortex are able to recognize their appropriate target cells.

The establishment of domains of axonal distribution in the developing nervous system is also profoundly influenced by activity. In the tectum of the frog, when axon potential propagation along regenerating retinotectal axons is blocked the regenerating fibers can still reach the tectum, but their terminal ramifications are unusually widespread and fail to establish the fine grain retinotopy which is normally observed (Schmidt, 1985) and which is dependent upon NMDA receptor activation of postsynaptic cells (Cline et al., 1987). In the establishment of connectivity in the mammalian cerebral cortex, the initial pattern of ingrowth of afferent axons is relatively diffuse and is only later refined into domains of influence of individual or groups of related axons, upon which topographic maps in the cortex depend. One of the best known examples of this is in the visual cortex of cats and monkeys in which ocular dominance columns representing alternating input regions of thalamocortical fibers bearing impulses from the left and right eyes segregate out from an initially diffuse, overlapping pattern (Hubel et al., 1977; LeVay et al., 1978). This process of segregation begins in utero but is strongly influenced by sensory input early in postnatal life. During a critical early postnatal period, segregation of thalamocortical fibers into ocular dominance columns is strongly dependent on matched patterns of input emanating from the two eyes. If this becomes unbalanced, e.g. if one eye is deprived of pattern vision, or impulse activity is blocked in one optic nerve, the more active inputs and thus the unaffected eye is at a competitive advantage and comes to acquire more synaptic space in the cortex. This is manifested anatomically by its widened ocular dominance columns and a greater number of cells than usual being driven preferentially by the undeprived eye (LeVay et al., 1980). There are numerous visual deprivation paradigms which can alter the degree of ocular dominance segregation during the critical period. All of these depend upon changes in the balance of inputs from the two eyes. There are comparable experiments which demonstrate the same kind of activity dependent influences upon the topographic organization of the somatic sensory cortex of rodents

(Van der Loos and Woolsey, 1973; Killackey et al., 1976).

Effective connection formation also involves the stabilization of synapses once made and in the cerebral cortex, as elsewhere, this requires the induction of membrane events (Wilson et al., 1977; Singer et al., 1977; Shaw and Cynader, 1984; Reiter and Stryker, 1988) and of gene expression for particular molecules in the postsynaptic cells. Among the latter are postsynaptic effects that involve the regulation of neurotransmitter and receptor function (reviewed in Jones, 1990). Although activity

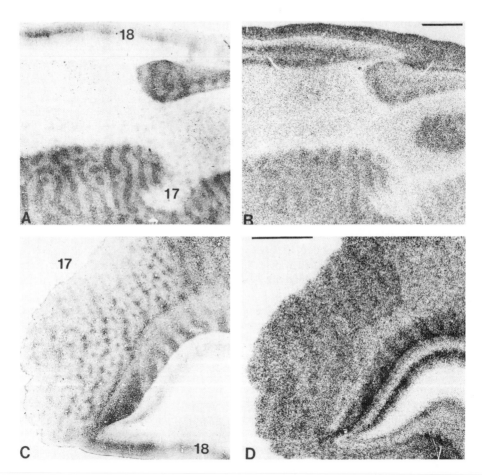

Figure 7. A Section through the visual cortex of an adult monkey in which impulse activity was blocked in one optic nerve for 48 hours by intravitreal injection of tetrodotoxin, stained for cytochrome oxidase and showing the pattern of alternating ocular dominance stripes related to the deprived (light) and non-deprived (dark) eye. B Autoradiogram from an adjacent section hybridized with a radioactive RNA probe complementary to the mRNA coding for CAM II kinase-a which shows increased expression in the deprived ocular dominance columns. Benson et al., 1991b. C,D Paired sections from another monkey, monocularly deprived for 8 days, showing the CO-stained deprivation effect (C) and a corresponding down regulation of labeling (D) for the mRNA coding for the a1 subunit of the GABA-A receptor. Huntsman et al., 1994.
Areas 17 and 18 indicated. Bars: 1mm.

dependent phenomena appear to be at work in the shaping of cortical connectivity during development, they are also involved in the maintenance of functional connectivity throughout the lifetime of the individual. This is probably best revealed by experiments that demonstrate the plasticity of representational maps in the somatic sensory, auditory and visual cortices of mature animals including primates. Large shifts in the position and extent of a portion of the cortex representing a particular part of the receptive periphery can be induced by reductions or enhancements of neural activity emanating from the peripheral receptors (Kaas et al., 1983; Wall et al., 1986; Clark et al., 1988; Jenkins et al., 1990; Allard et al., 1991). The exact nature of the mechanisms that induce shifts of several mms in parts of a representational map are incompletely understood but they are thought to involve to a large extent the silencing of certain synapses and the uncovering or enhancement of others that were previously silent, leading to changes in the previous balance of intracortical excitation and inhibition. This is associated with up- and down-regulation of gene expression for transmitter, receptor and other neuroactive molecules. Monocular visual deprivation, for as little as four days in an adult monkey, for example, will affect the visual cortex in such a way as to cause large decreases in the inhibitory transmitter, gaminobu-tyric acid and its receptors, and parallel increases in a calcium calmodulin dependent protein kinase, a postsynaptic density protein associated with excitatory synapses and synaptic learning (Hendry and Jones 1986,1988; Hendry and Kennedy 1986; Hendry et al;.,1990; Benson et al.,1991a, b, 1993; Huntsman et al.,1993) (Fig.7). Activity-dependent effects of this kind are likely to underlie changes in topographic maps under conditions of reduced, enhanced or perturbed inputs to the cortex.

The fact that neuronal activity is of crucial importance for the development and maintenance of neuronal circuitry in the brain raises the question of whether a defect of the cortical subplate in the schizophrenic brain, leading to some degree of alteration in the distribution of afferent axons, axonal pruning or the efficacy of connection formation in the overlying cortex could compromise this circuitry to the extent that interactions with other cortical and subcortical regions are compromised and may decompensate when stressed by life events, leading to the onset of symptoms. Altered or compromised circuitry should be manifested by the appearance of changes in the levels and distributions of neuroactive molecules whose expression is activity dependent. There are a number of observations that suggest, indirectly, that neural circuitry is compromised in the brains of schizophrenics and that this has had activity dependent consequences. Imaging studies in adult schizophrenics, show functional hypoactivity in widespread regions of the forebrain, particularly the prefrontal cortex, striatum and medial temporal lobe (Buchsbaum et al. 1992, Weinberger et al. 1992). These are regions that are highly interconnected with one another and with the mediodorsal thalamus and play an important role in representational memory (Goldman-Rakic, 1987). They are key elements in the psychosis circuitry proposed in virtually every circuit-based theory of schizophrenia. If this circuitry is hypoactive, are there any associated effects that can be attributed to activity-dependent down regulation of transmitter function? A number of observations suggest that this may be so. Many of these relate to the inhibitory GABAergic system. GABA is the transmitter used by 25% of the neurons of the primate cerebral cortex (Jones, 1993) and receptors for it are expressed by virtually every cell of the cortex (Huntsman et al., 1993). In schizophrenic brains, GABA function appears to be severely compromised, as measured by decreased GABA uptake in the temporal cortex (Simpson et al. 1992), by upregulation of GABA-A receptors as measured by radioactive ligand binding in superficial layers of the cingulate cortex (Benes et al. 1992b), and by decreased gene expression for glutamic acid decarboxylase (GAD), the enzyme that synthesizes GABA, as measured by in situ hybridization histochemistry in the prefrontal cortex (Bunney et al. 1993, Akbarian et al., 1993d) (Fig. 8). The down regulation of mRNA levels for GAD in the prefrontal cortex is of particular interest since it occurs in the absence of any loss of neurons in those areas (Fig. 5). Thus, it is probably best explained as an activity dependent change based upon hypoactivity and having parallels with the down regulation of GAD gene expression found under conditions of monocular deprivation in the visual cortex alluded to above. Up regulation of dopamine D_4 receptors observed in the brains of schizophrenics (Seeman et al., 1993) may be based on the same general mechanism although dopamine fibers appear to terminate preferentially on non-GABAergic neurons in the frontal cortex (Goldman Rakic et al., 1989). What is now required is to determine if the functional hypoactivity stems from altered circuitry that is developmentally based.

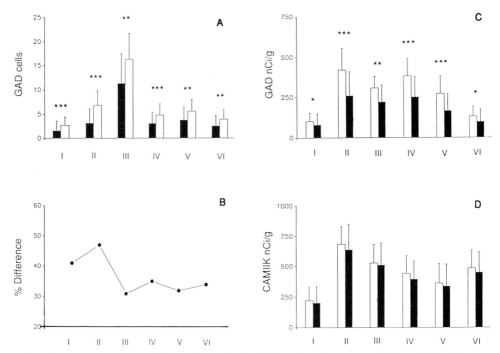

Figure 8. A Mean and SD of the number of GAD mRNA expressing neurons in layers I-VI of the prefrontal cortex in a cohort of 10 schizophrenic (filled symbols) and control (open symbols) brains. B Percentage decrease of GAD expressing neurons in layers I-V of the schizophrenic brains. *** $p < 0.0001$;** $p < 0.001$.C,D Mean levels of GAD (C) and CAM II kinase-a mRNAs across the six layers in the schizophrenic (filled symbols) and control (open symbols) cortex. *** $p < 0.0001$;** $p < 0.001$;* $p < 0.05$.cf Fig. 5. Akbarian et al., 1993d.

THE TIMING OF RISK DURING PREGNANCY AND EARLY POSTNATAL LIFE

Many dys- and hypoplasias of human tissues are determined by environmental factors that exert their influence only during a narrow time window of vulnerability in pregnancy (Graham, 1991). The phase specificity of environmental factors is given by the timing of the particular ontogenetic step with which they interfere. Is there evidence that in schizophrenia there is also a period of selective vulnerability during pregnancy and early postnatal life?

Epidemiological studies have identified a number of risk factors that act during pregnancy and increase the incidence of schizophrenia in offspring. These include viral illness, especially influenza (Mednick et al., 1988), obstetrical complications (Mednick and Cannon, 1991), and malnutrition (Susser and Lin, 1992). Infection with the influenza virus during pregnancy increases the incidence of schizophrenia only when the infection occurs during the second trimester (Mednick et al., 1988; Kendell and Kemp, 1989; Barr et al., 1990; Crow et al., 1991; O'Callaghan et al., 1991; Sham et al., 1992). By contrast, the effect of severe malnutrition, which increases the incidence of schizophrenia in female offspring only, seems to be limited to the first trimester (Susser and Lin, 1992). Obstetrical complications occurring around birth are another risk factor for the development of schizophrenia in offspring, especially in the presence of a genetic load as indicated by the diagnosis of schizophrenia in a first degree relative (Fish et al., 1992; Mednick and Cannon,1991). A yet incompletely understood observation is that births occurring in the spring quarter of the year are associated with an increased incidence of schizophrenia (Torrey and Bowler, 1990). The seasonality of birth hypothesis of schizophrenia has, however, been challenged on methodological grounds (Lewis, 1989).

A clear cut time window of vulnerability does not exist in schizophrenia, but all known risk factors affecting male offspring and the majority of risk factors affecting female offspring fall into the period extending from the second trimester of pregnancy to the time around birth. Influenza infection in the second trimester appears to be the most clear-cut example of a risk factor specifically acting during a relatively narrow time window.

What Steps of Forebrain Ontogenesis Are Most Likely to be Affected in Schizophrenia?

Morphological data, as presented in Part 2, have provided suggestive evidence that certain steps in brain ontogenesis, particularly neuronal migration, subplate function and axonal elimination may be affected in schizophrenia. Evidence for a disturbance of the earliest step, neuronal proliferation, and of the last step, synaptic pruning and myelination, is weak or absent. Two facts illustrate that any developmental pathology in schizophrenia is likely to be highly complex: First, no single major ontogenetic step may be affected. Second, each of the steps that have been postulated to be affected appear to be compromised only in selective forebrain regions, and not in the forebrain in general. Changes postulated to derive from defective neuronal migration, for example, are only apparent in limbic cortex of the medial temporal lobe (Scheibel and Kovelman, 1981; Jakob and Beckmann, 1986) and comparable changes cannot be detected in the remaining 85-90% of the cerebral cortex. By contrast, the changes that led to the hypothesis of an affection of the embryonic subplate were observed in prefrontal and lateral temporal neocortex but could not be detected in the medial temporal cortex (Akbarian et al., 1993a,b), although this may have been due to the thinness of the white matter in that region. Alterations in fiber architecture, possibly indicating a disturbance of axonal elimination, were found in cingulate cortex, but not in the adjacent prefrontal cortex (Benes et al., 1992). This heterogeneity of histological change and the difficulty of relating the changes directly to an overt disruption of any of the major steps in cortical histogenesis, make it unlikely that there is a single pathology demonstrable by conventional microscopic techniques in all schizophrenic brains. If a single developmental factor is involved, it may operate at a molecular level not identifiable with classical anatomical techniques. The various structural changes described may be secondary to this and differ from brain to brain. Individual schizophrenics may each have their own set of brain abnormalities, due to variations in the severity and anatomical location of the postulated primary developmental disturbance.

Despite the growing evidence for histological changes in the cerebral cortex of schizophrenics, it is clear that in the large majority of cases, the variations from normal do not result in major structural changes in the brain. Only a small subset of schizophrenics shows gross macroscopic alterations, such as partial agenesis of the corpus callosum (Swayze et al.. 1990; Degreef et al., 1992) or altered gyration in the insular and temporal cortex (Jakob and Beckmann, 1986) and it is not certain if these are in any way related to the pathophysiology of the disease. The most consistent macroscopic abnormality found in MRI studies of the schizophrenic brain is enlargement of the inferior horns of the lateral ventricles (Johnstone et al., 1976; Johnstone et al., 1989; Roberts and Bruton, 1990). The cause of this enlargement is not clear but, *a priori,* it would be expected to be associated with loss of cerebral substance, either of the white matter surrounding the ventricles or of adjacent gray matter structures such as the amygdala and hippocampus. Cell loss in one or other of these or loss of fibers joining them would clearly be of importance in advancing a connectionist view of schizophrenic symptomatology. It is difficult to explain the dilatation in the presence of the only equivocal changes in the volume of the white or gray matter that have been described.

In the absence of severe defects of brain structure in schizophrenics, it is likely that if developmental mechanisms are disrupted as a primary event in the disease, they will be those that govern the establishment and refinement of cortical connections. If the pattern of connectivity is not set up appropriately, it may play a major role in the symptomatology of the psychosis. The disintegration of orderly thought processes in schizophrenia can be likened to and may betoken a complex functional disconnection syndrome. Disruption of mechanisms involved in the formation and refinement of connections could stem from a disruption of interactions in the cortical subplate and of the process of axonal elimination. The normal range of timing of these two processes, extending from the second trimester to the early postnatal period, coincides well with the timing of most extraneous risk factors that appear to operate in schizophrenia.

Experimental studies have shown that the pattern of cortical connectivity can be altered by developmental perturbations without overt morphological changes. Selective destruction of the subplate by kainic acid injections beneath the developing visual cortex of fetal cats leads to failure of thalamo-cortical fibers, after entering the cortex, to segregate into ocular dominance columns. The cortex, however, appears entirely normal in terms of cytoarchitecture and gyration (Shatz et al., 1990; Gosh and Shatz, 1992). Similarly, critical period dependent changes in the distribution of retinogeniculate fibers in the visual cortex and many other experimental manipulations that cause aberrant connectivity of cortex (Sur et al., 1988; O'Leary and Koester, 1993) and of thalamocortical connections (Chang et al., 1986; Blakemore and Molnar, 1990; Molnar and Blakemore, 1991), are without overt morphological manifestations. This is not a universal finding; a notable exception is activity dependent alterations in the barrel cortex of developing rodents (Schlaggar et al., 1993). The massive reduction in the number of axons in the corpus callosum and loss of synapses in the course of normal cortical development (Rakic et al., 1986; La Mantia and Rakic, 1990; Lidow et al., 1991) are also not accompanied by overt changes in cortical architecture. These observations suggest that developmental defects that lead to a pathological wiring pattern in brains of schizophrenics could have serious consequences for cortical function, without being revealed by classical morphometric approaches such as cytoarchitectonics, cell counting or volumetry.

Although functional connectivity in the schizophrenic cortex, as manifested by

46

the symptoms of the disease, is obviously disorganized, defective connectivity has still not been identified morphologically. However, neurochemical alterations, such as down regulation of GAD gene expression and upregulation of dopamine D4 receptors, (that are not the result of neuroleptics), when taken in the light of knowledge about activity dependent regulation of neurotransmitter function in experimental animals, support the notion that altered connectivity may be an underlying element of the disease. Furthermore, this alteration of connectivity may have its origins in a developmental aberration.

Because major, morphologically detectable alterations of brain structure are absent in the majority of schizophrenics, we speculate that if a developmental disturbance is an operational factor in the causation of schizophrenia, it is most likely to be one involving mechanisms of orderly connection formation. The overt manifestations of this may stem from activity-dependent effects on transmitter- and receptor- related gene expression resulting from an imbalanced connectional pattern. Activity dependent effects may extend far beyond those on transmitter and receptor related molecule and include regulation of other neuronal components including structural proteins. This may explain the observation of Arnold et al. (1991b) that immunoreactivity for two microtubule associated proteins, MAP2 and MAP5, is reduced in the hippocampus of schizophrenic brains. Variations in the location and severity of a defect in connections or in the secondary effects resulting from it may help explain the heterogeneity of symptoms in schizophrenics. In the subpopulation of schizophrenics that shows morphological changes in the medial temporal lobe (Scheibel and Kovelman, 1981; Kovelman and Scheibel, 1986; Jakob and Beckmann, 1986; Arnold et al., 1991a), these changes may reflect major involvement of connections between the temporal cortex, hippocampus and frontal lobe. Whether this results from a primary defect of neuronal migration remains an open question.

Is There Altered Brain Ontogenesis in Schizophrenia and What Are Its Functional Consequences?

There are two possible relations between the putative developmental abnormalities in the brains of schizophrenics and the disease. In the first, the structural abnormalities that have been described may be caused by a defect in orderly brain development but by themselves may not be the underlying basis of schizophrenic psychopathology. That is, they may be only epiphenomena, perhaps deriving from the same genetic loading that leads to the brain dysfunction appearing in adolescence and adulthood that we term schizophrenia. However, the brain dysfunction and the ontogenetic alterations would not be causally related to one other. For example, a fundamental defect in neurotransmitter- or receptor-related gene expression could lead to defective functional circuitry in the adult and to developmental anomalies since a number of neurotransmitters and their receptors exert trophic influences on developing neurons. These include migratory guidance (Komuro and Rakic, 1992, 1993), neurite outgrowth (Mattson, 1988; Kater and Mills, 1991) and synaptogenesis (Jessell and Kandel, 1993).

The second possible relation between schizophrenia and putative developmental anomalies in the brain is that the two may be causally linked. In this case, psychopathological symptoms may be the final outcome of functional alterations that are triggered by particular developmental disturbances. That is to say, the developmental anomalies would cause disturbances of cortical connectivity that render the connections subject to functional decompensation when stressed by life events. Interference with a key structure such as the cortical subplate, potentially could lead to defective neuronal circuits that could under appropriate stress, decompensate and lead to schizophrenia - related psychopathology. The dysfunction of the adult brain would then be causally linked to a defective subplate. Subplate pathology could, however, be caused by a variety of genetic or toxic factors and these could vary from case to case. This could help explain the difficulty in identifying a single epidemiological cause of schizophrenia.

A causal linkage between a defect in the orderly establishment of forebrain connectivity and psychosis has been suggested by clinical investigations and in vivo imaging studies: Hyde et al. (1992) documented the similarities of psychopathological symptoms in schizophrenia and metachromatic leukodystrophy, a disorder characterized by diffuse demyelination of subcortical white matter (Alzheimer, 1910). The implication is, that abnormal connectivity is the underlying basis of the psychotic symptoms. While pathological connections in metachromatic leukodystrophy are obviously caused by demyelination, in schizophrenia this is less clear and they may derive from an ontogenetic defect. Anomalous connections between cortical and subcortical centers in brains of schizophrenics were suggested by Weinberger (1987) by correlating clinical observations with experimental anatomical studies (Mesulam, 1978) in monkeys. Functional imaging studies *in vivo* have demonstrated that in schizophrenia dysfunction of several forebrain regions such as prefrontal cortex, medial temporal cortex and basal ganglia may occur in an apparently interrelated fashion. This is manifested by simultaneous reductions in glucose metabolism in basal ganglia and prefrontal cortex (Buchsbaum et al., 1992), or by concurrent reductions in regional blood flow in the prefrontal and medial temporal cortex (Weinberger et al.,1992). These studies suggest a disturbed interaction between the prefrontal and medial temporal cortex and the basal ganglia as one basis of schizophrenic symptomatology. The basis of the disturbed interaction could be disorganized and/or decompensated connectivity. Decompensation may manifest itself by changes in expression of particular transmitters and their receptors and this in turn may be revealed by the psychopharmacology of the disease.

CONCLUSIONS

The lack of major morphological changes in brains of schizophrenics implies that the first steps of forebrain ontogenesis, that is proliferation and migration, are not profoundly affected, if at all, in the brains of most schizophrenics. The coincidence of timing at which most schizophrenia - related risk factors operate in pregnancy with the period during which patterns of normal connectivity are being established in the fetus, suggests that mechanisms involved in this complex, multidimensional process may be compromised in schizophrenia. Certain neuroanatomical findings such as corpus callosum abnormalities, described in brains of schizophrenics, and the results of functional imaging studies suggesting defective functional connectivity between forebrain centers tend to support this view. The results of our own investigations have led us to focus on the cortical subplate as a potential site of a lesion that may affect connectional development, and on the activity-dependent disturbances of functional circuitry that ensue from this.

In future research, it may be beneficial to concentrate upon the patterns of circuitry in brains of schizophrenics. Connection tracing methods that are applicable to post mortem material are now available and should enable the analysis of afferent, efferent and local connectivity in human adult and fetal brains (Burkhalter and Bernardo, 1989; Burkhalter et al., 1993). These should enable any alterations in circuitry to be detected. To them should be added studies of the mechanisms that enable key structures such as the subplate to determine the pattern of connections in the overlying cerebral cortex, and of the activity-dependent molecular and pharmacological consequences of an atypical pattern of connectivity, especially under conditions in which the connections are stressed.

ACKNOWLEDGMENTS

This work was supported by Grant number MH44188 from the National Institute of Mental Health, United States Public Health Service, by a Young Investigator Award from the National Alliance for Research on Schizophrenia and Depression to S.A. and by a Stanley Award from the National Alliance for the Mentally Ill to E.G.J.

REFERENCES

Akbarian, S., Bunney, W.E., Jr., Potkin, S.G., Wigal, S.B., Hagman, J.O., Sandman, C.A., and Jones, E.G., 1993a, Altered distribution of nicotinamide-adenine-dinucleotide-phosphate-diaphorase cells in frontal lobe of schizophrenics implies disturbances of cortical development, *Arch Gen Psychiatry* 50:169-177.

Akbarian, S., Viñuela, A., Kim, J.J., Potkin, S.G., Bunney, W.E., Jr., and Jones, E.G., 1993b, Distorted distribution of nicotinamide-adenine dinucleotide phosphate-diaphorase neurons in temporal lobe of schizophrenics implies anomalous cortical development *Arch Gen Psychiatry* 50:178-187.

Akbarian, S., Kim, J.J., Tafazzolli, A., Hagman, J.O., Potkin, S.G., Bunney, W.E. Jr., and Jones, E.G., 1993c, Altered neurocellular composition of prefrontal cortex in schizophrenia *Soc Neurosci Abstr.* 19:200.

Akbarian, S., Kim, J.J., Hagman, J.O., Potkin, S.G., Bunney, W.E., Jr., and Jones, E.G., 1993d, submitted, Gene expression for glutamic acid decarboxylase is reduced without loss of neurons in prefrontal cortex of schizophrenics.

Allard, T., Clark. SA., Jenkins W.M., and Merzenich, M.M., 1991, Reorganization of somatosensory area 3b representations in adult owl monkeys after digital syndactyly, *J Neurophysiol* 66:1048-1058.

Allendoerfer, K.L., Shelton, D.L., Shooter, E.M., and Shatz, C.J., 1990, Nerve growth factor immunoreactivity is transiently associated with the subplate neurons of the mammalian cerebral cortex, *Proc Natl Acad Sci USA* 87:187-190.

Altschuler, L.L., Conrad, A., Kovelman, J.A., and Scheibel, A., 1987, Hippocampal pyramidal cell orientation in schizophrenia, *Arch Gen Psychiatry* 44:1904-1098.

Altschuler, L.L., Casanova M.F., Goldberg T.E., and Kleinman, J.E., 1990, The hippocampus and parahippocampus in schizophrenic, suicide, and control brains, *Arch Gen Psychiatry* 47:1029-1034.

Alzheimer, A., 1910, Beitrag zur Kenntniss der pathologischen Neuroglia und ihrer Beziehungen zu Abbauvorgaengen im Nervengewebe, *in*: "Histologische und Histopathologische Arbeiten Ueber die Grosshirnrinde," F. Nissl, and A. Alzheimer, ed., Vol 3, pp 401-404. Jena, Germany: Gustav Fisher.

Arnold, S.E., Hyman, B.T., Van Hoesen, G.W., and Damasio, A.R., 1991a, Some cytoarchitectural abnormalities of the entorhinal cortex in schizophrenia, *Arch Gen Psychiatry* 48:625-632.

Arnold, S.E., Lee, V.M.-Y., Gur, R.E., and Trojanowski, J.Q., 1991b, Abnormal expression of two microtubule-associated proteins (MAP2 and MAP5, in specific subfields of the hippocampal formation in schizophrenia, *Proc Natl Acad Sci USA* 88:10850-10854.

Barr, C.E., Mednick S.A., and Munk-Jorgensen, P., 1990, Exposure to influenza during gestation and adult schizophrenia, *Arch Gen Psychiatry* 47:869-874.

Bender, L., 1947, Childhood schizophrenia: Clinical study of 100 schizophrenic children, *Am J Orthpsychiatry* 17:40-56.

Bender, L., and Freedman, A.M., 1952, A study of the first three years in the maturation of schizophrenic children, *QJ Child Behav* 1:245-272.

Benes, F.M., Davidson, J., and Bird, E.D., 1986, Quantitative cytoarchitectural analyses of the cerebral cortex of schizophrenics, *Arch Gen Psychiatry* 43:31-35.

Benes, F.M., and Bird, E.D., 1987, An analysis of the arrangement of neurons in the cingulate cortex of schizophrenic patients, *Arch Gen Psychiatry* 44:608-616.

Benes, F.M., and Bird, E.D., 1987, An analysis of the arrangement of neurons in the cingulate cortex of schizophrenic patients, *Arch Gen Psychiatry* 44:608-616.

Benes, F.M., 1989, Myelination of cortical-hippocampal relays during late adolescence, *Schizophr Bull* 15:585-593.

Benes, F.M., McSparren, J., Bird, E.D., SanGiovanni, J.P., and Vincent, S.L., 1991, Deficits in small interneurons in prefrontal and cingulate cortices of schizophrenic and schizoaffective patients, *Arch Gen Psychiatry* 48:996-1001.

Benes, F.M., Sorensen, I., Vincent, S.L., Bird, D., and Sathi, M., 1992a, Increased density of glutamate-immunoreactive vertical processes in superficial laminae in cingulate cortex of schizophrenic brain, *Cereb Cortex* 2:503-512.

Benes, F.M., Vincent, S.L., Alsterberg, G., Bird, E.D., and SanGiovanni, J.P., 1992b, Increased GABA A receptor binding in superficial layers of cingulate cortex in schizophrenia, *J Neurosci* 12:924-929.

Benson, D.L., Isackson, P.J., Hendry, S.H.C., and Jones, E.G., 1991a, Differential gene expression for glutamic acid decarboxylase and type II calcium-calmodulin-dependent protein kinase in basal ganglia, thalamus, and hypothalamus of the monkey, *J Neurosci* 11:1540-1564.

Benson, D.L., Isackson, P.J., Gall, C.M., and Jones, E.G., 1991b, Differential effects of monocular deprivation on glutamic acid decarboxylase and type II calcium-calmodulin-dependent protein kinase gene expression in the adult monkey visual cortex, *J Neurosci* 11:31-47.

Benson, D.L., Huntsman, M.M., and Jones, E.G., 1993, Activity dependent changes in GAD and preprotachykinin mRNAs in visual cortex of adult monkeys, *Cerebral Cortex*, in press.

Blakemore, C., and Molnar, Z., 1990, Factors involved in the establishment of specific interconnections between thalamus and cerebral cortex, *Cold Spring Harbor Symp Quant Biol* 55:491-504.

Bogerts, B., Hantsch, J., and Herzer, M., 1983, A morphometric study of the dopamine-containing cell groups in the mesencephalon of normals, Parkinson patients, and schizophrenics, *Biol Psychiatry* 18:952-969.

Bogerts, B., Meertz, E., and Schonfeldt-Bausch, R., 1985, Basal ganglia and limbic system pathology in schizophrenia, *Arch Gen Psychiatry* 42:784-791.

Bogerts, B., Falkai, P., Haupts, M., Greve, B., Ernst, S., Tapernon-Franz, U., and Heinzmann, U., 1990, Post-mortem volume measurements of limbic system and basal ganglia structures in chronic schizophrenics. Initial results from a new brain collection, *Schizophr Res* 3:295-301.

Breier, A., Buchanan, R.W., Elkashef, A., Munson, R.C., Kirkpatrick, B., and Gellad, F., 1992, Brain morphology and schizophrenia: a magnetic resonance imaging study of limbic, prefrontal cortex, and caudate structures, *Arch Gen Psychiatry* 49:921-926.

Buchsbaum, M.S., Haier, R.J., Potkin, S.G., Nuechterlein, K., Bracha, H.S., Katz, M., Lohr, J., Wu, J., Lottenberg, S., Jerabek, P.A., Trenary, M., Tafalla, R., Reynolds, C., and Bunney, W.E., Jr., 1992, Frontostriatal disorder of cerebral metabolism in never-medicated schizophrenics, *Arch Gen Psychiatry* 49:935-942.

Bunney, W.E., Jr., Akbarian, S., Kim J.J., Hagman, J.O., Potkin, S.G., and Jones, E.G., 1993, Gene expression for glutamic acid decarboxylase is reduced in prefrontal cortex of schizophrenics, *Neurosci Abstr* 19:199.

Burkhalter, A., and Bernardo, K.L., 1989, Organization of corticocortical connections in human visual cortex, *Proc Natl Acad Sci USA* 86:1071-1075.

Burkhalter, A., Bernardo, K.L., and Charles, V., 1993, Development of local circuits in human visual cortex, *J Neurosci* 13:1916-1931.

Carlsson, M., and Carlsson, A., 1990, Schizophrenia: a subcortical neurotransmitter imbalance syndrome? *Schizophr Bull* 16:425-432.

Casanova, M.F., Sanders, R.D., Goldberg, T.E., Bigelow, L.B., Christison, G., Torrey, E.F., and Weinberger, D.R., 1990, Morphometry of the corpus callosum in monozygotic twins discordant for schizophrenia: a magnetic resonance imaging study, *J Neurol Neurosurg Psychiatry* 53:416-421.

Caviness, V.S., Jr., and Williams, R.S., 1979, Cellular pathology of the developing human nervous system, *in*: "Congenital and Acquired Cognitive Disorders," R. Katzman, ed., pp 69-90. New York: Raven Press.

Caviness, V.S., Jr., Crandall, J.E., and Edwards, M.A., 1988, The reeler malformation: implications for neocortical histogenesis, *in*: "Cerebral Cortex," A. Peters, and E.G. Jones EG., eds., vol 7, pp 59-89. New York, New York: Plenum Press.

Chalupa, L.M., and Killackey, H.P., 1989, Process elimination underlies ontogenetic change in the distribution of callosal projection neurons in the postcentral gyrus of the fetal rhesus monkey, *Proc Natl Acad Sci USA* 86:1076-1079.

Chalupa, L.M., Killackey, H.P., Snider, C.J., and Lia, B., 1989, Callosal projection neurons in area 17 of the fetal rhesus monkey, *Brain Res, Dev Brain Res* 46:303-308.

Chang, F., Steedman J.G., and Lund, R.D., 1986, The lamination and connectivity of embryonic cerebral cortex transplanted into newborn rat cortex, *J Comp Neurol* 244:401-411.

Chou, I-H., Shenton M.E., Benes, F., Wible, C.G., Kikinis, R., Jolesz, F.A., and McCarley, R.W., 1993, A magnetic resonance imaging study of the cingulate gyrus in schizophrenia, *Biol Psychiatry* 33:317.

Christinson, G.W., Casanova, M.F., Weinberger, D.R., Rawlings, R., and Kleinman, J.E., 1989, A quantitative investigation of hippocampal pyramidal cell size, shape and variability of orientation in schizophrenia, *Arch Gen Psychiatry* 46:1027-1032.

Chun, J.J.M., and Shatz, C.J., 1989a, The earliest-generated neurons of the cat cerebral cortex: characterization by MAP2 and neurotransmitter immunohistochemistry during fetal life, *J Neurosci* 9:1648-1667.

Chun, J.J.M., and Shatz, C.J., 1989b, Interstitial cells of the adult neocortical white matter are the remnant of the early generated subplate neuron population, *J Comp Neurol* 282:555-569.

Clark, S.A., Allard, T., Jenkins, W.M., and Merzenich, M.M., 1988, Receptive fields in the body-surface map in adult cortex defined by temporally correlated inputs, *Nature* 332:444-445.

Cline, H.T., Debski, E.A., and Constantin-Paton, M., 1987, N-methyl-d-aspartate receptor antagonist desegregates eye specific stripes, *Proc Natl Acad Sci USA* 84:4342-4345.

Coger, R.W., and Serafetinides, E.A., 1990, Schizophrenia, corpus callosum, and interhemispheric communication: a review, *Psychiatry Res* 34:163-184.

Colon, E.J., 1970, Quantitative cytoarchitectonics of the human cerebral cortex in schizophrenic dementia, *Acta Neuropathol* 20:1-10.

Conrad, A.J., Abebe, T., Austin, R., Forsythe, S., and Scheibel, A.B., 1991, Hippocampal pyramidal cell disarray in schizophrenia as a bilateral phenomenon, *Arch Gen Psychiatry* 48:413-417.

Crow, T.J., Done, D.J., and Johnstone, E.C., 1991, Influenza and schizophrenia after prenatal exposure to 1957 A2 influenza epidemic, *Lancet* 337:1248-1250.

Crow, T.J., 1990, Temporal lobe asymmetrics as the key to the etiology of schizophrenia, *Schizophr Bull* 16:433-443.

Daviss, S.R., and Lewis, D.A., 1993, Calbindin- and calretinin-immunoreactive local circuit neurons are increased in density in the prefrontal cortex of schizophrenic subjects. *Neurosci Abstr* 19:201.

Deakin, J.F.W., Simpson, M.D.C., Gilchrist, A.C., Skan, W.J., Royston, M.C., Reynolds, G.P., and Cross, A.J., 1989, Frontal cortical and left temporal glutamatergic dysfunction in schizophrenia, *J Neurochem* 52:1781-1786.

Degreef, G., Lantos, G., Bogerts, B., Ashtari, M., and Lieberman, J., 1992, Abnormalities of the septum pellucidum on MR scans in first-episode schizophrenic patients, *Am J Neuroradiol* 13:835-840.

Dehay, C., Horsburgh, G., Berland, M., Killackey, H., and Kennedy, H., 1989, Maturation and connectivity of the visual cortex in monkey is altered by prenatal removal of retinal input, *Nature* 337:265-267.

Falkai, P., Bogerts, B., and Rozumek, M., 1988, Limbic pathology in schizophrenia: the entorhinal region: a morphometric study, *Biol Psychiatry* 24:515-521.

Feinberg, I., 1982, Schizophrenia: caused by a fault in programmed synaptic elimination during adolescence? *J Psychiat Res* 17:319-334.

Fish, B., 1957, The detection of schizophrenia in infancy, *J Nerv Ment Dis* 125:1-24.

Fish, B., Marcus, J., Hans, S.L., Auerbach, J.G., and Perdue, S., 1992, Infants at risk for schizophrenia: sequelae of a genetic neurointegrative defect, *Arch Gen Psychiatry* 49:221-235.

Flechsig, P., 1927, Meine myelogenetische hirnlehre. Mit biographischer einleitung. Springer, Berlin.

Friauf, E., McConnell, S.K., and Shatz, C.J., 1990, Functional synaptic circuits in the subplate during fetal and early postnatal development of cat visual cortex, *J Neurosci* 10:2601-2613.

Frost, D.O., and Moy, Y.P., 1989, Effects of dark rearing on the development of visual callosal connections, *Exp Brain Res* 78:203-213.

Galaburda, A.M., Sherman, G.F., Rosen, G.D., Aboitiz, F., and Geschwind, N., 1985, Developmental dyslexia: four consecutive patients with cortical anomalies, *Ann Neurol* 18:222-233.

Ghosh, A., and Shatz, C.J., 1992, Pathfinding and target selection by developing geniculocortical axons, *J Neurosci* 12:39-55.

Giguere, M., and Goldman-Rakic, P.S., 1988, Mediodorsal nucleus: areal, laminar, and tangential distribution of afferents and efferents in the frontal lobe of rhesus monkey, *J Comp Neurol* 277:195-213.

Goldman-Rakic, P.S., 1987, Circuitry of primate prefrontal cortex and regulation of behavior by representational memory, *in*: "Handbook of Physiology - The Nervous System V", J.M. Brookhart and V.B. Mountcastle, eds., pp 373-417. American Physiological Society, Bethesda, MD.

Goldman-Rakic, P.S., Leranth, C., Williams, S.M., Mons, N., and Geffard, M., 1989, Dopamine synaptic complex with pyramidal neurons in primate cerebral cortex, *Proc Natl Acad Sci USA* 86:9015-9019.

Graham, J.M., 1991, Clinical approach to human structural defects, *in*: "Seminars in Perinatology," vol. 15, R. Creasy, and W.J. Duluth, eds., W.B. Saunders, Philadelphia.

Grüsser, O-J., 1991, Impairment of perception and recognition of faces, facial expression and gestures in schizophrenic patients, *In*: "Visual Agnosias and Other Disturbances of Visual Perception and Cognition," O-J. Grusser, and T. Landis, eds., vol 12, pp 287-295, Macmillan Press, Houndsmill, London.

Gunther, W., Petsch, R., Steinberg, R., Moser, E., Streck, P., Heller, H., Kurtz, G., and Hippius, H., 1991, Brain dysfunction during motor activation and corpus callosum alterations in schizophrenia measured by cerebral blood flow and magnetic resonance imaging, *Biol Psychiatry* 29:535-555.

Hauser, P., Dauphinais, I.D., Berrettini, W., DeLisi, L.E., Gelernter, J., and Post, R.M., 1989, Corpus callosum dimensions measured by magnetic resonance imaging in bipolar affective disorder and schizophrenia, *Biol Psychiatry* 26:659-668.

Heckers, S., Heinsen, H., Geiger, B., and Beckmann, H., 1991a, Hippocampal neuron number in schizophrenia, *Arch Gen Psychiatry* 48:1002-1008.

Heckers, S., Heinsen, H., Geiger, B., and Beckmann, H., 1991b, Cortex, white matter, and basal ganglia in schizophrenia: a volumetric postmortem study, *Biol Psychiat* 29:556-566.

Hendry, S.H.C., Jones, E.G., and Emson, P.C., 1984, Morphology, distribution and synaptic relations of somatostatin- and neuropeptide Y-immunoreactive neurons in rat and monkey neocortex, *J Neurosci* 4:2497-2517.

Hendry, S.H.C., and Jones, E.G., 1986, Reduction in number of immunostained GABAergic neurons in deprived-eye dominance columns of monkey area 17, *Nature* 320:750-753.

Hendry, S.H.C., and Kennedy, M.B., 1986, Immunoreactivity for a calmodulin-dependent protein kinase is selectively increased in macaque striate cortex after monocular deprivation, *Proc Natl Acad Sci USA* 83:1536-1540.

Hendry, H.C., and Jones, E.G., 1988, Activity-dependent regulation of GABA expression in the visual cortex of adult monkeys, *Neuron* 1:701-712.

Hendry, S.H.C., Fuchs, J., DeBlas, A.L., and Jones, E.G., 1990, Distribution and plasticity of immunocytochemically localized GABA A receptors in adult monkey visual cortex, *J Neurosci* 10:2438-2450.

Hubel, D.H., Wiesel, T.N., and LeVay, S., 1977, Plasticity of ocular dominance columns in monkey striate cortex, *Phil Trans R Soc London*, B 278:377-409.

Huntley, G.W., Benson, D.L., Jones, E.G., and Isackson, P.J., 1992, Developmental expression of brain derived neurotrophic factor mRNA by neurons of fetal and adult monkey prefrontal cortex, *Dev Brain Res* 70:53-63.

Huntsman, M.M., Isackson, P.J., and Jones, E.G., 1993, Lamina-specific expression and activity-dependent regulation of seven GABA A receptor subunit mRNAs in monkey visual cortex, *J Neurosci*, in press.

Huttenlocher, P.R., 1979, Synaptic density in human frontal cortex: developmental changes and effects of aging, *Brain Res* 163:195-205.

Huttenlocher, P.R., and De Courten, C., 1987, The development of synapses in striate cortex of man, *Hum Neurobiol* 61:1-9.

Huttenlocher, P.R., 1990, Morphometric study of human cerebral cortex development, *Neuropsychologica* 28:517-527.

Hyde, T.M., Weinberger, D.R., 1990, The brain in schizophrenia, *Seminars in Neurol* 10:276-286.

Hyde, T.M., Ziegler, J.C., and Weinberger, D.R., 1992, Psychiatric disturbances in metachromatic leukodystrophy: insights into the neurobiology of psychosis, *Arch Neurol* 49:401-406.

Jakob, H., and Beckmann, H., 1986, Prenatal development disturbances in the limbic allocortex in schizophrenics, *J Neural Trans* 65:303-326.

Jakob, H., and Beckmann, H., 1989, Gross and histological criteria for developmental disorders in brains of schizophrenics, *J Roy Soc Med* 82:466-469.

52

Jenkins, W.M., Merzenich, M.M., Ochs, M.T., Allard, T., and Guic-Robles, E., 1990, Functional reorganization of primary somatosensory cortex in adult owl monkeys after behaviorally controlled tactile stimulation, *J Neurophysiol* 63:82-104.

Jernigan, T.L., Zisook, S., Heaton, R.K., Moranville, J.T., Hesselink, J.R., and Braff, D.L., 1991, Magnetic resonance imaging abnormalities in lenticular nuclei and cerebral cortex in schizophrenia, *Arch Gen Psychiatry* 48:881-890.

Jessell, T.M., Kandel, E.R., 1993, Synaptic transmission: A bidirectional and self-modifiable form of cell-cell communication, *Cell* 72:1-30.

Johnstone, E.C., Crow, T.J., Frith, C.D., Husband, J., and Kreel, L., 1976, Cerebral ventricular size and cognitive impairment in chronic schizophrenia, *Lancet* 2:924-926.

Johnstone, E.C., Owens, D.G.C., Bydder, G.M., Colter, N., Crow, T.J., and Frith, C.D., 1989, The spectrum of structural brain changes in schizophrenia: age of onset as a predictor of cognitive and clinical impairments and their cerebral correlates, *Psychol Med* 19:91-103.

Jones, E.G., Valentino, K.L., and Fleshman, J.W., Jr., 1982, Adjustment of connectivity in rat neocortex after prenatal destruction of precursor cells of layers II-IV, *Dev Brain Res* 2:425-431.

Jones, E.G., 1990, The role of afferent activity in the maintenance of primate neocortical function, *J Exp Biol* 153:155-176.

Jones, E.G., 1993, Gabaergic neurons and their role in cortical plasticity in primates, *Cerebral Cortex* 3:361-372.

Kaas, J.H., Merzenich, M.M., and Killackey, H.P., 1983, The reorganization of the somatosensory cortex following peripheral nerve damage in adult and developing mammals, *Ann Rev Neurosci* 6:325-356.

Karson, C.N., Garcia-Rill, E., Biedermann, J.A., Mrak, R.E., Husain, M.M., and Skinner, R.D., 1991, The brain-stem reticular formation in schizophrenia, *Psychiatry Res Neuroimaging* 40:31-48.

Kater, S.B., and Mills, L.R., 1991, Regulation of growth cone behavior by calcium, *J Neurosci* 11:891-899.

Kendell, R.E., Kemp, I.W., 1989, Maternal influence in the etiology of schizophrenia, *Arch Gen Psychiatry* 46:878-882.

Killackey, H.P., Belford, G., and Ryugo, D.K., 1976, Anomalous organization of thalamocortical projections consequent to vibrissae removal in the newborn rat and mouse, *Brain Res* 104:309-316.

Komuro, H., and Rakic, P., 1992, Selective role of N-type calcium channels in neuronal migration, *Science* 257:806-809.

Komuro, H., and Rakic P., 1993, Modulation of neuronal migration by NMDA receptors, *Science* 260:95-107.

Kostovic, I., and Rakic, P., 1990, Developmental history of the transient subplate zone in the visual and somatosensory cortex of the macaque monkey and human brain, *J Comp Neurol* 297:441-470.

Kovelman, J.A., and Scheibel, A.B., 1986, A neurohistologic correlate of schizophrenia, *Biol Psychiatry* 19:1601-1621.

Kraepelin, E., 1919, Dementia praecox and paraphrenia. Edinburgh, Scotland: E & L Livingstone.

LaMantia, A.S., and Rakic, P., 1990, Axon overproduction and elimination in the corpus callosum of the developing rhesus monkey, *J Neurosci* 10:2156-2175.

Lewis, M.S., 1989, Age incidence and schizophrenia: Part I. The season of birth controversy, *Schizophr Bull* 15:59-73.

LeVay, S., Stryker, M.P., and Shatz, C.J., 1978, Ocular dominance columns and their development in layer IV of cat's visual cortex. A quantitative study, *J Comp Neurol* 179:223-244.

LeVay, S., Wiesel, T.N., and Hubel, D.H., 1980, The development of ocular dominance columns in normal and visually deprived monkeys, *J Comp Neurol* 191:1-51.

Lidow, M.S., Goldman-Rakic, P.S., and Rakic, P., 1991, Synchronized overproduction of neurotransmitter receptors in diverse regions of the primate cerebral cortex, *Proc Natl Acad Sci USA* 88:10218-10221.

Marin-Padilla, M., 1988, Early ontogenesis of the human cerebral cortex, *in*: "Cerebral Cortex: Volume 7, Development and Maturation of Cerebral Cortex," A. Peters and E.G. Jones, eds., pp 1-30, Plenum Press, New York.

Mattson, M.P., 1988, Neurotransmitters in the regulation of neuronal cytoarchitecture, *Brain Res Rev* 13:179-212.

Mednick, S.A., Machon, R.A., Huttunen, M., and Bone, D., 1988, Adult schizophrenia following prenatal exposure to an influenza epidemic, *Arch Gen Psychiatry* 45:189-192.

Mednick, S.A., and Cannon, T.D., 1991, Fetal development, birth and the syndromes of adult schizophrenia, in: "Fetal Neural Development and Adult Schizophrenia," S.A. Mednick, T.D. Cannon, C.E. Barr, and M. Lyon, eds., pp 3-13, Cambridge University Press, New York.

Meinecke, D.L., and Rakic, P., 1993, Low-affinity p75 nerve growth factor receptor expression in the embryonic monkey telencephalon: timing and localization in diverse cellular elements. *Neurosci* 54:105-116.

Meissirel, C., Dehay, C., Berland, M., and Kennedy, H., 1991, Segregation of callosal and association pathways during development in the visual cortex of the primate, *J Neurosci* 11:3297-3316.

Mesulam, M.M., and Geschwind, N., 1978, On the possible role of neocortex and its limbic connections in the process of attention and schizophrenia: clinical cases of inattention in man and experimental anatomy in monkey, *J Psychiat Res* 14:249-259.

Miller, M.W., 1993, Migration of cortical neurons is altered by gestational exposure to ethanol. Alcohol, Clin Exp Res 17:304-314.

Missler, M., Wolff A., Merker, H.J., and Wolff, J.R., 1993, Pre- and postnatal development of the primary visual cortex of the common marmoset. II. Formation, remodeling, and elimination of synapses as overlapping processes, *J Comp Neurol* 333:53-67.

Molnar, Z., and Blakemore, C., 1991, Lack of regional specificity for connections formed between thalamus and cortex in coculture, *Nature* 351:475-477.

Nasrallah, H.A., Andreasen, S., Coffman, J., Olson, S., Dunn, V., Ehrhardt, J., and Chapman, S., 1986, A controlled magnetic resonance imaging study of corpus callosum thickness in schizophrenia, *Biol Psychiatry* 21:274-282.

Nasrallah, H.A., Schwarzkopf, S.B., Olson, S.C., and Coffman, J.A., 1991, Perinatal brain injury and cerebellar vermal lobules I-X in schizophrenia, *Biol Psychiatry* 29:567-574.

O'Callaghan, E., Sham, P., Takei, N., Glover, G., and Murray, R.M., 1991, Schizophrenia after prenatal exposure to 1957 A2 influenza epidemic, *Lancet* 337:1248-1250.

O'Leary, D.D., and Koester, S.E., 1993, Development of projection neuron types, axon pathways, and patterned connections of the mammalian cortex, *Neuron* 10:991-1006.

O'Neal, P., and Robins, L.N., 1958, Childhood patterns predictive of adult schizophrenia: a 30-year follow-up study, *Am J Psychiatry* 115:385-391.

Pakkenberg, B., 1990, Pronounced reduction of total neuron number in mediodorsal thalamic nucleus and nucleus accumbens in schizophrenics, *Arch Gen Psychiatry* 47:1023-1028.

Pakkenberg, B., 1992, The volume of the mediodorsal thalamic nucleus in treated and untreated schizophrenics, *Brain Res* 7:95-100.

Pfefferbaum, A., and Zipursky, R.B., 1991, Neuroimaging studies of schizophrenia, *Schizophr Res* 4:193-208.

Purohit, D.P., Davidson, M., Perl, D.P., Powchik, P., Haroutunian, V.H., Bierer, L.M., McCrystal, J., Losonczy, M., and Davis, K.L., 1993, Severe cognitive impairment in elderly schizophrenic patients: A clinicopathological study, *Biol Psychiatry* 33:255-260.

Raine, A., Harrison, G.N., Reynolds, G.P., Sheard, C., Cooper, J.E., and Medley, I., 1990, Structural and functional characteristics of the corpus callosum in schizophrenics, psychiatric controls, and normal controls. A magnetic resonance imaging and neuropsychological evaluation, *Arch Gen Psychiatry* 47:1060-1064.

Rakic, P., 1972, Mode of cell migration to the superficial layers of the fetal monkey neocortex, *J Comp Neurol* 145:61-84.

Rakic, P., 1974, Neurons in rhesus monkey visual cortex: systematic relationship between time of origin and eventual disposition, *Science* 183:425-427.

Rakic, P., 1975, Timing of major ontogenetic events in the visual cortex of the monkey, in: "Brain Mechanisms in Mental Retardation," N. A. Buckwald, and M. Brazier, eds., pp 3-40, Academic Press, New York.

Rakic, P., Bourgeois, J-P., Eckenhoff, M.F., Zecevic, N., and Goldman-Rakic, P.S., 1986, Concurrent overproduction of synapses in diverse regions of the primate cerebral cortex, *Science* 232:232-235.

Rakic, P., 1988, Defects of neuronal migration and the pathogenesis of cortical malformations, *Prog Brain Res* 73:15-37.

Reiter, H.O., and Stryker, M.P., 1988, Neural plasticity without postsynaptic action potentials: Less active inputs become dominant when kitten visual cortical cells are pharmacologically inhibited, *Proc Natl Acad Sci USA* 85:3623-3627.

Richman, D.P., Stewart, R.M., Hutchinson, J.W., and Caviness, V.S., 1975, Mechanical model of brain convolutional development, *Science* 189:18-21.

Roberts, G.W., Colter, N., Lofthouse, R., Johnstone, E.C., and Crow, T.J., 1987, Is there gliosis in schizophrenia? Investigation of the temporal lobe, *Biol Psychiatry* 22:1459-1468.

Roberts, G.W., and Bruton, C.J., 1990, Notes from the graveyard: neuropathology and schizophrenia, *Neuropathol Appl Neurobiol* 16:3-16.

Rosene, D.L., and Van Hoesen, G.W., 1987, The hippocampal formation of the primate brain: A review of some comparative aspects of cytoarchitecture and connections, *in*: "Cerebral Cortex," E.G. Jones and A. Peters, eds., vol 6, pp 345-456, Plenum Press, New York.

Rossi, A., Stratta, P., Gallucci, M., Passariello, R., and Casacchia, M., 1989, Quantification of corpus callosum and ventricles in schizophrenia with nuclear magnetic resonance imaging: a pilot study, *Am J Psychiatry* 146:99-101.

Scheibel, A.B., and Kovelman, J.A., 1981, Disorientation of the hippocampal pyramidal cell and its processes in the schizophrenic patient, *Biol Psychiatry* 16:101-102.

Schlaggar, B.L., Fox, K., and O'Leary, D.D.M, 1993, Postsynaptic control of plasticity in developing somatosensory cortex, *Nature* 364:623-625.

Schmidt, J.T., 1985, Formation of retinotopic connections: selective stabilization by an activity-dependent mechanisms, *Cell Molec Neurobiol* 5:65-84.

Schwartz, M.L., and Goldman-Rakic, P.S., 1990, Development and plasticity of the primate cerebral cortex, *Clin Perinatal* 17:83-102.

Schwartz, M.L., and Goldman-Rakic, P.S., 1991, Prenatal specification of callosal connections in rhesus monkey, *J Comp Neurol* 307:144-162.

Seeman, P., Guan, H-C., and VanTol, H.H.M, 1993, Dopamine D4 receptors elevated in schizophrenia, *Nature* 365:441-444.

Selemon, L.D., Rajkowska, G., and Goldman-Rakic, P.S., 1993, Cytologic abnormalities in area 9 of the schizophrenic cortex, *Neurosci Abstr* 19:200.

Sham, P.C., O'Callaghan, E., Takei, E., Murray, G.K., Hare, H., and Murray, R.M., 1992, Schizophrenia following prenatal exposure to influenza epidemics between 1939 and 1960, *Br J Psychiatry* 160:461-466.

Shatz, C.J., 1990, Impulse activity and the patterning of connections during CNS development, *Neuron* 5:745-756.

Shatz, C.J., Gosh, A., McConnell, S.K., Allendoerfer, K.L., Friauf, E., and Antonini, A., 1990, Pioneer neurons and target selection in cerebral cortical development. *In*: "Cold Spring Harbor Symposia on Quantitative Biology," vol LV, "The Brain," pp 469-480. Cold Spring Harbor: Laboratory Press.

Shaw, C., and Cynader, M., 1984, Disruption of cortical activity prevents ocular dominance changes in monocularly deprived kittens, *Nature* 308:731-734.

Shenton, M.E., Kikinis, R., Jolesz, F.A., Pollak, S.D., LeMay, M., Wible, C.G., Hokama, H., Martin, J., Metcalf, D., and Coleman, M., 1992, Abnormalities of the left temporal lobe and thought disorder in schizophrenia. A quantitative magnetic resonance imaging study, *N Eng J Med* 327:604-612.

Shetty, A.K., and Phillips, D.E., 1992, Effects of prenatal ethanol exposure on the development of Bergmann glia and astrocytes in the rat cerebellum: an immunohistochemical study, *J Comp Neurol* 321:19-32.

Simpson, M.D.C., Slater, P., Claier Royston, M., and Deakin, J.F.W, 1992, Reduced GABA uptake in the temporal lobe in schizophrenia, *Neurosci Let* 107:211-215.

Singer, W., Rauschecker, J., and Werth, R., 1977, The effect of monocular exposure to temporal contrasts on ocular dominance in kittens, *Brain Res* 134:568-572.

Sobel, D.E., 1961, Children of schizophrenic patients: preliminary observations on early development, *Am J Psychiatry* 118:512-517.

Suddath, R.L., Casanova, M.F., Goldberg, T.E., Daniel, D.G., Kelsoe, J.R., Jr., and Weinberger, D.R., 1989, Temporal lobe pathology in schizophrenia: a quantitative magnetic resonance imaging study, *Am J Psychiatry* 146:464-472.

Suddath, R.L., Christinson, G.W., Torrey, E.F., Casanova, M.F., and Weinberger, D.R., 1990, Anatomical abnormalities in the brains of monozygotic twins discordant for schizophrenia, *N Eng J Med* 322:789-794.

Sur, M., Garraghty, P.E., Roe, A.W., 1988, Experimentally induced visual projections into auditory thalamus and cortex, *Science* 242:1437-1441.

Susser, E.S., and Lin, S.P., 1992, Schizophrenia after prenatal exposure to the Dutch hunger winter of 1944-1945, *Arch Gen Pychiatry* 49:983-988.

Swayze, V.W., Andreasen, N.C., Ehrhardt, J.C., Yuh, W.T., Alliger, R.J., and Cohen, G.A., 1990, Developmental abnormalities of the corpus callosum in schizophrenia, *Arch Neurol* 47:805-808.

Swayze, V.W., Andreasen, N.C., Alliger, R.J., Yuh, W.T., Ehrhardt, J.C., 1992, Subcortical and temporal structures in affective disorder and schizophrenia: a magnetic resonance imaging study, *Biol Psychiatry* 31:221-240.

Torrey, E.F., and Bowler, A.E., 1990, The seasonality of schizophrenic births: a reply to Marc S. Lewis, *Schizophr Bull* 16:1-3.

Van der Loos, H., and Woolsey, T.A., 1973, Somatosensory cortex: structural alterations following early injury to sense organs, *Science* 179:395-398.

Wall, J.T., Kaas, J.H., Sur, M., Nelson, R.J., Felleman, D.J., and Merzenich, M.M, 1986, Functional reorganization in somatosensory cortical areas 3b and 1 of adult monkeys after median nerve repair: possible relationships to sensory recovery in humans, *J Neurosci* 6:218-233.

Webster, M.J., Ungerleider, L.G., and Bechevalier, J., 1991, Connections of inferior temporal areas TE and TEO with medial temporal-lobe structures in infant and adult monkeys, *J Neurosci* 11:1095-2116.

Weinberger, D.R., 1987, Implications of normal brain development for the pathogenesis of schizophrenia, *Arch Gen Psychiatry* 44:660-669.

Weinberger, D.R., Berman, K.F., Suddath, R., and Fuller Torrey, E., 1992, Evidence of dysfunction of a prefrontal-limbic network in schizophrenia: a magnetic resonance imaging and regional cerebral blood flow study of discordant monozygotic twins, *Am J Psychiatry* 149:890-897.

Wible, C.G., Shenton, M.E., Hokama, H., Kikinis, R., Jolesz, F.A., and McCarley, R.W., 1993, A magnetic resonance imaging study of the prefrontal cortex in schizophrenia, *Biol Psychiatry* 33:316.

Wilson, J.R., Webb, S.V., and Sherman, S.M., 1977, Conditions for dominance of one eye during competitive development of central connections in visually deprived cats, *Brain Res* 136:277-287.

Woodruff, PW., Pearlson, G.D., Geer, M.J., Barta, P.E., and Chilcoat, H.D., 1993, A computerized magnetic resonance imaging study of corpus callosum morphology in schizophrenia, *Psychol Med* 23:45-56.

Yakovlev, P.I., and Lecours, A., 1967, The myelogenetic cycles of regional maturation of the brain, *in*: "Regional Development of the Brain in Early Life," A. Minkowski, ed., pp 3-70. Blackwell, Oxford.

Yurkewicz, L., Valentino, K.L., Floeter, M.K., Fleshman, J.W., Jr., and Jones, E.G., 1984, Effects of cytotoxic deletions of somatic sensory cortex in fetal rats, *Somatosens Res* 1:303-327.

Zec, R.F., and Weinberger, D.R., 1986, Brain areas implicated in schizophrenia: a selective overview, *in*: "The handbook of schizophrenia, 1: The neurology of schizophrenia," H.A. Nasrallah, and D.R. Weinberger, eds., pp 175-206, Elsevier Science Publishers, Amsterdam, The Netherlands.

Zecevic, N., Bourgeois, J.P., and Rakic, P., 1989, Changes in synaptic density in motor cortex of rhesus monkey during fetal and postnatal life, *Brain Res, Dev Brain Res* 50:11-32.

Zipursky, R,B., Lim, K.O., Sullivan, E.V., Brown, B.W., and Pfefferbaum, A., 1992, Widespread cerebral gray matter volume deficits in schizophrenia, *Arch Gen Psychiatry* 49:195-205.

STRUCTURAL BRAIN ABNORMALITIES IN SCHIZOPHRENIA: DISTRIBUTION, ETIOLOGY, AND IMPLICATIONS

Lisa T. Eyler-Zorrilla[1] and Tyrone D. Cannon[2]

[1]Department of Psychology
[2]Departments of Psychology and Psychiatry
University of Pennsylvania
Philadelphia, Pennsylvania

INTRODUCTION

Structural brain abnormalities (SBAs) are now a widely-accepted feature of schizophrenia. More than 200 studies of schizophrenics have reported SBAs, with most implicating limbic system pathology and enlargement of the third and lateral ventricles (Bogerts, 1991; Cannon, 1991, Raz & Raz, 1990). However, many questions remain regarding the distribution, prevalence, etiology, and functional implications of SBAs in schizophrenia.

Three questions will be addressed in this chapter. The first regards the prevalence and distribution of SBAs in schizophrenia; specifically, **what proportion of patients show SBAs, and are the abnormalities limited to a subgroup of patients with a specific clinical profile?** The second issue to be addressed concerns the etiology of SBAs in schizophrenia; specifically, **what etiological factors predict the presence or degree of SBAs in schizophrenia?** The third question that we will begin to answer concerns the functional implications of the SBAs found in schizophrenics; specifically, **what particular neural system deficits are associated with the typical pattern of observed SBAs?**

DISTRIBUTION AND PREVALENCE

There are two main competing hypotheses about the distribution of SBAs in schizophrenia: 1) the subgroup model and 2) the continuum model. The subgroup model predicts that the distribution of SBAs should be multimodal, with the number of modes depending on the number of clinical subtypes of schizophrenia. According to this model, if an SBA distribution was found to be bimodal, patients with SBAs should present a *qualitatively* different clinical picture from those without SBAs. In contrast, the continuum model predicts a unimodal distribution of SBAs in

Neural Development and Schizophrenia, Edited by S.A. Mednick
and J.M. Hollister, Plenum Press, New York, 1995

schizophrenia, with patients at the upper and lower ends of the distribution differing in severity but not type of symptomatology.

How do the predictions of these two models stand up to the evidence? First it is clear that for the most well-studied SBA measure -- ventricle to brain ratio (VBR) -- the schizophrenic distribution is not multimodal but unimodal, with a positive skew (Weinberger, 1987). The shape of the SBA distribution in schizophrenia is thus more compatible with the continuum model. The issue of clinical differences is more difficult to test. Given that the schizophrenic distribution is not bimodal, where should the cut-off be placed to determine which patients have high levels of SBAs and which have low levels? One possibility is to define "high SBAs" as those patients who have SBAs greater than the mean of the normal distribution. Using this tactic, however, one includes in the "high SBA group" patients whose brain measures are equivalent to those of controls who have no clinical symptoms of the disorder. Another method is to define "high SBA" as those patients whose values fall outside the control distribution. For example, in a quantitative review of 93 studies, Raz and Raz (1990) found that there was a 43% non-overlap between the distributions of schizophrenics and controls for lateral ventricular enlargement. However, if we define the 43% of patients whose VBRs are beyond the control maximum as "high SBAs", how can we be certain that the difference between a subject who is one cm^3 above the cutoff and one who is one cm^3 below it is biologically- or clinically-meaningful? Despite this ambiguity, most studies have used the latter technique to search for clinical differences that distinguish "high SBA" patients from "low SBA" patients. Much of this work was motivated by Crow's (1989) typology, in which SBA patients are hypothesized to be those with poor premorbid adjustment, intellectual deficits, a poor response to neuroleptics, and prominent negative symptoms. However, in a review of studies that examined the relationship between ventricular enlargement and positive and negative symptoms, Cannon (1991) found that only 7 of 20 studies revealed significantly more negative symptoms in patients with enlarged ventricles. The results of studies of other clinical features were similarly equivocal (Cannon, 1991; Raz, 1989). Therefore, the prediction of the subgroup model of unique clinical findings in patients with SBAs also lacks support.

In contrast, the continuum model predicts that variation between patients in terms of SBAs should be reflected in variation along a single phenomenological dimension, such as severity of illness. Two recent quantitative reviews of the VBR distribution in schizophrenics support this prediction (Cannon, 1991; Raz and Raz, 1990). These studies found that severity of illness, as indexed by cumulative length of hospitalization, was a significant predictor of mean VBR and mean effect size. These correlations remained significant after accounting for the age of the subjects, suggesting that the relationship between severity of illness and VBR is present in both younger and older patients. The continuum model can also help to explain why some studies have been successful in demonstrating clinical differences between "high SBA" patients and "low SBA" patients. If an underlying construct such as severity of illness is associated with the distribution of SBAs in schizophrenia, then some studies, but not all, will find clinical differences by bifurcating the sample. That is, if the range of severity in a particular sample is high, the study will more likely demonstrate clinical differences, but if the range of severity is restricted, clinical differences will less likely be found. **According to this model, however, such differences would be observed on every symptom measure rather than on a particular illness dimension, such as negative symptoms.**

Note, however, that if the continuum model is correct, every schizophrenic patient should have some degree of SBAs. Why, then, is there a large degree of overlap between the schizophrenic and normal control distributions on SBAs? For instance, some normal individuals show a degree of ventricular enlargement that rivals that of severely schizophrenic patients. One possible reason for this lack of sensitivity may be that quantitative measures of brain morphology, such as VBR, have no clear threshold beyond which a clinical syndrome will always appear. In order to assess sensitivity, in the absence of a clear threshold for defining abnormality on the distribution of an SBA measure such as VBR or hippocampal volume, studies must attempt to match the patients and controls on all factors known to influence the control distribution for the measure in question. Past studies have matched the schizophrenic and control samples on age, gender, SES, education, and other known and suspected correlates of brain morphology in controls. However, using normal monozygotic (MZ) and dizygotic (DZ) twins, Reveley et al. (1982) found that 90% of the variance in ventricle size is between-family variance and that there is high heritability for the size of the very brain structures that are abnormal in schizophrenia. Given this high heritability, two demographically-identical but genetically-unrelated individuals may differ greatly from each other on VBR because they are from different families, regardless of their psychiatric status. Therefore, in order to determine the sensitivity of SBAs as a marker of the schizophrenic phenotype, the ideal control group consists of the healthy first-degree relatives of schizophrenics, especially co-twins and siblings (Cannon and Marco, 1994). In summation, using the family members' measures of brain structure as a comparison reduces the non-schizophrenia-related between-family sources of genetic and environmental variability, and may give a more accurate picture of what the patient's brain may have looked if he/she were not schizophrenic. Figure

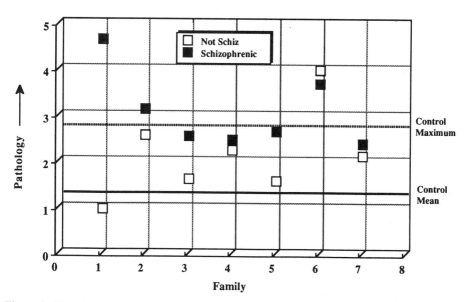

Figure 1. Hypothetical result of a study of SBAs in 7 families, each with one schizophrenic (closed squares) and one non-schizophrenic member (open squares). The solid line represents the control mean and the dashed line represents the control maximum. Note that whereas only 3 schizophrenics are deviant compared to the control maximum, 6 out of 7 are deviant compared to their own non-schizophrenic family member.

1 shows the theoretical result of a study of SBAs using multiple families, each with one sibling who has schizophrenia and one who does not. In this model, the distributions of scores for schizophrenics and non-schizophrenics overlap somewhat *across families*. However, *within families*, in almost every case, the schizophrenic family member is more impaired than the unaffected family member.

Four studies have used unaffected co-twins or siblings as controls to examine the prevalence and magnitude of an SBA (VBR) in schizophrenic patients (Table 1). In general, there is a large increase in sensitivity in these studies compared with studies using unrelated controls. Whereas the average sensitivity of the latter studies is around 50% (Raz and Raz, 1990), these four studies obtained an average sensitivity of 84% (71-100%). In addition, the magnitude of the difference in VBR between the affected and unaffected family member is quite large (50-100% pairwise difference).

Table 1. Results of studies examining differences in VBR between schizophrenics and their unaffected first-degree relatives.

Study	Imaging Method	Type of Relatives	N Probands	N Relatives	Sens-itivity[1]	Pair-wise % Difference[2]
Weinberger et al. (1981)	CT	Siblings	10	12	100%	122%
DeLisi et al. (1986)	CT	Siblings	25	10	71%	76%
Suddath et al. (1991)	MRI	MZ Twins	15	15	80%	NA[3]
Reveley et al. (1982)	CT	MZ Twins	7	7	86%	47%

[1]Sensitivity refers to the percentage of patients with more deviant values than their unaffected relatives.

[2]Pair-wise percent difference indicates the magnitude of difference (as a percentage of the relative's value) between each patient and each relative, averaged across pairs.

[3]NA indicates that data necessary to perform the calculation were not given in the referenced paper.

In conclusion, the answer to the question of the prevalence and distribution of structural brain abnormalities in schizophrenia appears to be, 1) given appropriate biological controls, all or nearly all patients show significant SBAs, and 2) brain pathology in schizophrenia is probably distributed on a continuum associated with increasing severity of the disorder. Of course, the existence of a unimodal distribution for the most studied SBA, ventricle-brain ratio, does not preclude the possibility that other areas are selectively affected in certain clinical subtypes or in certain families or both. In order to assess these possibilities, future post mortem and *in vivo* imaging studies are suggested to incorporate the within-family design -- comparison to co-twins or first-degree family members -- for revealing SBAs related specifically to the schizophrenic phenotype.

ETIOLOGY

Given that SBAs appear to be reliable markers of schizophrenia, we can go on to ask what sort of etiological factors might determine the presence or location of the abnormalities. The etiological model that we propose is derived from our more general diathesis-stress model of schizophrenia. Specifically, given that family and twin studies have provided evidence that nearly 80% of the liability for schizophrenia is due to genetic factors (Gottesman and Shields, 1982; Kendler, 1983; Kety, 1978), one can propose that there is an underlying genetic vulnerability for the disorder. However, the lack of full concordance between MZ twins (Kendler, 1983) indicates that environmental factors of some sort also play a role. Therefore, one can propose a diathesis-stress model of schizophrenia where the genotype predisposes to certain biological vulnerabilities that by themselves lead only to a borderline phenotype, such as schizotypy, but that in combination with an environmental stressor lead to schizophrenia itself. In this general form, the model is inadequate because it does not specify either the specific nature of the vulnerability, the nature or level of the stressor, or the mechanism of their interaction. However, it is useful as an heuristic for research on markers of schizophrenia in that it leads to the following testable predictions: 1) among first-degree relatives of schizophrenic patients, there should be increased psychiatric morbidity for spectrum disorders, but not other psychiatric disorders; 2) environmental stressors should be specific to those with schizophrenia; 3) biological characteristics related to the genotype for schizophrenia should be shared by those with schizophrenia and SPD; and 4) biological characteristics that require environmental input should be specific to those with schizophrenia.

These predictions have been tested using data from the Copenhagen High Risk Project. In 1962, Mednick and Schulsinger initiated a prospective, longitudinal study of 207 high-risk (HR) children (offspring of severely schizophrenic mothers) and 104 matched low-risk (LR) controls. The mean age of the children at the inception of the study was 15.1 years. There have since been two major follow-up assessments, one in 1972-1974 (mean age = 25 years), and one in 1986-89 (mean age = 42) when the subjects were nearly through the risk period for schizophrenia. At the later follow-up, diagnoses were made based on the Diagnostic and Statistical Manual of Mental Disorders, Version III, Revised (DSM-IIIR) criteria (American Psychiatric Association, 1987). In addition, in 1980-83, a diagnostic study of the subjects' biological fathers was conducted using interviews, or hospital records when the father was deceased. Those HR subjects whose fathers were diagnosed with a schizophrenic spectrum disorder (n=62) were designated as super high-risk (SHR).

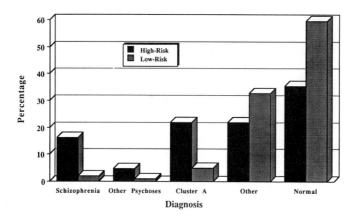

Figure 2. Lifetime DSM-III-R diagnoses in LR and HR groups. Hierarchical percentages of diagnoses in each risk group are given for schizophrenia, other psychoses (schizoaffective disorder, schizophreniform disorder, and atypical psychosis), cluster A personality disorders (SPD, paranoid personality, and schizoid personality), other Axis I and II disorders, and no Axis I or II disorder.

The first prediction of the diathesis-stress model, that genetic risk for schizophrenia should lead to increased psychiatric morbidity specific to schizophrenia spectrum disorders, was tested by comparing lifetime DSM-IIIR diagnoses in the LR and HR groups (Figure 2) (Parnas et al., 1993). As hypothesized, there was an increased risk for spectrum disorders, but not other disorders, among the offspring of schizophrenics.

The second prediction of the diathesis-stress model is that, among offspring of schizophrenic parents, those with schizophrenia, but not SPD, should show evidence of environmental stressors. One candidate for an environmental stressor which could interact with genetic liability, leading to full-blown schizophrenia, is pregnancy and birth complications (PBCs). At the beginning of the Copenhagen study, midwife reports on the pregnancy and birth experiences of the subjects were located and transcribed. When PBCs were examined in relation to diagnostic outcome, HR subjects with schizophrenia evidenced more PBCs than HR subjects with SPD or no mental illness (Parnas et al., 1982). In the LR group, however, there was no association between PBCs and diagnosis. These results suggest that an interaction of genetic risk and birth complications can lead to schizophrenia.

There are, of course, alternative models of the etiology of schizophrenia (and, relatedly, of SBAs in schizophrenia). One of the most influential is the familial-sporadic model (Lewis et al., 1987). This model proposes that there are two types of schizophrenia, one that arises primarily as a result of genetic factors (familial) and one that arises primarily as a result of environmental factors (sporadic). Some support for this model comes from studies finding an *inverse* relationship between the presence of SBAs and a positive family history of schizophrenia (Reveley et al., 1984; Oxenstierna et al., 1984; Owens et al., 1985; Reveley and Chitkara, 1985; Cazzullo et al., 1985; Turner et al., 1986). One problem with the family history approach is that the lack of a first-degree relative with schizophrenia does not necessarily imply the lack of a predisposing genotype. Given that only 10-15% of schizophrenics have first degree relatives with the disorder (Gottesman and Shields, 1982), but twin and adoption studies yield an estimate of 80.% heritability of liability, one would expect many patients to have relatives with the genetic predisposition, but not the clinical phenotype. Therefore, the family history method underestimates the number of schizophrenics with genetic liability, and, consequently, any relationship to genetic factors may be obscured using this approach. Other support for the familial-sporadic model comes from studies relating SBAs to environmental and obstetric insults (Lewis and Murray, 1987; Owen, Lewis, and Murray, 1988; Pearlson et al., 1985; Pearlson et al., 1989; Turner et al., 1986). However, the obstetric and childhood information in these studies was based on retrospective reports from the parents or the patients themselves, which may be biased or inaccurate. Although the familial-sporadic model may be a valid approach to schizophrenia and associated SBAs, we conclude that the model has not been adequately tested due to potential methodological flaws.

Given the support for the first two predictions of the diathesis-stress model of schizophrenia (i.e., that genetic factors create a diathesis for all spectrum disorders and that environmental stressors, such as PBCs, may increase risk for specific expression of schizophrenia), we can go on to ask about the specific nature of the gene-environment interaction. Because schizophrenia is a disorder of the brain, and because SBAs are so prevalent in schizophrenic patients, it is logical to ask what effects genetic predisposition and PBCs have on brain structure. One hypothesis, consistent with the third prediction of the diathesis-stress model, is that genetic predisposition to schizophrenia leads to specific SBAs which are shared by schizophrenics and schizotypes. These SBAs alone may result only in subclinical symptoms and mild cognitive deficits (e.g., the symptoms of SPD). Additional presence of obstetric complications may exacerbate the existing SBAs or create additional areas of abnormality, leading to full phenotypic expression of schizophrenia. According to the fourth general prediction of the diathesis-stress model, schizophrenics and schizotypes would not be expected to share these PBC-related SBAs.

An initial test of these predictions was performed using 34 HR subjects from the Copenhagen High-Risk sample, including 10 with schizophrenia, 10 with SPD, and 14 with no mental illness (NMI) (Schulsinger et al., 1984). Each of these subjects was given a CT scan to examine the width or area of the third and lateral ventricles in relation to whole brain width and area. Schizophrenics had significantly greater VBR than SPD or NMI subjects. In addition, the degree of ventricular enlargement was correlated with number and severity of PBCs. These results suggest that the genotype for schizophrenia may have increased susceptibility to the PBCs, which in turn increased the degree of brain pathology observed in the subjects as adults.

How might we explain the increased vulnerability to PBCs in individuals at genetic risk for schizophrenia? Many studies of the neuropathology of schizophrenia have demonstrated migratory and other developmental abnormalities in entorhinal cortex, hippocampus and prefrontal cortex (Bogerts, 1990). Nowakowski (1991) has demonstrated that similar deficits and ectopias in mutant strains of mice -- suggesting the possibility that natural genetic variation could lead to such problems. Therefore, it is possible that genetically-produced neurodevelopmental migratory deficits could interact with PBCs to increase structural pathology. Because the migration of cells to the cortex originates in the ventricular zone, a possible site of the interaction with perinatal insult is the periventricular region. Although migration takes place earlier than the potential complications occur, the abnormal migration may leave this periventricular region vulnerable to later insult. Thus, we would expect that genetic risk for schizophrenia would lead to cortical abnormalities and that an interaction between genetic risk and PBCs might lead to ventricular enlargement. Consequently, as an extension of the third and fourth predictions of the diathesis-stress model, two forms of neuropathology should be seen in individuals with schizophrenia, general cortical disruption and ectopias due to genetic factors, and periventricular disruptions due to the interaction of genes and PBCs. In contrast, individuals with SPD should only show the diathesis-related cortical SBAs.

In order to test these specific predictions, the CT data from the 34 HR subjects described above were factor analyzed (Cannon et al., 1989). Two factors emerged -- a cortical/cerebellar factor and a periventricular factor -- which differed in their relationships to genetic risk and PBCs. The cortical/cerebellar factor varied by level of genetic risk for schizophrenia, but not by presence or absence of PBCs. In contrast, the ventricular factor was predicted by an interaction between genetic risk and PBCs, such that ventricular enlargement increased with a greater level of genetic risk in the presence of PBCs. Given that cortical/sulcal enlargement was associated only with genetic factors, one would predict that schizophrenic and SPD subjects, who share a genetic risk, should show an equivalent degree of sulcal enlargement. In contrast, since ventricular enlargement appears to result from an interaction between genetic factors and PBCs, one would expect a greater degree of this SBA in schizophrenics (who, as shown previously, experienced more PBCs than HR subjects with other outcomes). Both of these predictions were supported by the data. Sulcal enlargement was present to equivalent degrees in schizophrenic and SPD subjects (but also in NMI subjects). Ventricular enlargement, however, was greater in schizophrenic subjects compared to those with SPD and no mental illness.

Cannon et al. (1989) was limited in several ways. Because of the small number of subjects, the effects of particular PBCs could not be examined separately, brain measurements were not examined by cortical lobe or hemisphere, no distinction was made between prenatal developmental disruptions and pregnancy complications, and we did not examine the relationship of anesthesias (some of which may have neurotoxic effects) to the brain measures. In addition, the sample did not include any subjects without genetic risk for schizophrenia. All of these issues were addressed in the most recent assessment of the Copenhagen project (i.e., 1986-89), during which CT scans were obtained on 60 LR subjects, 72 HR subjects and 25 SHR subjects. Another limitation of the pilot study was that we could not rule out the possibility that the relationship between PBCs and ventricular abnormalities was the result of covariation of PBCs with genetic risk. This was shown not to be the case in the expanded sample, where none of the obstetric factors varied systematically with genetic risk. A final limitation was the lack of control for age, gender, substance abuse, organic brain syndromes, and head injuries. In the expanded study, all of these secondary variables were entered first into the regression to ensure that their associations with the variables of interest were partialled out.

The results of the expanded study replicated and strengthened the pilot report. There was a main effect of risk on overall CSF-Brain ratio that was linear and dose dependent (Figure 3) (Cannon et al., 1993). That is, LR subjects showed the least abnormalities, SHR showed the most, and HR subjects fell exactly in between. In addition, there were main effects of both delivery complications (presence of complications associated with greater abnormality) and type of anesthesia (ether anesthesia associated with greater abnormality) (Figure 3). As was seen in the smaller sample, ventricular and sulcal enlargement differed in their associations with genetic risk and delivery complications (Figure 4). Sulcal enlargement varied by level of risk regardless of the presence of delivery complications (or the other PBCs examined). Ventricular enlargement, however, varied significantly by risk only in the presence of delivery complications. This variation again took the form of a step-wise increase in abnormality from LR to HR to SHR. These results therefore support the proposal that genetic risk alone is associated with cortical abnormalities, but that the *combination* of genetic risk and PBCs is associated with ventricular abnormalities. Given these findings, one would again predict that schizophrenics alone should show ventricular abnormalities, but that both schizophrenic and SPD subjects, by virtue of their shared genetic diathesis, should evidence cortical abnormalities. This pattern of results was confirmed in the larger sample (Figure 5) (Cannon, Mednick, et al., submitted).

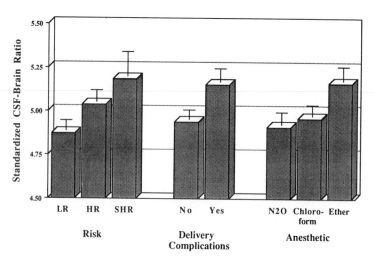

Figure 3. Relationship between overall, standardized CSF-Brain ratio and genetic risk for schizophrenia (left panel), delivery complications (center panel), and type of anesthetic (right panel).

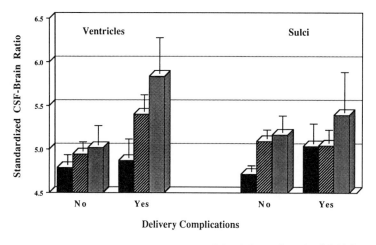

Figure 4. Standardized CSF-Brain ratio of the ventricles (left panel) and sulci (right panel) in LH (black bars), HR (striped bars), and SHR (gray bars) subjects, stratified by delivery complications.

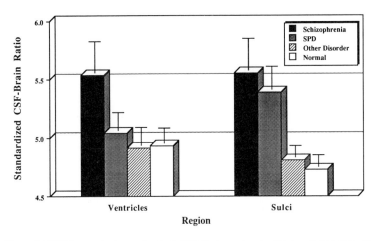

Figure 5. Mean (+SEM) ventricular and sulcal CSF-Brain ratios by lifetime DSM-IIIR diagnosis. Pairwise t-tests indicated that the schizophrenic group was significantly different from the other three groups on the ventricular measure and that the schizophrenic and SPD groups did not differ from each other and were significantly different from the other two groups on the sulcal measure.

In conclusion, the answer to the question of the etiology of SBAs in schizophrenia seems to be that 1) cortical abnormalities are associated with genetic risk for schizophrenia and are found in both schizophrenics and SPD subjects, but 2) ventricular abnormalities are associated with the interaction of genetic factors and PBCs and are greater in schizophrenics than individuals with SPD. This pattern of results helps to explain why the studies comparing VBR in twins discordant for schizophrenia were able to predict nearly perfectly which family member had the disorder. The pattern also suggests that cortical deficits will be difficult to demonstrate in schizophrenics in comparison to family members who share a predisposing genotype. Cortical deficits may, however, help to distinguish family members who "carry" the genotype from those who do not, and thus may ultimately be useful as endophenotypic markers in linkage studies of schizophrenia.

These findings must still be regarded as tentative, however, for two main reasons. The first is that the method of brain imaging used in these studies, CT scanning, has relatively low spatial and contrast resolution and therefore lacks the ability to resolve the specificity of the brain regions involved. The second is that, although secondary factors leading to brain abnormalities were all controlled statistically, one cannot know whether the abnormalities in the patients and SPD subjects were present at birth (as is implicated by the hypothesis). Repeated brain imaging studies of prospectively-identified subjects at risk for schizophrenia are needed to isolate the origins and time course of SBAs in schizophrenia.

IMPLICATIONS

The evidence we have presented thus far suggests that SBAs are quite prevalent in schizophrenia and may be linked to etiological factors involved in the disease itself. However, the question of the functional implications of SBAs in the manifestation of schizophrenia remains. The ideal design to study these implications is again one that compares individuals with schizophrenia to: 1) individuals who carry a predisposing genotype but do not show the full clinical phenotype (i.e., relatives with SPD), 2) relatives with no evidence of the genotype (e.g., those who lack sub-clinical signs and/or show no cortical SBAs), and 3) normal controls. In addition, the concomitants of SBAs may manifest themselves at many levels of analysis. Consequently, such studies should examine clinical presentation, neuropsychological performance, and neurophysiology (i.e., cerebral activation) using the family design.

We have initiated such a study at the University of Pennsylvania to examine cognitive functioning, brain structure, and neurophysiology in first-degree relatives of schizophrenics. In the first phase of this project, we used a comprehensive neuropsychological battery to examine cognitive functioning in 15 patients with DSM-IIIR diagnoses of schizophrenia, 16 of their non-schizophrenic siblings, and 31 demographically-balanced normal controls (Cannon, Eyler Zorrilla, et al., submitted). All subjects were screened for history of head injury, neurologic illness, major medical conditions, substance use, and Axis I psychiatric disorders other than schizophrenia. Test scores from the comprehensive battery were combined into seven cognitive domains based on factor-analytic studies. The scores of schizophrenics, their non-schizophrenic siblings, and normal controls (normalized to the control means and standard deviations) are presented in Figure 6. Multivariate analysis of variance confirmed that, as seen in the figure, both schizophrenics and their siblings were impaired neuropsychologically relative to normal controls, with the non-schizophrenic siblings' scores intermediate between those of the patients and controls on every domain of functioning. In addition, the shapes of the patient and sibling deficit profiles were similar. Specifically, schizophrenics showed the greatest deficits in verbal memory, abstraction, attention, and language functions and there was a non-significant trend toward a similar differential impairment in the siblings. This pattern of impairment suggests that both schizophrenics and their siblings may have functional deficits in the frontal and left temporal lobes. Among siblings, those with suspected or confirmed SPD were more impaired overall than those without schizophrenia spectrum diagnoses. This study also demonstrated high within-family sensitivity of neuropsychological deficits as illness markers. Four-fifths of schizophrenics obtained more deviant scores than the non-schizophrenic sibling in their own families, compared with one-third of patients with scores outside the range of unrelated controls and one-fourth of patients with scores outside the range of the siblings.

The findings of this study are preliminary in several respects. First, more subjects must be studied to confirm that the pattern of neuropsychological deficits in

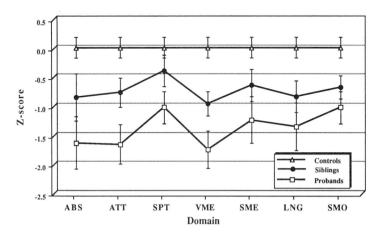

Figure 6. Neuropsychological profiles (mean z-scores± SEMs) of schizophrenic probands (open squares), non-schizophrenic siblings of probands (closed circles), and demographically-balanced normal controls (open triangles). Probands differed significantly from controls on all domains. Siblings differed significantly from controls on all domains except for spatial ability. Abbreviations: ABS-abstraction, ATT-attention, SPT-spatial, VME-verbal memory, SME-spatial memory, LNG-language, SMO-sensorimotor.

siblings parallels that found in schizophrenics. Second, more siblings with and without SPD must be evaluated in order to distinguish the patterns of deficits seen in these two subgroups of siblings. For example, based on the studies of SBAs in SPD and schizophrenia, one might expect that siblings with SPD would show similar cognitive deficits to their schizophrenic sibling on tasks of frontal lobe functioning (due to shared cortical abnormalities), but not show similar difficulties on tests sensitive to functioning of sub-cortical areas (because they do not share ventricular abnormalities). In contrast, non-SPD siblings might show relatively normal neuropsychological profiles. Finally, our initial study was based exclusively on the neuropsychological level of analysis. Our future studies will examine the brain structure of these subjects and how the size of structures relates to neuropsychological performance in various domains. In addition, we will examine patterns of brain activation in schizophrenics, siblings and normal controls during specific cognitive tasks. Through these studies, we will be able to compare patterns of blood flow in the three groups and relate physiological and structural indices of the targeted neural systems.

In summary, our perspective on the question of functional implications of SBAs in schizophrenia is still tentative. Our initial study comparing schizophrenics with their non-schizophrenic siblings and controls suggests that frontal and left temporal lobe function is disrupted in individuals with a schizophrenogenic genotype. It remains to be seen whether these disruptions are related to SBAs in either the patients or siblings and what neurophysiological disruptions might accompany or lead to these deficits. The goal of examining schizophrenics and their relatives at each of these levels of analysis is to refine the phenotype of schizophrenia by identifying "endophenotypes." Such patterns of characteristics, because they are likely to be more closely associated with genetic risk for the disorder than clinical diagnostic categories, may increase sensitivity and power in genetic linkage studies.

SUMMARY

Structural brain abnormalities are a prevalent feature of schizophrenia and appear to vary along a continuum associated with severity of the illness. The same factors which have been implicated as etiologic contributors to schizophrenia (i.e., genetic predisposition and PBCs) predict the degree of structural brain abnormalities observed in adult patient and at-risk groups. Specifically, our evidence suggests that genetic risk for schizophrenia leads to neural-developmental deficits, that by themselves lead to cortical abnormalities and SPD, but that in combination with birth complications lead to structural abnormalities in the ventricular region and the full-blown expression of schizophrenia. Finally, preliminary evidence suggests that schizophrenia is characterized by functional deficits in frontal and left temporal neural systems, which in turn may be related to structural and/or neurophysiological abnormalities in these same regions.

REFERENCES

American Psychiatric Association, 1987, "Diagnostic and Statistical Manual of Mental Disorders," Author, Washington, DC.

Bogerts, B., 1991, The neuropathology of schizophrenia: Pathophysiological and neurodevelopmental implications, in: "Fetal Neural Development and Adult Schizophrenia," S.A. Mednick, T.D. Cannon, C.E. Barr, and M. Lyon, eds., Cambridge University Press, Cambridge.

Cannon, T.D., 1991, Genetic and perinatal sources of structural brain abnormalities in schizophrenia, in: "Fetal Neural Development and Adult Schizophrenia," S.A. Mednick, T.D. Cannon, C.E. Barr, and M. Lyon, eds., Cambridge University Press, Cambridge.

Cannon, T.D., Eyler Zorrilla, L.T., Shtasel, D., Gur, R.E., Gur, R.C., Marco, E.J., Moberg, P., and Price, A., submitted, Neuropsychological functioning in siblings discordant for schizophrenia and in healthy volunteers, Arch Gen Psychiatry.

Cannon, T.D., and Marco, E.J., 1994, Structural brain abnormalities as indicators of vulnerability to schizophrenia, Schizophr Bull. 20:89-102.

Cannon, T.D., Mednick, S.A., Parnas, J., Schulsinger, F., Praestholm, J., and Vestergaard, A., 1993, Developmental brain abnormalities in the offspring of schizophrenic mothers. I. Contributions of genetic and perinatal factors, Arch Gen Psychiatry. 50:551-564.

Cannon, T.D., Mednick, S.A., Parnas, J., Schulsinger, F., Praestholm, J., and Vestergaard, A., submitted, Developmental brain abnormalities in the offspring of schizophrenic mothers. II. Structural brain characteristics of schizophrenia and schizotypal personality disorder, Arch Gen Psychiatry.

Cazullo, C.L., Vita, A. and Sacchetti, E., 1989, Cerebral ventricular enlargement in schizophrenia: Prevalence and correlates, in: "Schizophrenia: Scientific Progress," S.C. Schulz and C.A. Tamminga, eds., Oxford University Press, New York.

Crow, T.J., 1989, A current view of the type II syndrome: age of onset, intellectual impairment, and the meaning of structural changes in the brain, Br J Psychiatry. 7:15-20.

DeLisi, L.E., Goldin, L.R., Hamovit, J.R., Maxwell, E., Kurtz, D., and Gershon, E.S., 1986, A family study of the association of increased ventricular size with schizophrenia, Arch Gen Psychiatry. 43:148-153.

Gottesman I.I. and Shields, J., 1982, "Schizophrenia: The Epigenetic Puzzle," Cambridge University Press, Cambridge.

Kendler, K.S., 1983, Overview: A current perspective on twin studies of schizophrenia, *Am J Psychiatry*. 140:1413-1425.

Kety, S.S., 1987, The significance of genetic factors in the etiology of schizophrenia: Results from the national study of adoptees in Denmark, *J Psychiatr Res*. 4:423-429.

Lewis, S.W. and Murray, R.M., 1987, Obstetric complications, neurodevelopmental deviance, and risk of schizophrenia, *J Psychiatr Res*. 21:413-421.

Lewis, S.W., Reveley, A.M., Reveley, M.A., Chitkara, B., and Murray, R.M., The familial/sporadic distinction as a strategy in schizophrenia research, *Br J Psychiatry*. 151:306-313.

Nowakowski, R.S., 1991, Genetic disturbances of neuronal migration: Some examples from the limbic system of mutant mice, *in*: "Fetal Neural Development and Adult Schizophrenia," S.A. Mednick, T.D. Cannon, C.E. Barr, and M. Lyon, eds., Cambridge University Press, Cambridge.

Owen, M.J., Lewis, S.W., and Murray, R.M., 1988, Obstetric complications and schizophrenia: A computed tomographic study, *Psychol Med*. 18:331-339.

Oxenstierna, G., Bergstrand, G., Bjerkenstedt, L., Sedvall, G., and Wik, G., 1984, Evidence of disturbed CSF circulation and brain atrophy in cases of schizophrenic psychosis, *Br J Psychiatry*, 144:654-61.

Parnas, J., Cannon, T.D., Jacobsen, B., Schulsinger, H., Schulsinger, F., and Mednick, S.A., Lifetime DSM-III-R diagnostic outcomes in the offspring of schizophrenic mothers: Results from the Copenhagen high-risk study, *Arch Gen Psychiatry*. 50:707-714.

Pearlson, G.D., Garbacz, D.J., Moberg, P.J., Ahn, H.S., and DePaulo, J.R., 1985, Symptomatic, familial, perinatal, and social correlates of computerized axial tomography (CAT) changes in schizophrenics and bipolars, *J Nerv Ment Dis*. 173:42-50.

Pearlson, G.D., Kim, W.S., Kubos, K.L., Moberg, P.J., Jayaram, G., Bascom, M.J., Chase, G.A., Goldfinger, A.D., and Tune, L.E., Ventricle-brain ratio, computed tomographic density, and brain area in 50 schizophrenics, *Arch Gen Psychiatry*. 46:690-697.

Raz, S., 1989, Structural brain abnormalities in the major psychoses, *in*: "Neuropsychological Function and Brain Imaging," E.D. Bigler, R.A. Yeo, and E. Turkheimer, eds., Plenum Press, New York.

Raz, S. and Raz, N., 1990, Structural brain abnormalities in the major psychoses: A quantitative review of the evidence from computerized imaging, *Psychol Bull*. 108:93-108.

Reveley, A.M., Reveley, M.A., Clifford, C.A., and Murray, R.M., 1982, Cerebral ventricular size in twins discordant for schizophrenia, *Lancet*. 1:540-541.

Reveley, A.M., Reveley, M.A., and Murray, R.M., 1984, Cerebral ventricular enlargement in nongenetic schizophrenia: A controlled twin study, *Br J Psychiatry*. 144:89-93.

Reveley, M.A. and Chitkara, B., 1985, Subgroups in schizophrenia, *Lancet*. 1:1503.

Schulsinger, F., Parnas, J., Petersen, E.T., Schulsinger, H., Teasdale, T.W., Mednick, S.A., Moller, L., and Silverton, L., 1984, Cerebral ventricular size in the offspring of schizophrenic mothers: a preliminary study, *Arch Gen Psychiatry*. 41:602-606.

Suddath, R.L., Christison, G.W., Torrey, E.F., Casanova, M.F., and Weinberger, D.R., 1990, Anatomical abnormalities in the brains of monozygotic twins discordant for schizophrenia, *New England J Med*. 322:789-794.

Turner, S.W., Toone, B.K., and Brett-Jones, J.R., 1986, Computerized tomographic scan changes in early schizophrenia - preliminary findings, *Psychol Med*. 16:219-225.

Weinberger, D.R., 1987, Implications of normal brain development for the pathogenesis of schizophrenia, *Arch Gen Psychiatry*. 44:660-669.

Weinberger, D.R., DeLisi, L.E., Neophytides, A.N., and Wyatt, R.J., 1981, Familial aspects of CT scan abnormalities in chronic schizophrenic patients, *Psychiatr Res*. 4:65-71.

CEREBRAL ASYMMETRIES IN SCHIZOPHRENIA: FURTHER EVIDENCE FOR A LATERALIZATION HYPOTHESIS

Alessandro Rossi and Paolo Stratta

Institute of Experimental Medicine
Department of Psychiatry, University of L'Aquila
L'Aquila, Italy

INTRODUCTION

After Broca's (Broca, 1861) confirmation of Dax's (Dax, 1836) hypothesis of lateralization of speech, numerous observations demonstrated that the human brain is not a single homogeneous organ and the two cerebral hemispheres are generally not the mirror images of each other in either structure or function (Geschwind, 1968; Galaburda, 1978).

The notion that schizophrenia could be a disease of cerebral asymmetry was initially posed by Flor-Henry formulations based on the study of patients with left-lateralized temporal lobe epilepsy developing schizophrenia- like psychosis (Flor-Henry, 1969); subsequently direct studies of patients with schizophrenia generated a range of hypotheses which can still be considered as quite current (Flor-Henry, 1983; Flor-Henry, 1991).

However, it was not really until the 1970's and the initial application of new brain imaging techniques that the search for a "neuropathology of schizophrenia" was revitalized leading to substantial support to the hypothesis that the schizophrenic disease process is in some way related to an anomaly of the mechanisms that determine morpho-functional lateralization in the human brain (Crow, 1993).

EVIDENCE FOR PATHOLOGICAL CEREBRAL ASYMMETRIES

Using Computed Tomography (CT) Luchins et al. (1979) found higher frequencies of reverse asymmetries in right-handed schizophrenic patients without evidence of brain atrophy, as compared to a control sample. In a later study, Luchins et al. (1992) confirmed this finding regarding the occipital lobes in a schizophrenic population, also noting an increased frequency of aspecific human leukocyte antigen (HLA-A2) in the patient group without lateral ventricular enlargement (Luchins et al., 1980; Luchins et al., 1981). Naeser et al. (1981) reported a similar reversal of occipital

Neural Development and Schizophrenia, Edited by S.A. Mednick
and J.M. Hollister, Plenum Press, New York, 1995

cerebral asymmetry in a sample of schizophrenic patients treated with leucotomy. And Tsay et al. (1983) observed reversed occipital asymmetry was observed more frequently in schizophrenics than in manic-depressives. Other studies, however, reported no differences in pattern or type of asymmetry between schizophrenics and controls (Jernigan et al., 1982; Andreasen et al., 1982).

Results from brain density by CT investigation of brain structure in schizophrenia showed lower numbers in the anterior left hemisphere (Golden et al., 1981) and laterality differences in white matter density (Largen et al., 1984; Rossi et al., 1989). Reveley et al. (1987), in a carefully- controlled study, reported that the left hemisphere was less dense than the right in schizophrenics, while the reverse was found for the co-twins and controls. On the other hand, Jernigan et al. (1982) noted that although there was no significant difference in density between their schizophrenic and control groups, "several schizophrenic patients seemed to have somewhat higher CT values than normal subjects".

Clinical correlate of abnormal asymmetry was the finding of lower Verbal than Performance IQ in schizophrenics (Luchins et al., 1979). Absent or reversed hemispheric asymmetry was observed to be associated with greater psychopathology in terms of hallucination and dysfunction of language competence and communication abilities within the schizophrenic group (Luchins et al., 1983). These observations suggest that anomaly in the normal hemispheral lateralization may underlie defects of language that may be manifest as symptoms of conceptual disorganization.

Differences in composition of the control groups, methodological discrepancies in asymmetry measurement and the technical limitations of CT studies may account for the inconsistency of results reported by different investigators (Jernigan et al., 1982). As more accurate and comprehensive radiological assessments by Magnetic Resonance (MR) are made and as patient control comparisons become more precise, further suggestion of a derangement of brain lateralization has emerged from the investigation of brain structures previously impossible or difficult to visualize.

In a schizophrenic sample with lateral ventricular enlargement and smaller corpus callosum compared with healthy volunteers, Stratta et al. (1989) failed to find differences in hemispheric measurements between groups; nevertheless, marked differences between left and right hemispheres were evidenced in schizophrenics due to reduction of left frontal dimensions.

Rossi et al. (1987) reported significant differences between left/right prefrontal white matter and temporal white and grey matter in schizophrenics detected by MR image intensity. Several MR studies reported evidence of lateralized changes of the Temporal Lobe (TL): Johnstone et al. (1989) in an investigation at Northwick Park found that compared with age-matched controls and patients with affective disorder, the area (on the left side) of the TL was relatively reduced in schizophrenics. Rossi et al. (1990; 1990a) also reported significant diagnosis by side interactions with reduction of the left TL in schizophrenia. From a neuropsychological point of view, the schizophrenic group with significant TL abnormalities as assessed by MR, showed an abnormal Luria Nebraska Neuropsychological profile (Di Michele et al., 1992). Compared with a sample of bipolar patients, Rossi et al. (1991) reported a reduction of TL areas in those sections corresponding to the hippocampal region. This finding was more pronounced for the left side, although no diagnosis by side interaction was present. Coffman et al. (1989) reported similar findings and DeLisi et al. (1991) found a reduction in TL size in their chronic patients that was greater on the left side. Suddath et al. (1990) in the NIMH study of discordant monozygotic twins, reported that relative to the well twin, the brain of the proband showed bilateral TL abnormalities; however, an interesting asymmetry with respect to the total volume of grey matter in the TL was seen on the left but not on the right side.

However, no hypotheses more than on a descriptive, morphofunctional level had been made to explain the preponderance of these anomalies in the left side of the brain of the schizophrenic patients (Flor-Henry, 1991).

In the search for identifying the structure within the temporal lobe which would be primarily affected, particularly if the damage is left lateralized, several researchers focused their attention on exploring the Planum Temporale (PT) and related structures.

The PT is the temporal structure which, according to Geschwind & Levitsky (1968), has the most prominent asymmetry in the human brain. Since Geschwind and Levitsky's original (1968) observation of planum temporale asymmetry, further supporting evidence has come from post-mortem, and more recently from neuroimaging studies (Damasio & Frank, 1992; Steinmetz et al., 1989; Steinmetz et al., 1991; Steinmetz et al., 1991a; Kulynych, 1993; Rossi et al., in press). Moreover the PT is considered covered by cortical association areas putatively involved in the production of speech and auditory processing, which can be seen as relevant to the clinical picture of schizophrenia.

The PT lies on the superior surface of the posterior part of the superior temporal gyrus and is situated within the Sylvian fossa. It is a relatively flat surface and lies posterior to the transverse temporal gyrus (Heschl gyrus) or gyri which contain the primary auditory sensory cortex. The left planum is within the general region described as Wernicke's region, which is crucial for the comprehension of language (Witelson, 1982; Witelson & Kigar, 1988). Recent neuromorphological studies suggest that a reduction in lateralization of the left posterior regions related to Wernicke's area might have pathophysiological significance in schizophrenia (Falkay et al., 1992; Rossi et al., 1992; Crow et al., 1992; Hoff et al., 1992).

The PT constitutes an interesting experimental area for the detection of a left temporal lobe involvement in schizophrenia; in fact, PT shows an inverse asymmetry to that of the global TL, so that, if a diffuse TL involvement in schizophrenia is present, PT would be a region primarily affected.

As suggested by studies on developmental learning disorders, pathological agents that interfere with PT lateralization, resulting in a disruption of the physiological left-right PT asymmetry could influence the development of highly lateralized cognitive functions such as language processing (Steinmetz et al., 1991). Recent work supports the hypothesis of frontal lobe dysfunction in language communication disturbances (Barr et al., 1989; Morice, 1986). Other studies suggest a possible role for posterior association cortex in neurobehavioral disorders associated with language deficits (Pennington, 1991).

A recent MR study found a strong negative correlation between the left posterior temporal gyrus and a measure of thought disorder (Shenton et al., 1992). Barta et al. (1990) reported a shrinkage of the left anterior superior temporal gyrus strongly correlated to the severity of auditory hallucinations. Both regions are considered to be covered mostly by the auditory association cortex. Recent findings of a lack of asymmetry between the left and right PT further suggest a possible abnormality in the development and/or lateralization of the auditory association cortex of schizophrenics with severe language disorder (Rossi et al., in press).

These findings give some preliminary evidence of Crow's "lateralization hypothesis" (1993) which predicts that a pathological process elicits abnormal development of lateralization in schizophrenia. Similar conclusions have been drawn by recent post-mortem and MR studies (Falkay et al., 1992; Rossi et al., 1992; Crow et al., 1992; Hoff et al., 1992) measuring PT related regions. Hoff et al. (1992) found a reduction of the lateral sulcus asymmetry - a PT related region- significant in female patients only. However the two papers reporting positive findings in the left posterior brain region (Hoff et al., 1992; Shenton et al., 1992) did not measure PT area but related regions such as the posterior superior temporal gyrus and the lateral sulcus and found these abnormalities in both males and females. At present, there are no studies reporting correlations between these variables and the PT; thus these studies may not be comparable.

As further suggested by Bilder and Degreef (1991) a failure in the normal process of asymmetric cerebral specialization may limit the growth of widespread tertiary neocortical regions, including the prefrontal and posterior association cortices. Moreover a mechanism causing the aberration in brain development during the latter half of pregnancy will inevitably affect the left more than the right temporal cortex since the development of the left temporal cortex lags behind the right (Roberts, 1991; Bracha, 1991). This may be the case for the PT abnormalities.

Further neuropsychological studies are needed to test the hypothesis that the absence or reduction of asymmetry in language-related regions may be related to a failure in the development of specialized language abilities and, from a phenomenological perspective, to language disturbances. Neuromorphological studies should address the issue of the possible independence of the PT findings from other structural abnormalities (Bilder, 1992) in schizophrenia.

CALLOSAL ANATOMY AND CEREBRAL ASYMMETRY

Evidence derived from both neuropsychological and neurophysiological studies have suggested defects of interhemispheric communication in schizophrenia. Since the Corpus Callosum (CC) provides the major conduit for association bundles connecting the two hemispheres, there have been several morphometric studies searching for abnormalities of this structure in schizophrenia with not unambiguous results (for a review see Casanova, 1990).

More recently, another body of research suggests that the development of cerebral lateralization may be abnormal in schizophrenia (Falkay et al., 1992; Rossi et al., 1992; Crow et al., 1992; Hoff et al., 1992).

A quantification of the relationship between callosal connections and brain asymmetry in normal individuals comes from recent studies that report the posterior part of the body of the CC, particularly the isthmus, that interconnects the right and left perisylvian regions, depends on the size and asymmetry of perisylvian regions only in males, with a negative correlation between perisylvian asymmetries and the size of callosal isthmus (Aboitiz, 1992). The issue of corpus callosum morphometry in relationship to brain asymmetry seems relevant for neuroanatomy of schizophrenia (Flor-Henry, 1991).

A recent post-mortem study in normal individuals showed that the reduction in callosal area and some of its callosal regions occurs in the brain with normal aging and differs between the sexes, being significant in males only (Witelson, 1991). As the area of the CC may reflect the number of axons, a reduction in callosal area may reflect a loss of axons with aging, possibly due to the death of callosal neurons in the neocortex.

In a recent MR study (personal communication) we confirm the previous Witelson finding (1991) and we add the observation that normal subjects showed a significant correlation between the posterior part of the corpus callosum, i.e. the isthmus, and the degree of asymmetry in planum temporale, with larger isthmus corresponding to less PT asymmetry. This correlation is significant for males only, confirming similar findings in literature (Aboitiz, 1992; Witelson, 1992). When the patient group is analyzed, both these correlations disappear, in other words the variation in callosal anatomy does not relate to age or perisylvian asymmetry.

We can hypothesize that abnormal callosal axon loss during brain development may cause variation in functional asymmetry with the atypical pattern of neuropsychological and neurophysiological testing in schizophrenia, as suggested by Beaumont and Dimond (1973). This view is compatible either with an acquired or inheritable misconnection (Goodman, 1989).

As to the issue of the clinical correlate of our neuroanatomical finding, we found that only formal thought disorder (TD) correlates with PT asymmetry (i.e. the less the asymmetry, the more severe the disorder). Interestingly, the TD group showed reduced PT asymmetry _and_ smaller isthmus.

Our findings suggest a possible abnormality in the development of lateralization of the PT region with related callosal abnormalities in a group of schizophrenics with severe language disorder. A disorganization syndrome, which includes formal thought disorder, has been reported (Bilder & Degreef, 1991) within a three-dimensional structure of schizophrenia.

These findings stimulate new interest in the "old" lateralization hypothesis of schizophrenia. The embryological and callosal connectivity literature could add further clues about the nature of the neurodevelopment of cerebral asymmetry and sex differences in interhemispheric organization in schizophrenia.

ACKNOWLEDGMENTS

This work was partly supported by a 40% grant in 1991 to Professor Massimo Casacchia from the Ministero della Pubblica Istruzione, Italy - (A.F. 1991 n.93020903074).

REFERENCES

Aboitiz, F., Scheibel, A.B., Zaidel, E., 1992, Morphometry of the sylvian fissure and the corpus callosum, with emphasis on sex differences, Brain 115:1521-1541.

Andreasen, N.C., Dennert, J.W., Olsen, S.A., Damasio, A.R., 1982, Hemispheric asymmetries and schizophrenia, Am J Psychiatry 139:427-430.

Barr, W.B., Bilder, R.M., Goldberg, E., Kaplan, E., Mukherjee, S., 1989, The neuropsychology of schizophrenic speech, J Comm Disord 22:327-349.

Barta, P.E., Pearlson, G.D., Powers, R.E., Richards, S.S., 1990, Tune Auditory hallucinations and smaller superior temporal gyral volume in schizophrenia, Am J Psychiatry 147: 1457-1462.

Beaumont, J., Dimond, S., 1973, Brain disconnection and schizophrenia, Br J Psychiatry 123:661-662.

Bilder, R.M., Degreef, G., Morphologic markers of neurodevelopmental paths to schizophrenia, in: Developmental Neuropathology of schizophrenia. Edited by S.A. Mednick et al. Plenum Press, New York (1992).

Bilder, R.M., 1992, Structure-function relations in schizophrenia: brain morphology and neuropsychology, in: Walker, E.F., Dworkin, R.H., Cornblatt, B.A., (eds), Progress in Experimental Personality and Psychopathology Research, Vol.15, Springer Publishing Company, New York.

Bracha, H.S., 1991, Etiology of Structural Asymmetry in Schizophrenia: an Alternative Hypothesis, Schizophr Bull 17:551.

Broca, P., 1861, Nouvelle observation d'aphèmie produite par une lèsion de la moitiè postèrieure des deuxième et troisième circonvolutions frontales, Bulletins de la Sociètè Anatomique de Paris 6:398-407.

Casanova, M.F., Sanders, R.D., Goldberg, T.E., Bigelow, L.B., Christison, G., Bigelow, G.C., Torrey, E.F., Weinberger, D.R., 1990, Morphometry of the corpus callosum in monozygotic twins discordant for schizophrenia: a magnetic resonance imaging study, Journal of Neurology, Neurosurgery, and Psychiatry, 53:416-421.

Coffman, J.A., Schwarzkopf, S.B., Olson, S.C., et al., 1989, Temporal lobe asymmetry in schizophrenics demonstrated by coronal MRI brain scans, Schizophr Res 2:117.

Crow, T.J., Brown, R., Bruton, C.J., Frith, C.D., Gray, V., 1992, Loss of sylvian fissure asymmetry in schizophrenia: findings in the Runwell 2 series of brain, Schizophr Res 6 Special Issue:152-153.

Crow, T.J., 1993, Sexual selection, Machiavellian intelligence, and the origins of psychosis, Lancet 342:594-598.

Damasio, H., Frank, R, 1992, Three-dimensional in vivo mapping of brain lesion in humans, Arch Neurol 49:137-143.

Dax, M., 1836, Lèsions de la moitiè gauche de l'encèphale coincidait avec l'oubli des signes de la pensee (Lu a Montpellier en 1836), Gazette Hebdomadaire de Mèdicine et de Chirurgie 33:259-262.

DeLisi, L.E., Hoff, A.L., Schwartz, J.E., et al., 1991, Brain morphology in first episode schizophrenic-like psychotic patients: a quantitative magnetic resonance imaging study, Biol Psychiatry 29:159-175.

Di Michele, V., Rossi, A., Stratta, P., Schiazza, G., Bolino, F., Giordano, L., Casacchia, M., 1992, Neuropsychological and clinical correlates of temporal lobe anatomy in schizophrenia, Acta Psychiatr Scand 85:484-488.

Falkai, F., Bogerts, B., Benno, G., Pfeiffer, U., Machus, B., Folsch-Reetz, B., Majtenyi, C., Ovary, I., 1992, Loss of sylvian fissure asymmetry in schizophrenia: a quantitative post-mortem study, Schizophr Res 7:23-32.

Flor-Henry, P., 1969, Psychosis and temporal lobe epilepsy: a controlled investigation, Epilepsia 10:363-395.

Flor-Henry, P., 1983, Cerebral basis of psychopathology, John Wright, Bristol.

Flor-Henry, P., 1991, The future of neuropsychological research in schizophrenia, in: Handbook of Schizophrenia, Vol 5: neuropsychology, psychophysiology and information processing, S.P. Steinhauer, J.H. Gruzelier and J. Zubin, eds, Elsevier Science Publishers B.V., Amsterdam.

Geschwind, N., Levitsky, W., 1968, Human brain:left-right asymmetries in the temporal speech region, Science 161:186-187.

Galaburda, A.M., Le May, M., Kemper, T.L., Geschwind, N., 1978, Right-left asymmetries in the brain, Science 199:852-856.

Golden, C.J., Graber, B., Coffman, J., Berg, R.A., Newlin, D.B., Bloch, S., 1981, Structural brain deficits in schizophrenia: identification by computed tomographic scan density measurements, Arch Gen Psychiatry 38:1014-1017.

Goodman, R., 1989, Neuronal Misconnections and Psychiatric Disorder Is There a Link?, Br J Psychiatry 154: 292-299.

Hoff, A.L., Riordan, H., O'Donnell, D., Stritzke, P., Neale, C., Boccio, A., Anand, A.K., DeLisi, L.E., 1992, Anomalous lateral sulcus asymmetry and cognitive function in first- episode schizophrenia, Schizophr Bull 18:257-272.

Jernigan, T.L., Zatz, L.M., Moses, J.A., Cardellino, J.P., 1982, Computed tomography in schizophrenics and normal volunteers. II. Cranial asymmetry, Arch Gen Psychiatry 39:771-773.

Johnstone, E.C., Owens, D.C.G., Bydder, G.M., Colter, N., Crow, T.J., Frith, C.D., 1989, The spectrum of structural brain changes in schizophrenia: age of onset as a predictor of cognitive and clinical impairments and their cerebral correlates, Psychol Med 19:91-103.

Kulynych, J.J., Vlador, K., Jones, D.W., Weinberger, D.R., 1993, Three- dimensional surface rendering in MRI morphometry: a study of the planum temporale, J Comput Assist Tomogr 17(4):529-535.

Largen, J.W., Smith, R.C., Calderon, M., Baumgartner, R., Lu, R.B., Schoolar, J.C., Ravichandran, G.K., 1984, Abnormalities of brain structure and density in schizophrenia, Biol Psychiatry 19:991-1013.

Luchins, D.J., Weinberger, D.R., Wyatt, R.J., 1979, Schizophrenia: evidence of a subgroup with reversed asymmetry, Arch Gen Psychiatry 36:1309-1311.

Luchins, D.J., Torrey, E.F., Weinberger, D.R., Zalcman, S., DeLisi, L., Johnson, A., Rogentine, N., Wyatt, R.J., 1980, HLA antigen in schizophrenia: differences between patients with and without evidence of brain atrophy, Br J Psychiatry 136:243-248.

Luchins, D.J., Weinberger, D.R., Torrey, E.F., Johnson, A., Rogentine, F., Wyatt, R.J., 1981, HLA-A2 antigen in schizophrenic patients with reversed cerebral asymmetry, Br J Psychiatry 138:240-243.

Luchins, D.J., Weinberger, D.R., Wyatt, R.J., 1982, Schizophrenia and cerebral asymmetry detected by computed tomography. Am J Psychiatry 139:753-757.

Luchins, D.J., Meltzer, H.Y., 1983, A blind, controlled study of occipital asymmetry in schizophrenia, Psychiatr Res 10:87-95.

Morice, R., 1986, Beyond language-Speculations on the prefrontal cortex and schizophrenia, Australian and New Zealand Journal of Psychiatry 20:7-10.

Naeser, M.A., Levine, H.L., Benson, D.F., et al., 1981, Frontal leukotomy size and hemispheric asymmetries on computerized tomographic scans of schizophrenics with variable recovery, Arch Neurol 38:30-37.

Pennington, B., 1991, Genetic and neurological influences on reading disability: An overview, in: Reading Disabilities:Genetic and Neurological Influences. B. Pennington, ed., Kluwer Academic Publisher.

Reveley, M.A., Reveley, A.M., Baldy, R., 1987, Left cerebral hemisphere hypodensity in discordant schizophrenic twins, Arch Gen Psychiatry 44:625-632.

Roberts, G.W., 1991, Schizophrenia: A Neuropathological Perspective, Br J Psychiatry 158:8-17.

Rossi, A., Stratta, P., Gallucci, M., Amicarelli, I., Passariello, R., Casacchia, M., 1987, Standardized magnetic resonance image intensity study in schizophrenia, Psychiatr Res 25:223-231.

Rossi, A., Stratta, P., D'Albenzio, L., et al., 1989, Quantitative computed tomographic study in schizophrenia: cerebral density and ventricle measures, Psychol Med 19:337-342.

Rossi, A., Stratta, P., D'Albenzio, L., Tartaro, A., Schiazza, G., di Michele, V., Bolino, F., Casacchia, M., 1990, Reduced temporal lobe areas in schizophrenia: preliminary evidence from a controlled multiplanar magnetic resonance study, Biol Psychiatry 27:61-68.

Rossi, A., Stratta, P., D'Albenzio, L., Tartaro, A., Schiazza, G., Di Michele, V., Ceccoli, S., Casacchia, M., 1990a, Reduced temporal lobe area in schizophrenia by magnetic resonance imaging: preliminary evidence, Psychiatr Res 29:261-263.

Rossi, A., Stratta, P., Di Michele, V., Gallucci, M., Splendiani, A., de Cataldo, S., Casacchia, M., 1991, Temporal lobe structure by magnetic resonance in bipolar affective disorders and schizophrenia, J Affective Disorders 21:19-22.

Rossi, A., Stratta, P., Mattei, P., Cupillari, M., Bozzao, A., Gallucci, M., Casacchia, M., 1992, Planum Temporale in Schizophrenia: a magnetic resonance study, Schizophr Res 7:19-22.

Rossi, A., Serio, A., Stratta, P., Petruzzi, C., Schiazza, G., Mancini, F., Casacchia, M., in press, Three dimensional in vivo planum temporale reconstruction, Brain and Language.

Rossi, A., Serio, A., Stratta, P., Petruzzi, C., Schiazza, G., Mancini, F., Casacchia, M., in press. Planum temporale asymmetry and thought disorder in schizophrenia, Schizophr Res.

Steinmetz, H., Rademacher, J., Huang, Y., Hefter, H., Zilles, K., Thron, A., Freund, H.J., 1989, Cerebral Asymmetry: MR Planimetry of the Human Planum Temporale, J Comput Assist Tomogr. 13:996-1005.

Steinmetz, H., Volkmann, J., Jancke, L., Freund, H.J., 1991, Anatomical Left-Right Asymmetry of Language-related Temporal Cortex is Different in Left- and Right-Handers, Ann. Neurol. 29:315-319.

Steinmetz, H., Galaburda, A.M., 1991, Planum temporale asymmetry: In-vivo morphometry affords a new perspective for neuro-behavioral research. Reading and Writing 3:329-341. Selected re-republication in: B.F. Pennington, ed., Reading Disabilities: Genetic and Neurological Influences, Kluwer, Dordrecht (Holland): 143-155.

Stratta, P., Rossi, A., Gallucci, M., Amicarelli, I., Passariello, R., Casacchia, M., 1989, Hemispheric asymmetries and schizophrenia: a preliminary magnetic resonance imaging study, Biol Psychiatry 25:275-284.

Shenton, M.E., Kikinis, R., Jolesz, F.A., et al., 1992, Abnormalities of the left temporal lobe and Thought Disorder in Schizophrenia. A quantitative Magnetic Resonance Imaging Study, N England J Med 327:604-612.

Suddath, R.L., Christison, G.W., Torrey, E.F., Casanova, M.F., Weinberger, D.R., 1990, Cerebral anatomical abnormalities in monozygotic twins discordant for schizophrenia, N. Engl J Med 322:789-794.

Tsay, L.Y., Nasrallah, H.A., Jacoby, C.G., 1983, Hemispheric asymmetries on computed tomographic scans in schizophrenia and mania. A controlled study and critical review, Arch Gen Psychiatry 40:1826-1289.

Witelson, S.F., 1992, Bumps on the Brain: Right-Left Anatomic Asymmetry as Key to Functional Lateralization. In: Language Functions and Brain Organization, Academic Press Inc., pp. 117-144.

Witelson, S.F., Kigar, D.L., 1988, Asymmetry in brain function follows asymmetry in anatomical form: gross, microscopic, postmortem and imaging studies, in: Handbook of Neuropsychology, Vol 1, chapter 6, Elsevier Science Publisher.

Witelson, S.F., 1991, Sex differences in neuroanatomical changes with aging. NEJM 325:211-212.

Witelson, S.F., 1992, Cognitive Neuroanatomy: a new era, Neurology 42:709-713.

MORPHOLOGIC MARKERS OF NEURODEVELOPMENTAL PATHS: REVISITED

Robert M. Bilder

Hillside Hospital Division of Long Island Jewish Medical Center
Glen Oaks, New York

INTRODUCTION

"Morphology . . . is the largest single basis of behavior."
(G. Edelman, 1992, **Bright Air, Brilliant Fire**, Basic Books, NY, p. 49).

Recent decades have seen a transformation in attitudes, both lay and scientific, about the causes of schizophrenia. There is no longer much debate that schizophrenia reflects brain dysfunction, but there remain many questions about the nature of this dysfunction and its basic causes. Gerald Edelman (1988) presented compelling arguments that all function (or dysfunction) is ultimately rooted in structure (or dysmorphology). Functioning of the brain may be altered by structural abnormalities at the level of individual molecules (i.e., those comprising receptors and membrane elements), at the level of molecular aggregates comprising cells and their interactions, or at the level of interconnected networks of cells, comprising functional anatomic systems. To understand the causes of schizophrenia it is important to determine what structural anomalies exist at the molecular, cellular, and gross anatomic levels, and how these structural abnormalities are related to physiologic abnormalities. Although ultimately even gross anatomic features are explicable in terms of more microscopic processes, it is striking that in schizophrenia, we have clues to pathophysiology that are so obvious -- on a scale that they may be observed by the unaided eye. Characterizing the gross anatomic abnormalities in schizophrenia therefore offers a useful starting point in our attempts to appreciate the fundamental causes of schizophrenia. Once abnormalities on the macroscopic level are more clearly understood, in terms of their population distributions, antecedents, and associated features, organized searches for the more molecular changes underlying these abnormalities may be conducted.

In a chapter contributed to this volume's predecessor three years ago, we speculated that the most widely studied morphologic abnormalities in schizophrenia reflect independent pathologic processes (Bilder and Degreef, 1991). Further, we hypothesized that morphologic "markers" may help define syndromes with unique developmental trajectories or "paths," with distinctive courses and modes of symptom

Neural Development and Schizophrenia, Edited by S.A. Mednick
and J.M. Hollister, Plenum Press, New York, 1995

expression, neuropsychological deficit patterns, and a range of other features. This speculation was designed to help constrain the range of hypotheses to be tested in a research program that often risks suffering from "data toxicity"; we typically study such a large number of morphologic, neuropsychologic, physiologic, symptomatic, and historical variables that there are far too many opportunities to detect chance associations in exploratory analyses.

We offered a set of hypotheses, suggesting that at least three independent neurodevelopmental paths to schizophrenia could be identified. These were: 1. a medial fronto-limbic path; 2. a periventricular path; and 3. a cerebral specialization path. Some further development of these hypotheses has been published elsewhere (Bilder, 1992; Bilder and Szeszko, in press). The goal of this chapter is to review the status of the hypotheses given data collected in our laboratory and elsewhere. Given that the key advantage of any specific hypothesis is its falsifiability, it is unfortunate to report that most of the key elements of these hypotheses have not been disconfirmed. This could, of course, suggest that the hypotheses are ill framed and untestable. Alternatives include the probability that critical data needed to disconfirm the hypotheses are not available, and the possibility that the hypotheses have elements of truth. In the meantime, some additional supporting evidence has come to light.

MEDIAL FRONTO-LIMBIC PATH

This "path" was hypothesized to reflect a neurodevelopmental abnormality in the growth or migration of cellular elements within the dorsal or medial cytoarchitectonic trend (also know as the archicortex, following the nomenclature of Sanides, 1969, and elaborated by Pandya and Barnes, 1987; Yeterian and Pandya, 1988). This archicortical trend includes the hippocampus, cingulate gyrus, and the medial and dorsal aspects of the neocortex, including both posterior and frontal cortices. We had hypothesized that this trend may be marked by two types of abnormality: (a) volume reductions in the mesiotemporal (MT) lobe (specifically in the anterior hippocampal formation); and (b) prominence of cortical sulci, especially on the dorsal aspects of the frontal and parietal lobes. The hypothesis that they may be linked was based on the possibility that a basic neuromigratory defect affecting the core element of this cytoarchitectonic trend (namely, the hippocampal formation), might also disturb the organization of other dorsomedial structures (i.e., cingulate gyrus, the dorsal interhemispheric fissure, the dorsal and medial frontal and parietal sulci).

The simplest element of this hypothesis to test is that a unitary process might lead to both volume reductions in the anterior hippocampal formation, and to multi-site cortical abnormalities (in the sense used by Cannon and his colleagues, 1989; 1993), and that both of these features should be independent of other morphologic abnormalities, such as ventricular enlargement, or abnormal hemispheric asymmetries. Thus these morphologic abnormalities should be correlated. We are not aware of any published data either supporting or disconfirming the association of mesiotemporal volume reductions with multisite cortical abnormalities. In our studies using Magnetic Resonance (MR), preliminary analyses have failed to detect significant correlations of anterior hippocampal volume with either the volume of the CSF or ratings of sulcal prominence on a single slice at the level of the anterior commissure in sample of patients with first-episode schizophrenia (Bilder et al., 1994b). If this observation is supported through further research, then it could suggest either that there is not a unitary process affecting both hippocampal volume and cortical sulcal prominence, or that the features we are measuring are not adequate indices of this process.

There has been some partial and indirect support for other elements of this hypothesis. First, it was hypothesized that sulcal enlargement and reductions in anterior hippocampal volume would be most associated with positive (florid, active, and "paranoid") forms of psychotic decompensation. There are two studies suggesting that positive symptoms may be associated with reduced volume of the superior temporal gyrus (Barta et al., 1990; Shenton et al., 1992), although it is unclear from these studies whether the volume reduction in the STG is in fact accompanied by enlargement of the Sylvian fissure or other superior temporal sulcal spaces. We reported an association of positive psychotic symptoms with anterior hippocampal volume reductions in patients with chronic schizophrenia (Bogerts et al., 1993). A comparable pattern was not observed in patients in the first episode of schizophrenia (Bogerts et al., 1990), perhaps because fewer of the first episode patients had such severe hippocampal pathology. It remains unclear how many will go on to have chronic positive symptoms as was true of the samples studied by Bogerts et al. (1993) and Shenton et al. (1992). Other labs have reported hippocampal volume reductions, but only a few find correlations between hippocampal structure volume and symptoms (Breier et al., 1992; Barta et al., 1990; Shenton et al., 1992). Whether the differences between studies that found hippocampal volume-symptom correlates are best explained by differences in samples, differences in methods for assessing volume (i.e., the anterior part of hippocampus does appear most relevant), low statistical power due to small sample sizes, or a combination of factors, is unclear.

There have unfortunately been few reports of sulcal enlargement and its clinical correlates in the MR imaging literature, perhaps because newer studies have emphasized measurement of soft tissue structure volumes. Among these are reports that structural brain abnormality in patients with schizophrenia is best characterized as a diffuse reduction of cortical gray matter (Zipursky et al., 1992; 1994; Harvey et al., 1993). The relation of this finding to reports of cortical sulcal enlargement remains unclear. While it is in some ways intuitively appealing to see this diffuse tissue reduction as the structural substrate of sulcal prominence, to our knowledge that association has not been demonstrated. It is also intriguing to note that the findings of diffuse cortical gray matter reduction were seen in the context of overall tendencies for patients with schizophrenia to have relatively <u>larger</u> volumes of white matter. The combination of less gray with more white matter suggests that these findings may reflect a fundamental developmental trend more related to "cerebral specialization" as discussed in the section below.

Another component of the hypothesis was that medial fronto-limbic defects would lead to executive and motor deficits most frequently associated with the functioning of the frontal lobes. This hypothesis was based on a modest association observed between multisite cortical deficits (sulcal enlargement) and attentional/executive functions, in a sample of patients with chronic schizophrenia (Bilder et al., 1988; Bilder 1985). In support of this hypothesis, there have been some extremely interesting reports relating anterior hippocampal volume reductions to functional impairments implicating the frontal lobes. Weinberger and his colleagues, in their studies of monozygotic twins discordant for schizophrenia, have reported that smaller volume of the pes hippocampi (anterior hippocampus) strongly predicts the failure to "activate" the frontal lobes (as observed in patterns of cerebral blood flow) while performing the Wisconsin Card Sorting Test (Weinberger et al., 1992). We recently reported that anterior hippocampal volume reduction predicts executive and motor deficits, but not memory deficits, in a sample of first episode patients (Bilder et al., 1994a). These findings converge in suggesting that structural abnormalities in the hippocampal formation may predict abnormalities of functions usually associated with the frontal lobes. Moreover, the finding that hippocampal volume is associated with executive and motor deficits, but not memory deficits, suggests that some of the functional roles classically assigned to the hippocampal formation need careful reassessment, particularly when the hippocampus is affected early in development (Bilder et al., 1994a).

The importance of this developmental perspective is highlighted by recent work from the laboratory of Dr. Jocelyne Bachevalier. These investigators examined the effects of early lesions to the hippocampus and other temporal lobe structures in primates. These animals tend to show relatively modest impairment on the usual tests of memory function, but do show deficits on the classic tests for "frontal lobe" dysfunction (e.g.,delayed alternation). Of particular importance is the observation that these animals tended to show these deficits not during infancy, but only after they matured (Bachevalier, 1993; Bachevalier 1994; Beauregard et al., 1992). Comparable findings have been reported by Dr. Barbara Lipska and her colleagues, where rats with neonatal lesions in the ventral hippocampus (the rat equivalent of the anterior hippocampus in humans) show a pattern of pharmacologic and behavioral response to stress that is characteristic of the adult animals receiving lesions to the frontal lobes (Lipska et al., 1994). These findings may help reconcile theories of early neurodevelopmental defect with the fact that schizophrenic symptoms only emerge during late adolescence or early adulthood. The findings suggest that early developmental defects in the hippocampal formation may remain relatively quiescent until subsequent development takes place, and then these defects may be expressed in the form of frontal lobe dysfunction.

The original hypothesis did not consider the possibility that adequate morphologic markers of the medial frontolimbic defect might be observed within the frontal lobes themselves, and sulcal prominence over the dorsal frontal region was proposed as a "proxy"index of integrity within the frontal component of this structural system. The hypothesis suggested that the developmental defect would lead to morphologic abnormalities within the "...medial and dorsal motor, premotor, and prefrontal cortices..."(Bilder and Degreef, 1991, p. 177), but it was unclear whether the defects would lead to gross volume reductions in these regions, or whether these frontal subregions could be reliably parcellated, particularly given the tremendous variability of sulco-gyral patterns in the frontal lobes. There is more recent evidence that such parcellation may be feasible (Rademacher et al., 1992; Wible et al., 1993), and a recent report suggests that this parcellation may be important to observe structure-function correlations relevant to the frontal system (Seidman et al., 1994). Seidman and his colleagues studied 17 patients with schizophrenia, using a battery of Neuropsychological (NP) tests that included tests of "frontal" function, and reported areas of frontal subdivisions (dorsolateral and orbital frontal) measured on a single MR image slice at the level of the genu of the corpus callosum. They reported robust correlations between the dorsolateral measure (especially on the left) and NP measures of frontal function (e.g., left dorsolateral area correlated with Wisconsin Card Sorting Test, Categories achieved score; r = .65). In contrast to these findings, there were no significant correlations with orbitofrontal areas, or with total temporal lobe volumes. The functional specificity of the frontal lobe correlations was supported by the observation that the dorsolateral area was not correlated with either finger-tapping scores or psychosis/motivation ratings. Although the findings must be considered with caution given the large number of correlations, and a tendency for the frontal-executive tasks to correlate with overall measures of brain size, these findings are encouraging. Specifically with respect to the hypothesis about the medial fronto-limbic path, the findings may be seen as supporting the idea that the more dorsal frontal subregion (i.e., within the archicortical trend) is more relevant to the executive deficits in schizophrenia.

PERIVENTRICULAR PATH

Since the publication of this volume's predecessor, there have been multiple replications of the finding that ventricular volumes are increased in schizophrenia (see Bilder et al., 1994c, for a review). While in general these studies served to further confirm knowledge available from the era of CT-scanning, some advances in our knowledge about ventricular enlargement (VE) in schizophrenia have come from the application of the methods for magnetic resonance imaging, which enable multiplanar reconstruction of the entire ventricular system. For example, Degreef et al. (1992a) examined the volumes of each of the ventricular compartments in a sample of patients in first episode schizophrenia compared to healthy controls. They found enlargement of all ventricular subdivisions among the patients, and further showed that volumes of the temporal horns of the lateral ventricle were correlated with psychotic symptoms. This provides support for the hypothesis, namely that syndromal correlates of ventricular enlargement may be most related to the regions where the enlargement is observed; it was predicted specifically that temporal horn enlargement would be associated most with the positive symptoms of schizophrenia (Bilder and Degreef, 1991).

We previously hypothesized that both developmental and deteriorative processes are important in schizophrenia, and had suggested, based on the neuropsychological correlates of ventricular enlargement observed on CT scans, that VE may be linked to NP deterioration, while patients without VE were hypothesized to be more likely to have NP profiles suggesting poor early cognitive development (Bilder et al., 1988; Bilder, 1992). While such findings are likely to be sample dependent, it was striking that patients who had more VE had higher scores on NP measures, usually considered indexes of premorbid ability, along with evidence of detenoration from previously higher levels. In contrast, those with smaller ventricles had NP profiles suggesting failure in the development of basic NP competencies. These effects were of sufficient magnitude that a surprising correlation of higher IQ with larger ventricle size was observed. The associations of larger ventricle size with higher IQ and higher estimates of premorbid ability (which in the absence of such a hypothesis might be considered paradoxical), and with test-based estimates of deterioration, as reported by Bilder et al. (1988) was recently replicated by Dequardo et al. (1994). Dequardo et al. (1994) also argue that the evidence supports independent developmental processes, with VE more pronounced in a later onset group of patients who are more likely to have adequate early development of cognitive competencies. These studies provide at best indirect assessment of the possibility that there is progressive enlargement of ventricular spaces in schizophrenia. While several studies are attempting to document the longitudinal stability and possible change of brain morphologic features in samples of first episode schizophrenia (see DeLisi and Lieberman 1991), so far the results of these studies are equivocal.

We have conducted some additional preliminary analyses of ventricular volumes and their NP correlates in the same sample studied by Degreef et al. (1992a). In these analyses, we aimed first to reduce the number of ventricular volume variables using principal components analysis (Bilder et al., 1991). This revealed two principal components, one reflecting the dorsal ventricular system (i.e., the frontal horns, body, and occipital horns of the lateral ventricles), while the other reflected the ventral parts (temporal horns, third ventricle). We then assessed the NP correlates of these dorsal and ventral ventricular factors. Replicating the CT-scan study ventricular size and NP function in chronic patients (Bilder et al., 1988), we found the paradoxical association of better functioning with larger size of the ventricles. This was generally true for both the dorsal and ventral components. As we had done previously, an NP index of premorbid ability was used as a statistical control (i.e., forced to enter in a multiple regression approach) in predicting VE from NP measures. In the previous CT scan study, we had also found an association of VE with memory impairment, after controlling for premorbid ability. In the MR study of first episode patients, we found a similar result only for the dorsal part of the ventricular system, while enlargement of the ventral part was associated with more widespread impairments (Bilder et al., 1991).

The hypothesis presented in this volume's predecessor about the independence of different morphologic markers also noted that VE might be distinguished from sulcal prominence based on historical antecedents, following the initial findings of Cannon et al. (1989), who showed that the sulcal abnormalities were predicted by genetic risk, while VE was predicted by a combination of genetic risk and obstetric complications. In a substantially expanded replication study, Cannon et al. (1993) found that genetic risk has a nonspecific effect on ventricular and sulcal measures, but that the effect of delivery complications on VE was significantly greater than the corresponding effect on sulcal enlargement. While these findings indicate that VE is multiply determined, they reinforce the concept that obstetric complications may selectively be associated with increases in ventricular size.

Another interesting set of findings was reported by T.J. Crow and his colleagues (Crow et al., 1989a). Based on an analysis all ventricular compartments in a post-mortem series, they reported greatest relative enlargement of the temporal horns. Since the temporal horns are the last part of the ventricular system to assume their final position during development, they suggested that this illustrates failure in the developmental progression and descent of the temporal lobes. They have further linked this to the process of failure in the development of normal hemispheric asymmetries, as is discussed in the next section.

CEREBRAL SPECIALIZATION: HEMISPHERIC ASYMMETRIES AND SIZE

We had originally suggested that "cerebral specialization failure" may comprise one of several independent pathologic processes, and that this process may be marked by absence or reversal of the normal asymmetries (Bilder and Degreef, 1991). Since then there has been renewed interest in the possible relevance of altered lateral asymmetries in schizophrenia (Crow et al., 1989a,b; Crow 1990). This interest comes largely from two independent research foci. On one hand are suggestions that the structural abnormalities in schizophrenia are asymmetric, and that particularly the left hemisphere is the target of pathologic change (for a review see Bilder et al., 1994c). On the other hand are suggestions that there may be an absence or reversal of the normal asymmetry in the brain. Findings of absent or reversed asymmetries in the frontal and/or occipital regions were originally reported in CT-scan studies, but there were subsequent replication failures (see Bilder et al., 1994c). Some more recent studies have suggested that normal asymmetries of the Sylvian fissure or superior temporal plane may be altered in schizophrenia, as assessed on MR images (Hoff et al., 1992) and in post-mortem material (Falkai et al., 1992), although already there have been failures to replicate these findings (Bartley et al., 1993; Kleinschmidt et al., 1994).

We recently completed a comprehensive study of regional hemispheric volumes in a sample of 70 patients experiencing their first episode of schizophrenia, and 51 healthy comparison subjects (Bilder et al., 1994c). In this study, overall volumes of the major cortical regions (prefrontal, premotor, sensorimotor, occipitoparietal, and temporal) were measured in each hemisphere on 3.1mm thin contiguous T1-weighted magnetic resonance images.

The controls showed a striking pattern of hemispheric asymmetries, with occipitoparietal and sensorimotor regions larger on the left, and with prefrontal, premotor, and temporal regions larger on the right. Patients lacked lateral asymmetries at every region, and differed significantly from the healthy comparison group in prefrontal, premotor, and occipitoparietal asymmetries (see Figure 1).

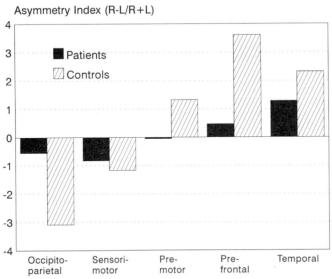

Figure 1. Asymmetry index scores in first episode schizophrenia (n = 70) and healthy control (n = 51) groups. Note that the controls have significant asymmetries at each region, and that patients do not. (Adapted from Bilder et al., 1994c.)

While most studies of cerebral asymmetries have emphasized lateral differences in occipital and frontal regions using linear or area measures, or examined differences localized to the anterior and posterior speech zones (Geschwind and Galaburda, 1987), these findings show that there is a systematic pattern of volumetric asymmetries across contiguous anterior-posterior (A-P) levels of the telencephalon in healthy individuals, and that this pattern of asymmetry is more likely to be absent or reversed in patients with schizophrenia or schizoaffective disorder.

The overall pattern of larger anterior right and posterior left cortical size was referred to by LeMay as "developmental **torque**", a term she attributed to Yakovlev, who noted similar asymmetries even at the spinal level (LeMay, 1976; Yakovlev and Rakic, 1966). We found posterior (occipitoparietal) and sensorimotor regions larger on the left, while premotor, prefrontal, and temporal regions were larger on the right. The normal lateral asymmetries in frontal and occipital regions have been well documented, although most studies relied only on linear or area rather than volumetric measures (Geschwind and Galaburda, 1987). The asymmetries in total temporal lobe volume are further consistent with some recent findings from other laboratories (Dauphinais et al., 1990; Rossi et al., 1991; Altshuler et al., 1991; DeLisi et al., 1991; Jack et al., 1989). To our knowledge, morphometry of the sensorimotor and premotor regions has not been reported previously, although methods for the detailed parcellation of cortical regions have been described, and applied in a single subject (Rademacher et al., 1992). The findings reported here for these structures are consistent with the hypothesis that the maturational processes leading to developmental torque yield a continuum of asymmetry in the A-P axis, with the shift from right-larger to left-larger occurring near the central sulcus. These findings of developmental torque in healthy controls are consistent with existing data, and are predicted by Catherine Best's neuroembryologic model of hemispheric specialization, which posits that these gross morphologic asymmetries reflect the operation of three interacting developmental gradients: (1) a general anterior-to-posterior gradient; (2) a ventro-dorsal gradient; and (3) a gradient from primary to secondary to tertiary neocortices (Best, 1988).

Sex and handedness effects in our study supported the validity of the torque construct. Although these effects did not distinguish patients from controls, we did find a pattern of results across these groups suggesting that dextrals and males are more likely than nondextrals and females to have more laterally asymmetric brain volumes, as has been suggested elsewhere (Kertesz et al., 1990; LeMay and Kido, 1978). These effects are illustrated in Figure 2. The figure shows that dextral males had significantly more asymmetry than nondextral males, and that dextral males had more asymmetry than dextral females. Nondextral females had high mean asymmetry that did not differ from the other groups, but the sample size was so small in this subgroup (n=7) that it cannot be considered a stable estimate.

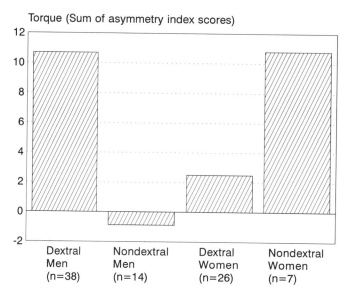

Figure 2. Torque (the composite index of cortical volume asymmetries) in subgroups defined by sex and hand preference (adapted from Bilder et al., 1994c).

We have obtained preliminary data suggesting that "torque" can be observed in healthy individuals not only at the cortical level, but also at the mesiotemporal and cerebellar levels, and that patients with schizophrenia show deviations from the normal pattern in all areas studied. The findings about mesiotemporal asymmetry are apparent in an earlier report about the first episode sample from Hillside Hospital, although asymmetries were not an explicit focus of that paper (Bogerts et al., 1990). That paper reported relative volume reductions among patients in the left posterior and right anterior mesiotemporal volume components, while differences were less pronounced in the right posterior and left anterior parts (in fact, the left anterior mesiotemporal part was larger in absolute terms among patients compared to controls). Among the controls, the right anterior mesiotemporal volume was larger than the left, and the left posterior part was larger than the right. However, the two sides were almost identical among patients. In the same sample, we also conducted some preliminary studies of cerebellar volume asymmetries (Snyder, et al. 1994). The volume of the cerebellum was computed separately for each hemisphere, and each cerebellar hemisphere was divided into anterior and posterior parts using a midline landmark. Analyses revealed that controls showed a pattern of cerebellar torque similar to those seen in the cortex and mesiotemporal lobe structures, with larger right anterior and left posterior subregions, and that this pattern was more frequently absent or reversed among patients.

Another possibly interesting pattern of associations was noted between the measures of torque and hand preference. There were relatively weak associations of handedness with cortical asymmetries (Bilder et al., 1994c). The correlations of handedness with MT asymmetries was somewhat more robust, and the correlations of handedness with cerebellar asymmetries were the most robust. In fact, the degree of right handedness was more significantly more strongly correlated with cerebellar torque than with cortical torque (Snyder, 1994). This set of findings suggests that handedness may be more closely related to structures that are lower in the neuraxis.

The specific processes underlying development of normal asymmetries in the brain are not yet well understood, but it has been assumed that there are both genetic and hormonal influences (Geschwind and Galaburda, 1987; Best, 1988). Gross anatomic differences between the hemispheres have been observed in newborns, and in fetal brains by week 20 of gestation (LeMay, 1976; Witelson and Pallie, 1973; Weinberger et al.,1982). Asymmetry of the Sylvian fissure, with the right Sylvian point higher than the left, was detected as early as the 16th week of gestation (LeMay and Culebras, 1972). Geschwind and Galaburda (1987) suggested that asymmetries may develop as early as the period of neural induction, even prior to differentiation of the neural plate, and it has been speculated that anatomic asymmetry may be inherent even in the ovum (Corballis and Morgan, 1978). Regardless of the precise time at which the program of asymmetric development is established, the gross anatomic asymmetries observed in the current study among controls, but not among patients, probably reflect neurodevelopmental events occurring early in ontogeny, and perhaps culminating by the second trimester of gestation. The extent to which these anatomic asymmetries may be modified during later development remains unclear. It is further unknown whether the timing of lateralized hemispheric growth in people who later develop schizophrenia follows the same time-course that is documented for healthy individuals. Studying "high risk" samples might clarify this issue. In the meantime, it is noteworthy that several hypotheses developed principally to help explain the unique features of schizophrenia closely parallel those used to explain the normal and pathologic development of cerebral asymmetries. For example, there are hypotheses that schizophrenia is associated with disturbances in the genetic controls over cerebral dominance (Crow et al., 1989a,b; Crow, 1988; 1990), and that the syndrome may be critically modulated by the timing of hormonal influences in the developing brain (Bogerts 1989, 1990; Saugstad, 1990).

Geschwind and Galaburda (1987) contrasted "linked" asymmetries, implying a common developmental process, with independent asymmetries, implying control by different developmental processes. The strong correlations in our data among asymmetries at different A-P levels suggest that these asymmetries are linked, and that a unitary process may underlie their development. The strength of these correlations also justifies referring to the composite observation of these asymmetries as "torque." It is possible also that the anatomic asymmetries observed in this study are linked to more localized asymmetries, such as those that characterize the speech and language areas in the temporal planum and frontal operculum. There is evidence that occipital asymmetry is correlated with asymmetries in the temporal planum (Pienadz and Naeser, 1984). The observation that these two asymmetries are linked in healthy individuals, however, does not necessarily mean that they are linked in schizophrenia or other neuropsychiatric syndromes. Although our findings may be seen as consistent with those reported recently from studies of the Sylvian fissure (Hoff et al., 1992; Falkai et al., 1992), these findings have not been easy to replicate (Bartley et al., 1993). There have been several studies also of the superior temporal plane, which have failed to show clear deviations from the highly asymmetric pattern seen in controls (Kleinschmidt et al., 1994; Shenton et al., 1994). It will therefore be important to determine empirically whether these different types of morphologic asymmetries covary in schizophrenia as they appear to in healthy subjects.   Indeed, finding that these asymmetries are **not** linked in schizophrenia might give important clues to pathophysiology.

The results of our study suggested that absence or reversal of normal hemispheric asymmetries may mark a pathologic process that is independent of other morphologic abnormalities.   Specifically, we found no significant association of abnormal cortical asymmetries with mesiotemporal volume reductions, ventricular enlargement, or cavum septi pellucidi, which were reported previously in patients from this sample (Degreef et al., 1992a, b; Bogerts et al., 1990). These results are compatible with those of Luchins et al. (1979) who found reversals of the normal asymmetry were most prevalent among patients who **did not** have ventricular or sulcal enlargement. Moreover, in the current study there were not significant associations of hemispheric asymmetries with cortical volumes, suggesting that brain size and asymmetry may also be independent.

Earlier studies had suggested that patients with schizophrenia might lack normal asymmetry in the occipital or frontal regions (Luchins et al., 1979, 1982; Tsai et al., 1983), but some controlled studies failed to replicate this finding (Naeser et al., 1981; Andreasen et al., 1982; Jernigan et al., 1982; Luchins et al., 1983).   Methodologic differences in imaging should be considered a major possible source of discrepancies. In prior studies that used linear or areal measures, the indices of asymmetry may have been less reliable and valid than the volumetric measures we used, because measured asymmetry depends critically on the plane of section in both anterior-posterior and superior-inferior planes (Zipursky et al., 1990; Kertesz et al., 1990; Best, 1988). Zipursky et al. (1990) further pointed out the importance of computing appropriate indexes of asymmetry, rather than simple hemisphere differences or ratios.

Our finding of an overall hemispheric asymmetry, with the left hemisphere larger than the right, is compatible with results from a volumetric analysis of CT-scan data (Kertesz et al., 1990), but superficially at odds with the recent report of Gur et al. (1991), who found larger right compared to left hemispheric volume using MR imaging. This difference may reflect the regions measured, with our study focusing more selectively on convexital cortical regions, while the study of Gur et al. included the uppermost portion of the brain stem and all subcortical gray and white matter structures, comprising an additional 11% to 16% of brain tissue, the asymmetry of which remains unknown. Supporting this possibility, we recently measured total hemispheral cerebral volume in 10 cases, using a method that includes all subcortical tissue, and found slightly larger right compared to left hemisphere volumes. It should be recognized also that the magnitudes of these overall hemispheric asymmetries in each study are quite subtle, with volume differences of less than 1%.

There is evidence that abnormal asymmetry may be associated with functional abnormalities in some schizophrenic samples. In prior studies of occipital asymmetry, Luchins and colleagues (1979, 1982) found that patients with reversed asymmetry had lower Verbal IQ compared to Performance IQ (which is atypical in samples of patients with schizophrenia), and poorer "quality of interview" (rated on the Present State Exam), compared to patients with normal asymmetry. Together these findings suggested that abnormal development of language and communication abilities might characterize patients who lacked normal asymmetry. This idea gains further support from findings that hemispheric asymmetries may be absent or reversed in patients with language disorders or developmental dyslexia (Hier et al., 1978; Rosenberger et al., 1980; LeMay and Kido, 1978).

In our sample, there were very few clinical or historical correlates of cortical asymmetries (Bilder et al., 1994c). Exploratory analyses revealed that patients with absence or reversals of the normal asymmetry were more likely to have initial diagnoses of undifferentiated than paranoid schizophrenia, and among males, absence of the normal asymmetries was related to negative symptoms measured during an initial baseline assessment. These findings could be seen as compatible with the results of Luchins et al. (1983), and with our hypothesis that patients with normal asymmetries are more likely to have florid, active, and paranoid psychotic symptoms (Bilder and Degreef, 1991). These initial observations will be more convincing if we are able to document persistent syndromal differences that are related to cerebral asymmetries during our longitudinal assessments of these patients.

We had suggested previously that overall brain size might offer another marker of failure in the normal pattern of cerebral specialization (Bilder and Degreef, 1991). Although the patients in our study of hemispheric asymmetries tended to have smaller brains, we found no significant differences in the volumes of any of the hemispheric regions after controlling for body size (this was important because male patients were shorter than the male controls)(Bilder et al., 1994c). There are several plausible explanations for the differences between studies. First are sampling issues. Since our study sampled patients during their first episode of psychosis, we might not have detected smaller cerebral volumes in a subgroup of chronic, more severely affected patients. Group differences also are critically dependent on the criteria used to select controls (Andreasen et al., 1986; 1990). Among key subject variables, our controls and patients differed significantly in race and education. We examined effects of both variables and found these not to alter the findings. We also controlled for age, height, and parental class in the calculation of adjusted cortical volumes; none of these factors altered the results with respect to cortical volume differences. Despite the absence of effects in this study, we would stress the importance of large-scale studies of healthy controls, to provide more adequate sampling of individual differences in brain morphology that may be associated with demographic factors.

Second, it is possible that degenerative changes cause cerebral volume reductions as the illness progresses, and that we sampled patients before this process could occur. As noted earlier, preliminary follow-up data from MR imaging studies of first episode schizophrenic patients do not provide much support for this possibility (DeLisi and Lieberman, 1991). Prior CT studies were mixed, and earlier pneumoencephalographic studies suggested that progression occurred and was associated with clinical deterioration; unfortunately all these studies had methodological flaws and limited statistical power to detect subtle effects (for a review, see Bilder, 1992). It seems likely that this issue will remain unresolved until larger numbers of patients have been followed longitudinally, preferably in high risk samples, and at least from the beginning of overt signs of illness, using measures of brain tissue volumes that are sensitive, reliable, and valid.

Third, our study examined volumes of tissue on contiguous slices through the entire A-P axis of the brain, while some reports of localized or lateralized volume reductions were based on single slice measures, which may be inaccurate indices of overall structure volume because they depend critically on the plane of section. Thus group differences may emerge on single slice studies if there are: (a) differences in the shape of the structure; or (b) differences between the hemispheric cross-sectional volume of that structure at a particular plane of section. If groups differ in asymmetry, single slice data at the same apparent A-P level may spuriously suggest unilateral volume reductions at that level.

Finally, it should be recognized that the regional volumes measured in the current study were relatively large (approximating definitions of the major cortical lobes), and that these regions included both gray and underlying white matter. These results are therefore not incompatible with those indicating regional cortical gray matter volume reductions in more specific regions (Suddath et al., 1989; Barta et al., 1990; Shenton et al., 1992), or over a more widespread distribution (Zipursky et al., 1992; Zipursky et al., 1994). It is also possible that more localized tissue volume reductions, or volume reductions specific to gray matter are present in our patients, but that these differences were outweighed by the magnitude of the overall gray-white volume composites. Further study using detailed parcellation of cortical regions, including gray-white segmentation, should be able to resolve these questions (Rademacher et al., 1992).

SUMMARY AND CONCLUSIONS

In the three years that have passed since the publication of this volume's predecessor, the study of brain morphology in schizophrenia has benefitted much from the application of new MR scanning and image analysis methods, that enable the measurement of multiple, small tissue structures that are presumed to be relevant to the syndrome. We previously advanced a speculative hypothesis, suggesting that at least three distinct pathologic processes might be identified using gross anatomic "markers." Findings in our lab and elsewhere have so far failed to disconfirm the essential elements of this hypothesis. If anything, more recent data have served to illustrate that the situation may be still more complex, in that the range of morphologic abnormalities identified in people with schizophrenia continues to grow, while the number of putative mechanisms underlying these anatomic abnormalities has not been convincingly narrowed. The suggestion made previously still appears tenable: namely that the single most salient vulnerability to psychosis may be a defect in the early development of the medial frontolimbic cytoarchitectonic (archicortical) trend, and that other morphologic abnormalities such as ventricular enlargement and failures in the normal pattern of cerebral specialization are more epiphenomenal, contributing to the syndromal presentation and course of the disorder, but not comprising a fundamental diathesis. With the continued development of both structural and functional brain imaging methodologies, there is hope that the next volume in this series will offer more definitive conclusions about the causes and correlates of morphologic abnormalities in the schizophrenia syndrome.

ACKNOWLEDGEMENTS

This work was supported by USPHS grants MH-41646 and MH-41960 from the National Institute of Mental Health, Bethesda, MD; and by a grant from the National Alliance for Research on Schizophrenia and Depression, Chicago, IL.

REFERENCES

Altshuler, L.L., Conrad, A.J., Hauser, P., Li, X., Guze, B.H., Denikoff, K., Tourtellotte, W., and Post, R.M., 1991, Reduction of temporal lobe volume in bipolar disorder: A preliminary report of magnetic resonance imaging, *Arch. Gen. Psychiatry* 48:482.

Andreasen, N.C., Dennert, J.W., Olsen, S.A., and Damasio, A., 1982, Hemispheric asymmetries and schizophrenia, *Am. J. Psychiatry* 139:427.

Andreasen, N.C., Nasrallah, H.A., Dunn, V., Olsen, S.C., Grove, W.M., Ehrhardt, J.C., Coffman, J.A., and Crossett, J.H.W., 1986, Structural abnormalities in the frontal system in schizophrenia, *Arch. Gen. Psychiatry* 43:136.

Andreasen, N.C., Ehrhardt, J.C., Swayze, V.W., Alliger, R.J., Yuh, W.T.C., Cohen, G., and Ziebell, S., 1990, Magnetic resonance imaging of the brain in schizophrenia, *Arch. Gen. Psychiatry* 47:35.

Bachevalier, J., 1993, Cognition, localization, and schizophrenia, Paper presented at the Intl. Congress Schiz. Res., Colorado Springs, CO, April. (Abstract)

Bachevalier, J., 1994, Medial temporal lobe structures and autism: a review of clinical and experimental findings, *Neuropsychologia* (in press).

Barta, P.E., Pearlson, G.D., Powers, R.E., Richards, S.S., and Tune, L.E., 1990, Auditory hallucinations and smaller superior temporal gyral volume in schizophrenia, *Am. J. Psychiatry* 147:1457.

Bartley, A.J., Jones, D.W., Torrey, E.F., Zigun, J.R., and Weinberger, D.R., 1993, Sylvian fissure asymmetries in monozygotic twins: a test of laterality in schizophrenia, *Biol. Psychiatry* 34:853.

Beauregard, L., Malkova, L., and Bachevalier, J., 1992, Is schizophrenia a result of early damage to the hippocampal formation? A behavioral study in primates, Paper presented at the Society for Neuroscience Annual Meeting, Anaheim, CA, November. (Abstract)

Best, C.T., 1988, The emergence of cerebral asymmetries in early human development: A literature review and a neuroembryological model, *in*: "Brain lateralization in children: Developmental implications," D.L. Molfese and S.J. Segalowitz, eds., Guilford Press, New York.

Bilder, R.M., 1985, "Subtyping in chronic schizophrenia: Clinical, neuropsychological, and structural indices of deterioration," University Microfilms, Ann Arbor, MI.

Bilder, R.M., Degreef, G., Pandurangi, A.K., Rieder, R.O., Sackeim, H.A., and Mukherjee, S., 1988, Neuropsychological deterioration and CT-scan findings in chronic schizophrenia, *Schizophr. Res.* 1:37.

Bilder, R.M., Degreef, G., Ashtari, M., Lipschutz-Broch, L., Wu, H., and Lieberman, J.A., 1991, Ventricular enlargement in schizophrenia: Association with a "deterioration profile", *J. Clin. Exp. Neuropsychol.* 13:99.(Abstract)

Bilder, R.M., 1992, Structure-function relations in schizophrenia: Brain morphology and neuropsychology, *in*: "Progress in Experimental Personality & Psychopathology Research, Vol. 15," E.F. Walker, R.H. Dworkin and B.A. Cornblatt, eds., Springer Publishing Company, New York.

Bilder, R.M., Lipschutz-Broch, L., Reiter, G., Geisler, S.H., Mayerhoff, D.I., and Lieberman, J.A., 1992, Intellectual deficits in first-episode schizophrenia: Evidence for progressive deterioration, *Schizophr. Bull.* 18:437.

Bilder, R.M., Bogerts, B., Ashtari, M., Wu, H., Alvir, J.Ma., Jody, D., Reiter, G., Bell, L., and Lieberman, J.A., 1994a, Anterior hippocampal volume reductions predict "frontal lobe" dysfunction in first episode schizophrenia, *Schizophr. Res.* (in press)

Bilder, R.M., Bogerts, B., Wu, H., Degreef, G., Ashtari, M., and Lieberman, J.A., 1994b, Independence of morphologic markers in schizophrenia, *Biol. Psychiatry* 35:720.(Abstract)

Bilder, R.M., Wu, H., Bogerts, B., Degreef, G., and Ashtari, M., 1994c, Absence of regional hemispheric volume asymmetries in first episode schizophrenia, *Am. J. Psychiatry* (in press)

Bilder, R.M., and Degreef, G., 1991, Morphologic markers of neurodevelopmental paths to schizophrenia, *in*: "Developmental neuropathology of schizophrenia," S.A. Mednick, T.D. Cannon, C.E. Barr and J.M. LaFosse, eds., Plenum Press, New York..

Bilder, R.M., and Szeszko, P.R., 1993, Structural neuroimaging and neuropsychological impairments, *in*: "The Neuropsychology of Schizophrenia," C. Pantelis, H.E. Nelson, and T.R.E. Barnes, eds., John Wiley & Sons, New York (in press).

Bogerts, B., 1989, Limbic and paralimbic pathology in schizophrenia: interaction with age- and stress-related factors, *in*: "Schizophrenia: Scientific Progress," S.C. Schulz and C.A. Tamminga, eds., Oxford University Press, New York.

Bogerts, B., 1990, The neuropathology of schizophrenia: pathophysiological and neurodevelopmental implications, *in*: "Fetal neural development and adult schizophrenia," S.A. Mednick, T.D. Cannon, C.E. Barr, and M. Lyon, eds., Cambridge University Press, Cambridge.

Bogerts, B., Ashtari, M., Degreef, G., Alvir, J.Ma.J., Bilder, R.M., and Lieberman, J.A., 1990, Reduced temporal limbic structure volumes on magnetic resonance images in first episode schizophrenia, *Psychiatry Research: Neuroimaging* 35:1.

Bogerts, B., Lieberman, J.A., Ashtari, M., Bilder, R.M., Degreef, G., Lerner, G.S., Johns, C., and Masiar, S., 1993, Hippocampus-amygdala volumes and psychopathology in chronic schizophrenia, *Biol. Psychiatry* 33:236.

Bogerts, B., and Lieberman, J., 1993, Neuropathology in the study of psychiatric disease, *in*: "International Review of Psychiatry," N.C. Andreasen and M. Sato, eds., American Psychiatric Press, Washington, DC.

Breier, A., Buchanan, R.W., Elkashef, A., Munson, R.C., Kirkpatrick, B., and Gellad, F., 1992, Brain morphology and schizophrenia. A magnetic resonance imaging study of limbic, prefrontal cortex, and caudate structures, *Arch. Gen. Psychiatry* 49:921.

Brown, R., Colter, N., Corsellis, J.A.N., Crow, T.J., Frith, C.D., Jagoe, R., Johnstone, E.C., and Marsh, L., 1986, Postmortem evidence of structural brain change in schizophrenia: Differences in brain weight, temporal horn area, and parahippocampal gyrus compared with affective disorders, *Arch. Gen. Psychiatry* 43:36.

Cannon, T.D., Mednick, S.A., Parnas, J., Schulsinger, F., Praestholm, J., and Vestergaard, A., 1993, Developmental brain abnormalities in the offspring of schizophrenic mothers. I. Contributions of genetic and perinatal factors, *Arch. Gen. Psychiatry* 50:551.

Cannon, T.D., Mednick, S.A., and Parnas, J., 1989, Genetic and perinatal determinants of structural brain deficits in schizophrenia, *Arch. Gen. Psychiatry* 46:883.

Corballis, M.C., and Morgan, M.J., 1978, On the biological basis of human laterality, *Behavioral and Brain Sciences* 2:261.

Crow, T.J., 1988, Sex chromosomes and psychosis. The case for a pseudoautosomal locus, *Br. J. Psychiatry* 153:675.

Crow, T.J., Ball, J., Bloom, S.R., Brown, R., Bruton, C.J., Frith, C.D., Johnstone, E.C., Owens, D.G.C., and Roberts, G.W., 1989a, Schizophrenia as an anomaly of development of cerebral asymmetry, *Arch. Gen. Psychiatry* 460:1145.

Crow, T.J., Colter, N., Frith, C.D., Johnstone, E.C., and Owens, D.G.C., 1989b, Developmental arrest of cerebral asymmetries in early onset schizophrenia, *Psychiatry. Res.* 29:247.

Crow, T.J., 1990, Temporal lobe asymmetries as the key to the etiology of schizophrenia, *Schizophr. Bull.* 16:433.

Dauphinais, I.D., DeLisi, L.E., Crow, T.J., Alexandropoulos, K., Colter, N., Tuma, I., and Gershon, E.S., 1990, Reduction in temporal lobe size in siblings with schizophrenia: a magnetic resonance imaging study, *Psychiatry. Res.* 35:137.

Degreef, G., Ashtari, M., Bogerts, B., Bilder, R.M., Jody, D.N., Alvir, J.Ma.J., and Lieberman, J.A., 1992a, Volumes of ventricular system subdivisions measured from magnetic resonance images in first-episode schizophrenic patients, *Arch. Gen. Psychiatry* 49:531.

Degreef, G., Bogerts, B., Falkai, P., Greve, B., Lantos, G., Ashtari, M., and Lieberman, J.A., 1992b, Increased prevalence of the cavum septum pellucidum in MRI scans and postmortem brains of schizophrenic patients, *Psychiatry Research: Neuroimaging* 45:1.

DeLisi, L.E., Hoff, A.L., Schwartz, J.E., Shields, G.W., Halthore, S.N., Gupta, S.M., Henn, F.A., and Anand, A.K., 1991, Brain morphology in first-episode schizophrenic-like psychotic patients: A quantitative magnetic resonance imaging study, *Biol. Psychiatry* 29:159.

DeLisi, L.E., and Lieberman, J.A., 1991, American College of Neuropsychopharmacology Satellite Meeting: Longitudinal perspectives on the pathophysiology of schizophrenia: Examining the neurodevelopmental versus neurodegenerative hypotheses, *Schizophr. Res.* 5:183.

DeQuardo, J.R., Tandon, R., Goldman, R., Meador-Woodruff, J.H., McGrath-Giroux, M., Brunberg, J.A., and Kim, L., 1994, Ventricular enlargement, neuropsychological status, and premorbid function in schizophrenia, *Biol. Psychiatry* 35:517.

Edelman, G., 1988, "Topobiology," Basic Books, New York.

Edelman, G., 1992, "Bright Air, Brilliant Fire," Basic Books, New York.

Falkai, P., Bogerts, B., Greve, B., Pfeiffer, E., Machus, B., Fölsch-Reetz, B., Majtenyi, C., and Ovary, I., 1992, Loss of sylvian fissure asymmetry in schizophrenia. A quantitative post-mortem study, *Schizophr. Res.* 7:23.

Geschwind, N., and Galaburda, A.M., 1987, "Cerebral Lateralization. Biological Mechanisms, Associations, and Pathology," MIT Press, Cambridge.

Gur, R.E., Mozley, P.D., Resnick, S.M., Gottlieb, G.L., Kohn, M., Zimmerman, R., Herman, G., Atlas, S., Grossman, R., Berretta, D., and Erwin, R., 1991, Gender differences in age effect on brain atrophy measured by magnetic resonance imaging, *Proc. Natl. Acad. Sci., USA.* 88:2845.

Harvey, I., Ron, M.A., du Bouley, G., Wicks, D., Lewis, S.W., and Murray, R.M., 1993, Reduction of cortical volume in schizophrenia on magnetic resonance imaging, *Psychol. Med.* 23:591.

Hier, D.B., LeMay, M., Rosenberger, P.B., and Perlo, V.P., 1978, Developmental dyslexia. Evidence for a subgroup with a reversal of cerebral asymmetry, *Arch. Neurology* 35:90.

Hoff, A.L., Riordan, H., O'Donnell, D.W., Stritzke, P., Neale, C., Boccio, A., Anand, A.K., and DeLisi, L.E., 1992, Anomalous lateral sulcus asymmetry and cognitive function in first-episode schizophrenia, *Schizophr. Bull.* 18:257.

Jack, C.R., Twomey, C.K., Zinsmeister, A.R., Sharbrough, F.W., Peterson, R.C., and Cascino, G.D., 1989, Anterior temporal lobes and hippocampal formations: normative volumetric measurements from MR images in young adults, *Radiology* 172:549.

Jernigan, T.L., Zatz, L.M., Moses, J.A., and Cardellino, J.P., 1982, Computed tomography in schizophrenics and normal volunteers: II. Cranial asymmetry, *Arch. Gen. Psychiatry* 39:771.

Kertesz, A., Polk, M., Black, S.E., and Howell, J., 1990, Sex, handedness, and the morphometry of cerebral asymmetries on magnetic resonance imaging, *Brain. Res.* 530:40.

Kleinschmidt, A., Falkai, P., Huang, Y., Schneider, T., Furst, G., and Steinmetz, H., 1994, In-vivo morphometry of planum temporal asymmetry in first-episode schizophrenia, *Schizophr. Res.* (in press).

LeMay, M., 1976, Morphological cerebral asymmetries of modern man, fossil man, and nonhuman primate, *Annals of the New York Academy of Sciences* 280:349.

LeMay, M., and Culebras, R., 1972, Human brain morphological differences in the hemispheres demonstrable by carotid arteriography, *New England J. Med.* 287:168.

LeMay, M., and Kido, D.K., 1978, Asymmetries of the cerebral hemispheres on computed tomograms, *J. Comput. Assist. Tomogr.* 2:471.

Lipska, B.K., Jaskiw, G.E., and Weinberger, D.R., 1994, Postpubertal emergence of augmented exploration and amphetamine supersensitivity after neonatal deafferentation of the rat ventral hippocampus, *Neuropsychopharmacology* (in press).

Luchins, D.J., Weinberger, D.R., Torrey, E.F., Johnson, A., Rogentine, N., and Wyatt, R.J., 1981, HLA-A2 antigen in schizophrenic patients with reversed cerebral asymmetry, *Br. J. Psychiatry* 138:240.

Luchins, D.J., and Meltzer, H.Y., 1983, A blind, controlled study of occipital asymmetry in schizophrenia, *Psychiatry. Res.* 10:87.

Luchins, D.J., Weinberger, D.R., and Wyatt, R.J., 1979, Schizophrenia: Evidence of a subgroup with reversed cerebral asymmetry, *Arch. Gen. Psychiatry* 36:1309.

Luchins, D.J., Weinberger, D.R., and Wyatt, R.J., 1982, Schizophrenia and cerebral asymmetry detected by computed tomography, *Am. J. Psychiatry* 139:6:753.

Naeser, M.A., Levine, H.L., Benson, D.F., Stuss, D.T., and Weir, W.S., 1981, Frontal leukotomy size and hemispheric asymmetries on computerized tomographic scans of schizophrenics with variable recovery, *Arch. Neurology* 38:30.

Pandya, D.N., and Barnes, C.L., 1987, Architecture and connections of the frontal lobe, *in*: "The Frontal Lobes Revisited," E. Perecman, ed., IRBN Press, New York.

Pienadz, J.M., and Naeser, M.A., 1984, Computed tomographic scan cerebral asymmetries and morphologic brain asymmetries. Correlation in the same cases post mortem, *Arch. Neurology* 41:403.

Rademacher, J., Galaburda, A.M., Kennedy, D.N., Filipek, P.A., and Caviness, V.S., 1992, Human cerebral cortex: localization, parcellation, and morphometry with magnetic resonance imaging, *J. Cogn. Neurosci.* 4:352.

Rosenberger, P.B., and Hier, D.B., 1980, Cerebral asymmetry and verbal intellectual deficit, *Ann. Neurol.* 8:300.

Rossi, A., Stratta, P., di Michele, V., Gallucci, M., Splendiani, A., and Casacchia, M., 1991, Temporal lobe structure by magnetic resonance imaging in bipolar affective disorders and schizophrenia, *J. Affect. Disord.* 21:19.

Sanides, F., 1969, Comparative architectonics of the neocortex of mammals and their evolutionary interpretation, *Annals of the New York Academy of Sciences* 167:404.

Saugstad, L.F., 1989, Social class, marriage, and fertility in schizophrenia, *Schizophr. Bull.* 15:9.

Seidman, L.J., Yurgelun-Todd, D., Kremen, W.S., Woods, B.T., Goldstein, J.M., Faraone, S.V., Tsuang, M.T., 1994, Relationship of prefrontal and temporal lobe MRI measures to neuropsychological performance in chronic schizophrenia, *Biol. Psychiatry* 35:235.

Shenton, M.E., Kikinis, R., McCarley, R.W., Metcalf, D., Tieman, J., and Jolesz, F.A., 1991, Application of automated MRI volumetric measurement techniques to the ventricular system in schizophrenics and normal controls, *Schizophr. Res.* 5:103.

Shenton, M.E., Kikinis, R., Jolesz, F.A., Pollak, S.D., LeMay, M., Wible, C.G., Kokama, H., Martin, J., Metcalf, D., Coleman, M., and McCarley, R.W., 1992, Abnormalities of the left temporal lobe and thought disorder in schizophrenia: A quantitative magnetic resonance imaging study, *New England J. Med.* 327:604.

Shenton, M.E., Hokama, H., Kikinis, R., Ballard, M., Holinger, D.P., Galaburda, A., Jolesz, F.A., and McCarley, R.W., 1994, Use of 3D MR surface renderings for measuring planum temporal, *Biol. Psychiatry* 35:721. (Abstract)

Snyder, P.J., Wu, H., Bogerts, B., Bilder, R.M., and Lieberman, J.A., 1994, Cerebellar volume asymmetries are related to handedness: A quantitative MRI study, INS Program and Abstracts 90.(Abstract)

Suddath, R.L., Casanova, M.F., Goldberg, T.E., Daniel, D.G., Kelsoe, J.R., and Weinberger, D.R., 1989, Temporal lobe pathology in schizophrenia: A quantitative magnetic resonance imaging study, *Am. J. Psychiatry* 146:464.

Tsai, L., Nasrallah, H.A., and Jacoby, C.G., 1983, Hemispheric asymmetries on computed tomographic scans in schizophrenia and mania, *Arch. Gen. Psychiatry* 40:1286.

Weinberger, D.R., Luchins, D.J., Morihisa, J.M., and Wyatt, R.J., 1982, Asymmetric volumes of the right and left frontal and occipital regions of the human brain, *Ann. Neurol.* 11:97.

Weinberger, D.R., Berman, K.F., Suddath, R., and Torrey, E.F., 1992, Evidence of dysfunction of a prefrontal-limbic network in schizophrenia: A magnetic resonance imaging and regional cerebral blood flow study of discordant monozygotic twins, *Am. J. Psychiatry* 149:890.

Wible, C.G., Shenton, M.E., Hokama, H., Kikinis, R., Jolesz, F.A., and McCarley, R.W., 1993, A magnetic resonance imaging study of the prefrontal cortex in schizophrenia, *Biol. Psychiatry* 33:123A. (Abstract)

Witelson, S.F., and Pallie, W., 1973, Left hemisphere specialization for language in the newborn. Neuroanatomical evidence of asymmetry, *Brain* 96:641.

Yakovlev, P.I., and Rakic, P., 1966, Patterns of decussation of bulbar pyramids and distribution of pyrimidal tracts on two sides of the spinal cord, *Trans. Amer. Neurol. Assoc.* 91:366.

Yeterian, E.H., and Pandya, D.N., 1988, Architectonic features of the primate brain, in: "Information Processing by the Brain," H.J. Markowitsch, ed., Hans Huber Publishers, Switzerland.

Zipursky, R.B., Lim, K.O., Sullivan, E.V., Brown, B.W., and Pfefferbaum, A., 1992, Widespread cerebral gray matter volume deficits in schizophrenia, *Arch. Gen. Psychiatry* 49:195.

Zipursky, R.B., Marsh, L., Lim, K.O., DeMent, S., Shear, P.K., Sullivan, E.V., Murphy, G.M., Csernansky, J.G., and Pfefferbaum, A., 1994, Volumetric MRI assessment of temporal lobe structures in schizophrenia, *Biol. Psychiatry* 35:501.

Zipursky, R.B., Lim, K.O., and Pfefferbaum, A., 1990, Volumetric assessment of cerebral asymmetry from CT scans, *Psychiatry Research: Neuroimaging* 35:71.

FETAL DEVELOPMENTAL ANIMAL MODEL OF SCHIZOPHRENIA WITH DOPAMINE, ACETYLCHOLINE, AND NITRIC OXIDE PERSPECTIVES

Melvin Lyon[1] and William O. McClure[2]

[1]University of Arkansas for Medical Sciences
Department of Psychology and Behavioral Sciences
Little Rock, Arkansas

[2]University of Southern California
Department of Biological Sciences and Department of Neurology
Los Angeles, California

INTRODUCTION

The interest in finding an animal model of schizophrenia began with the report of Mednick et al. (1988), that schizophrenia risk for the offspring was doubled by maternal exposure to a viral epidemic in the second trimester of pregnancy (Barr et al., 1990). Additional evidence suggests that not only viral exposure, but also emotional trauma in the pregnant mother, or exposure to intense radioactivity may have a similar effect (Huttunen and Niskanen, 1978; Otake and Shull, 1984). The common feature in all these cases is that the changes almost certainly have been initiated during the fetal stages of brain growth and in particular during the last part of the first trimester or in the second trimester (Gilles et al., 1983).

In support of this, although there are structural and cellular differences in the brains of schizophrenic patients (Bogerts et al., 1985; Bogerts, 1993; Roberts, 1990; Pakkenberg, 1990; Pakkenberg, 1992; Karson et al., 1991), there is relatively little evidence of glial proliferation or increases in glial fibrillary acidic protein (GFAP) in subcortical regions of the brain in schizophrenia (Pakkenberg, 1990; Karson et al., 1993). Since glial proliferation rises rapidly during the third trimester of fetal development (Gilles et al., 1983), any alterations in brain structure involving the death of cells, and occurring later than the second trimester, would almost certainly leave some evidence of glial disturbance.

Furthermore, in addition to reports of decreases or increases in neuronal numbers in the brains of schizophrenic patients, there are also several reports indicating misplacement or incorrect orientation of neurons in the hippocampus and entorhinal cortex, which could only have occurred during early brain development (Kovelman and Scheibel, 1984; Jakob and Beckmann, 1986).

Neural Development and Schizophrenia, Edited by S.A. Mednick
and J.M. Hollister, Plenum Press, New York, 1995

The value of developing a fetal growth model for schizophrenia that uses animals derived from the obvious difficulties of relying solely upon data from the excellent, but extremely long-term, developmental investigations of children at a genetic high risk for schizophrenia, as for example in the work of Mednick and Schulsinger (1968). Such studies require 20 to 30 years of human development, whereas in the rat this same growth period may be investigated in as little as two years. Among the advantages of choosing the rat for a potential model of schizophrenia are the following:

1. Control of subjects genetically and behaviorally.
2. Ability to follow lifetime developments in a period of two-three years.
3. Small physical size and economy of maintenance.
4. Many physiological similarities to humans, including basic brain structure, neurotransmitters, and response to pharmacological agents.

On the other hand, the main problems in accepting a rat model include:

1. Difficulty in comparing rats and humans behaviorally.
2. Absence of immediately recognizable correlates to some classic human schizophrenic symptoms, such as hallucinations and delusions.
3. The widespread belief that schizophrenia is a specifically human illness.
4. Differences in pre- and postnatal developmental times for brain structures (i.e. in rats a greater degree of brain development takes place after birth than in humans).

In the rat, the developmental phase in the brain parallel to that of the human second trimester begins approximately at the 12th gestational day (GD) of the 21-22 day gestational period, and continues until about the fifth postnatal day (PND). The postnatal period overlaps with some of the human third trimester brain development (Gilles et al., 1983), which occurs almost completely after birth in the rat. The period of the 11-14th (or 12-15th) GD used in the present studies coincides with birth and earliest development of cells in subcortical regions of particular importance in schizophrenia, such as the corpus striatum, thalamus and hippocampal formation (see Figure 1). The newly born cells then migrate toward their final location, with regions appearing later in phylogeny also being among the last to complete their functional connections (Bayer and Altman, 1991).

Some neurotransmitters of importance in schizophrenia, such as dopamine (DA) and norepinephrine (NE), are already present in cells between the 12-15th days, but the receptors and functional synaptic structure are not completed until after birth (Coyle and Campochiaro, 1976). Acetylcholine (ACh), and several other neurotransmitters, appear even later than NE and DA, and their systems are also not completely functional until after birth.

The importance of this is that during the prenatal treatment periods used here (GD 11-14; 12-15), d-amphetamine, and other dopaminergic and cholinergic agents, cannot act in their typical manner upon synapses and nerve cells. On the other hand, given the importance often assigned to DA activity in schizophrenia (Carlsson, 1988), it seemed logical to test the effect of a well-known dopaminergic agent on fetal development at a stage when the cells bearing that neurotransmitter were first beginning to appear.

Our first choice for an agent with which to challenge mothers was d-amphetamine. The advantages of amphetamine (AM) include:

1. Its stability, solubility, known pharmacodynamics, and several other qualities:
2. Ability to cross the placental barriers to the fetus.
3. Known influence on early brain growth processes (Muller et al., 1977; Van Eden, 1986).

4. Close relationship to DA systems thought to be important in schizophrenia (Carlsson, 1988).
5. Extensive use in attempts to model schizophrenia in both humans and rats (see reviews in Lyon, 1991a,b)
6. Use in previous studies of prenatal effects upon later development and behavior in rats (Holson et al, 1985).

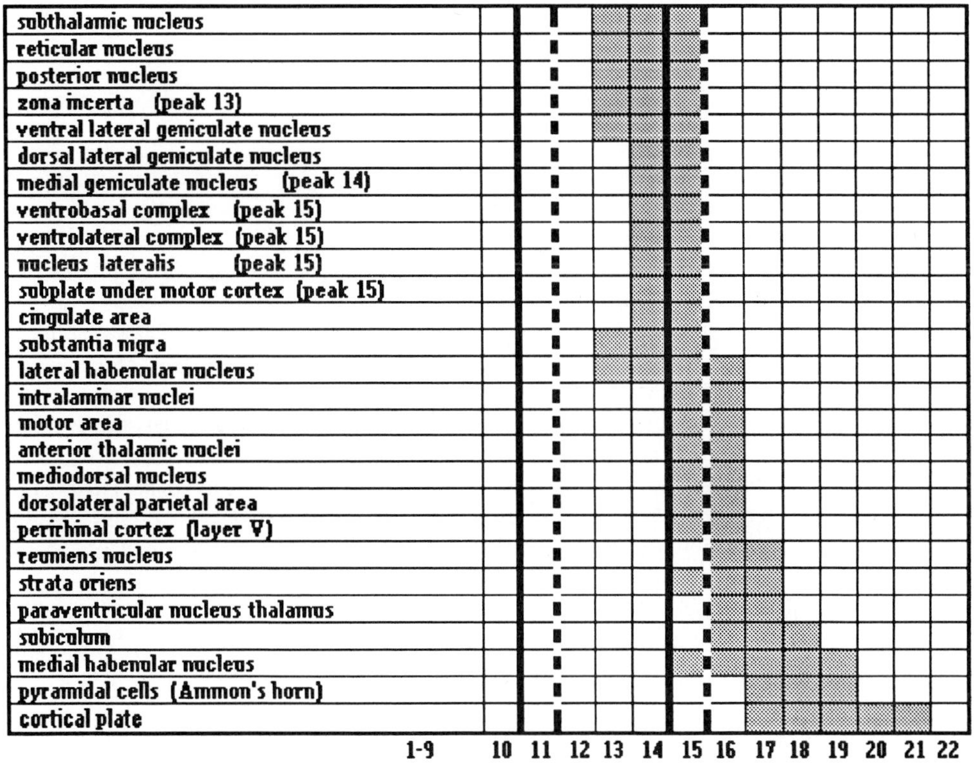
subthalamic nucleus
reticular nucleus
posterior nucleus
zona incerta (peak 13)
ventral lateral geniculate nucleus
dorsal lateral geniculate nucleus
medial geniculate nucleus (peak 14)
ventrobasal complex (peak 15)
ventrolateral complex (peak 15)
nucleus lateralis (peak 15)
subplate under motor cortex (peak 15)
cingulate area
substantia nigra
lateral habenular nucleus
intralaminar nuclei
motor area
anterior thalamic nuclei
mediodorsal nucleus
dorsolateral parietal area
perirhinal cortex (layer V)
reuniens nucleus
strata oriens
paraventricular nucleus thalamus
subiculum
medial habenular nucleus
pyramidal cells (Ammon's horn)
cortical plate
1-9
10 11 12 13 14 15 16 17 18 19 20 21 22

Figure 1. Approximate dates of birth of cells in various regions of the rat brain. Dates of birth of cells are indicated by the shaded days. The day of maximal cell birth is indicated specifically in selected cases. Data from Altman and Bayer (1979) and Bayer and Altman (1991).

PROTOCOL OF THE AMPHETAMINE MODEL

The typical plan of experiments with this model (Lyon and McClure, 1994) has been to treat the pregnant Sprague-Dawley female rats once per day on either GD 11-14 or GD 12-15 with d-amphetamine (AM) at 2.0 or 5.0 mg/kg s.c., or with saline control (CO) injections. In later experiments, two additional control groups were added. In an undernutritional control group (UN), pregnant females were not injected and were fed only the mean amount of food per day eaten by mothers treated with d-amphetamine; in an unhandled control group (UH), pregnant females were fed *ad lib* and were not handled on the days when the experimental animals were injected.

Animals were then allowed to give birth and, on PND 2, pups were culled to N=8 per litter and either left with their mothers to mimic the normal developmental course, or fostered to surrogate mothers to control for postnatal maternal influences.

On PND 20, pups were weaned and placed in social cage groups consisting of 2-4 siblings of the same sex. These offspring were then given several types of behavioral tests before they were sacrificed and their brains removed for histological analysis.

Because of the known difficulties with reduced variance within litters (Holson and Pearce, 1992), the results reported here are generally based on litter statistics, where a single mean value was used to represent the sibling scores. Data have been obtained describing both the behavior and the neuroanatomy of these treated animals.

BEHAVIORAL METHODS AND RESULTS

The Holeboard

Most of the data reported here were collected from behavioral observations in a holeboard with 16 holes, 4 of which were baited with food (KIX corn cereal or Hershey's Milk Chocolate Chips). The choice of this apparatus was suggested by the work of Oades (1982) who considered responding on the holeboard as a possible test of thought disorder, which is a cardinal symptom of schizophrenia. The measures obtained in these experiments were: *hole-pokes, locomotion, turning direction on leaving the startbox, latency for leaving the startbox, baits taken, time to last bait, eating (chewing) time, rearing against the wall, rearing in the field without support.*

Several derived scores were obtained from the basic measures given above: *Lateral preference strength* - turns on leaving the startbox to the side least frequently chosen subtracted from those to the side most frequently chosen; *Entries into the mid-field squares or holes*; *Perseverative hole poking* - this refers to the number of pokes >2 into the same hole; *Switching ratio* - this ratio equals the number of holes entered divided by the total number of hole pokes.

Using all of these measures, we could use the holeboard to test the following features of learning which might have relevance to schizophrenia and to behavioral abnormality in general.

Acquisition and retention of food location knowledge. In this case, the animal must gradually acquire learning about the position of the baited holes and must retain the memory of these locations between trials on alternate days. Such basic learning functions may be disturbed by a shorter attentional span, which is also presumed here to be a major cause of thought disorder in schizophrenia. Aside from this type of disturbance, learning and conditioning appear to progress in an orderly fashion in schizophrenia (Ayllon and Azrin, 1969; Bellack and Hersen, 1993).

Perseveration and switching of holepoke responses. This measure refers to perseveration in poking into the same hole many times, even when it no longer contains bait, or perseveration in switching constantly from one hole to another regardless of the relevance of this behavior to obtaining baits. Both are significant signs of abnormality also seen in the responses of schizophrenic patients when facing a choice response situation (Armitage et al., 1964; Lyon and Gerlach, 1988).

Turning direction and lateral preference can be tested in the holeboard as the animal repeatedly leaves the startbox and explores the field to the left or right side, and in the direction of rotation in the field or startbox. Bodily rotation and side preference are thought to be related to the dopaminergic balance in the striatum (Glick and Shapiro, 1985; Brown and Robbins, 1989). Changes in the preferred direction of bodily rotation toward the left side have been described in both schizophrenia and mania (Bracha, 1987; Lyon et al., 1992).

Response to reversal of a baiting pattern can be tested in the holeboard. For example, by reversing the field pattern of baited holes from a left- to a right-sided bias after initial training has occurred, one can test for the flexibility of responding to an altered "cognitive set". Such reversals in "set" are demonstrably more difficult for schizophrenic patients and account for their poor showing on the Wisconsin Card Sort

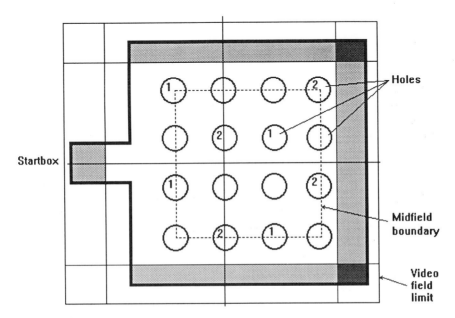

Figure 2. Holeboard apparatus. 1, holes baited with the original pattern; 2, holes baited with the reversal pattern. Activity was monitored in the marked areas using a suspended video camera.

Test, which has frequently been used in assessing cognitive deficits in schizophrenia (Daniel et al, 1991; Berman and Weinberger, 1990). Furthermore, the ability to deal with reversal learning is known to be related to the mediodorsal thalamic nucleus and the prefrontal cortex (Zola-Morgan and Squire, 1985), both of which are structurally disturbed in schizophrenia (Pakkenberg, 1990; Akbarian et al, 1993a).

Response to extinction. The failure to find reinforcements in the holeboard where they have previously been available induces in normal animals an increased number of responses for a time, followed by a complete cessation of responding. In keeping with their relatively normal conditioning process, schizophrenic individuals in extinction would be expected to show the same initial increase in responding. However, their responding, once started, might be expected to continue beyond the normal range, with continuing signs of response perseveration and switching, despite the complete lack of reinforcement (Lyon and Gerlach, 1988).

Results of Holeboard Testing

Animals from the prenatal treatment groups were tested twice as they grew up, first during an Early Juvenile (PND 25-31) period, and then in a Late Juvenile/Early Adult (PND 53-59) period.

In the Early Juvenile tests, the food bits were in the same four holes (see Figure 2) for three single trials on alternate days. These trials were identified as H1-H3. The results were analyzed as noted above by taking the mean for each litter group and comparing the treatments by litters, with results as shown in Figure 3.

Early Juvenile Test Period. The main points to be noted for the Early Juvenile period showed both non-gender- and gender-specific differences. On the first trial (H1) there was generally decreased activity in the AM animals, especially in the females. The AM females, compared to CO controls, had longer start latencies before entering the field, longer average times to find baits, and a decreased number of holepokes, rearings, and mid-field entries. AM females also showed a later (H3) development of increased holepoking that was not required to find baits and appeared to be a sign of increasing non- reinforcement-related ("adjunctive") activity.

AM males, on the other hand, did *not* show any decrease in mid-field time on the first holeboard trial, and even showed a significant increase in rearing out in the field, compared to CO animals. They also showed a first trial (H1) increase in perseverative holepokes (>2), which, however, reversed to significantly less than control values by the third trial (H3). Although this might seem to indicate increased efficiency in holepoking on H3, the time required to find the last bait did not change. This is the result of continued higher switching between holes in the AM animals, while switching has been gradually reduced in CO controls. Thus the AM animals go from significant increases in perseverative holepokes in the same hole to perseverative switching between holes as trials progress. This change from relatively simple repetitive activity to greater response switching is also frequently seen in the behavior of schizophrenic patients (Lyon and Gerlach, 1988).

Results from the Late Juvenile/Early Adult Test Period. Approximately three weeks after completion of the Early Juvenile trials, the animals were again tested in a larger, but topographically similar, holeboard for another three trials, again on alternate days. Behavioral measures on these trials included a new derived score: Lateral preference, which was defined as the right/left turning direction chosen most frequently when leaving the startbox. The H4-H6 trials in this test period were used to measure retention, reversal, and extinction. The major results were as follows (see also Figure 4).

Retention testing (H4). On this trial, the baits remained in the same position as on H1-3 to test both for memory and for generalization of the earlier learning to the larger field. The results were as follows:

AM animals of both sexes showed fewer different holes poked, fewer total holepokes, less mid-field time, but more time eating (chewing) and a much greater lateral preference in turning right or left when leaving the startbox. Their lateral preference, whether to right or left, was approximately twice as strong as in control animals. It is interesting, in this connection, to note that non-psychotic humans do not show a consistent left/right direction of bodily rotation, whereas in never-medicated schizophrenic patients Bracha (1987) has reported a significant tendency to turn more often toward the left side.

Reversal testing (H5). On this trial, the pattern of baits in the field was reversed from a left- to a right-sided bias (see Figure 1) with the following results: The time spent eating continued to be higher in the AM animals. The reason for this is not entirely clear. Either the AM animals were not such efficient eaters, which might suggest some midbrain trigeminal nerve deficit, or they were reacting as if to a low dose of d-amphetamine, which in adult animals may increase eating time as a function of increased dopaminergic activity (Blundell and Latham, 1978).

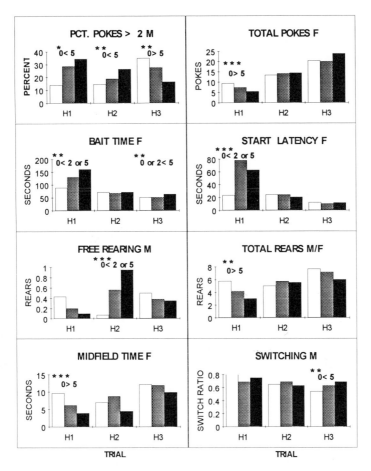

Figure 3. Activity of treated animals during the early juvenile test period. M, male; F, female. Dose of amphetamine: 0 mg/kg, open bars; 2 mg/kg, gray bars; 5 mg/kg, black bars. Significance: ***, p < 0.01; **, p < 0.05; *, p < 0.05 (one-tailed).

AM animals spent less time in mid-field, which usually is considered a sign of increased nervousness or anxiety, especially in a relatively unfamiliar environment. However, in these otherwise normally active animals responding in an environment that is already familiar, a tendency to remain near, or in contact with, the enclosure wall may simply be the result of increased dopaminergic activity, as in amphetamine stimulation (Schiørring, 1971). The fact that female AM animals showed increased numbers of squares entered, with no gain in foraging efficiency, suggests that the latter interpretation may be correct (see also Lyon and Robbins, 1975). Once more, there is evidence of increased adjunctive (non-reinforcement-related) responding, which is also characteristic of schizophrenia.

AM males continued to show high levels of switching between holes as they holepoked, and this tendency was now matched by CO males on the reversal trial, perhaps since these animals were also now trying to find an appropriate response to the reversed pattern. However, the AM group was the only group that maintained a consistently high switching ratio across trials. The difference in strength of lateral preference was no longer significantly greater in AM animals on the reversal trial, but this may be expected in view of the tendency to try alternative behaviors when faced with the reversed baiting pattern. Meanwhile, CO animals showed a significantly increased number of right turns (toward the now-baited side) compared with both the low- and the high-dose AM groups. This probably indicates a failure on the part of the AM animals to adapt as readily to the reversed baiting pattern. This type of difficulty in changing cognitive "set" from previous

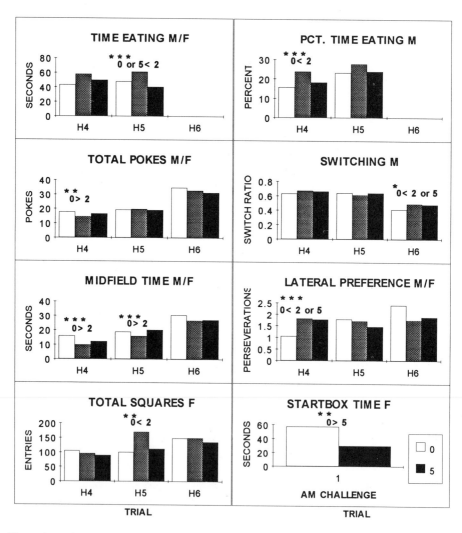

Figure 4. Activity of treated animals during the early adult test period. See Fig. 3 for information concerning symbols.

training is seen in schizophrenic patients on the Wisconsin Card Sort Test (Daniel et al., 1991), and in animals with reduced cell numbers in the mediodorsal thalamic nucleus (Zola-Morgan and Squire, 1985; Mair et al., 1992; Robinson and Mair, 1992), a neuroanatomical deficit which has also been reported in schizophrenia (Pakkenberg, 1990; 1992).

Extinction testing (H6). During extinction, no baits were accessible but food under the floor kept the olfactory cues similar and the trial period was five minutes in length, regardless of activity level. As expected, all animals increased their total holepokes during extinction, but AM males now again showed a significantly higher switching ratio than control animals, which remains similar to the findings in schizophrenia (Armitage et al., 1964; Lyon et al., 1986; Lyon and Gerlach, 1988).

Challenge Experiments

Since the behavioral evidence above suggested that AM animals were more sensitive to dopaminergic influences, it seemed important to test AM animals for changes in response to dopaminergic stimulation.

Neuroanatomical evidence (see below) indicated that AM animals might have more cholinergic cells in brainstem nuclei with projections to the nigrostriatal DA system. This suggested, in turn, a possible increase in sensitivity to cholinergic stimulants in the AM animals. A combined DA/ACh imbalance interaction has been suggested as a causal basis for many schizophrenic symptoms (Tandon and Greden, 1989), with dopaminergic overstimulation leading to the "positive" symptoms in schizophrenia, while a cholinergic overbalance might result in more negative symptomatology (Tandon et al., 1993).

In order to test for the effects of various agents on dopaminergic and cholinergic systems in particular, challenge experiments were carried out with several drugs in the offspring of AM and CO animals.

Dopaminergic Challenge

d-Amphetamine. The DA system was challenged with d-amphetamine by injecting AM and CO animals with 1.0 mg/kg d-amphetamine 30 minutes before a three minute trial in an open field. The results showed that the AM females were significantly more sensitive to the stimulant effects of the drug since their startbox time was considerably less than that of the CO females. Male AM animals showed a decided tendency in the same direction, but the difference did not reach statistical significance.

Apomorphine. Experiments were conducted in a counter-balanced series with apomorphine (0.5 or 1.0 mg/kg, s.c.) and saline injections on alternate days in AM, CO, and undernutritional control (UN) animals. The UN group had been prenatally exposed to maternal undernutrition based on the less-than-normal amount eaten by AM-treated mothers, and thus controlled specifically for any fetal effects of limiting maternal food intake during pregnancy. This is of concern here because of the suggestion by Susser and Lin (1992) that maternal starvation during pregnancy may increase the incidence of schizophrenia (see also Lyon and Bracha, 1994).

Following saline injections, AM animals showed significantly increased locomotion compared to CO animals, thus indicating a higher level of dopaminergic stimulation under control conditions. Under apomorphine, the CO animals showed an increase in locomotion which would be expected from the stimulant effects of the drug, but the AM animals showed a *decrease* in locomotion at this point so that the differences between the two groups AM and CO became non-significant. Such a reduction in locomotion is one of the first signs of an increased tendency toward high-dose apomorphine stereotypy (Robbins et al., 1990). Furthermore, the female AM animals also showed increased licking behavior, which is one of the prime signs of apomorphine stereotypy in the rat. It may be significant to note that the UN animals, especially the females, did not show the increased licking and floor contact with the snout that AM animals showed. These results indicate that the AM animals in particular were more sensitive to the dopaminergic stimulation, in agreement with the other behavioral evidence.

Cholinergic Challenge

Physostigmine. Physostigmine is a cholinesterase inhibitor with relatively specific stimulant effects upon muscarinic cholinergic receptors (Clarke et al., 1993). Animals were tested with a counterbalanced series of physostigmine (0.1 and 0.6 mg/kg, s.c.) and control saline injections given on alternate days as with apomorphine. Interestingly, the UN animals showed significant *decreases* in activities such as grooming, rearing, and locomotion, as compared with both AM and CO treatment groups. This would appear to indicate that the UN animals' general motor activity was in some way inhibited by the increased cholinergic stimulation. The AM animals, on the other hand, demonstrated significantly greater teeth chattering than CO or UN animals at the 0.1 mg/kg dose level, while both AM and UN animals showed more teeth chattering than CO control animals at the 0.6 mg/kg dose level. This indicates both that the AM animals were significantly more sensitive to the stimulant effects of acetylcholine than either CO or UN animals, and also that the UN animals could attain this level of stimulation when the dose was raised to 0.6 mg/kg.

Since teeth chattering has been closely associated with increased cholinergic activity (Ushijima et al., 1984; 1985), the above finding indicates an increased sensitivity to cholinergic stimulation in the AM animals, which also appears consistent with the larger number of cholinergic cells found in their brain stem nuclei (Nielsen et al., 1992). The fact that the UN animals also showed more teeth chattering than control animals, at the upper physostigmine dose level, suggests that undernutrition, which is known to induce changes in dopaminergic activity (Marichich et at., 1979), may also produce changes in the cholinergic system of these animals, although they appear to be less sensitive to this effect than AM animals.

Further Experiments

These experiments were performed in the same manner with the holeboard as in the original series, except that prenatal treatment days were GD 12-15 (instead of 11-14), trials were run in a well-lighted room rather than in semi-darkness, trials were five minutes in length even if all baits had been taken earlier, and the control comparisons included treatment groups with three dose levels of haloperidol (0.5, 1.5, and 2.5 mg/kg) as well as UN animals. The results from the haloperidol animals will not be discussed here, but, as expected, they were significantly different on many measures from the AM, CO and UN treatment groups.

It may be of importance to point out that changing the treatment days from GD 11-14 to 12-15 may have significant consequences for the types of cell birth and migration which are affected. It may be seen from Figure 1 that on days 14 and 15, in particular, there are many more cells whose birth may be affected by a prenatal treatment. Even one day more in development may also allow different populations of migrating cells to be affected in their passage to their intended functional location.

Despite the above differences in procedure, the results of this experimental series generally tended to confirm the findings from the first series. Lateral preference was again found to be significantly higher in the AM animals. Perseverative responses (greater than two) in hole-poking were again significantly higher in AM animals. In these experiments, in contrast to the first set of experiments, this result was found in later trials as well as in the first holeboard trial. In addition to these points, there were now clear signs of hyperactivity in AM and UN animals (more in females than in males - but present in both) in the extinction trials which occurred at the Late Juvenile/Early Adult stage of development.

This is an important addition to the evidence from the original experiments because it has been suggested that hyperactivity at this developmental age is an important marker of increased adult dopaminergic activity such as may occur in schizophrenia. Such hyperactivity is also one of the behavioral alterations noted following ventral hippocampal lesions in the young rat, which appear to model some symptoms related to schizophrenia (Lipska et al., 1993). The present evidence provides a distinct parallel to the findings of Lipska et al. and demonstrates that the increased activity can also be elicited in the young adult rat following early prenatal treatment as well as postnatal lesions. The increased lateral preference, perseverative responding, and Late Juvenile signs of hyperactivity, all found in the prenatal treatment model, are also suggestive of changes in dopaminergic activity similar to those apparently occurring in schizophrenia.

Comments on Undernutritional Controls (UN). The UN animals were significantly different from both CO and AM animals on many points, but were similar to AM animals on others. In general, UN animals were much more active than the AM animals, not only in observation cages but also in activity wheel and holeboard tests. The finding of greater activity is therefore quite general. There were also sex differences in UN animals, as well as in the AM animals. Some of these differences were parallel in both treatment conditions. The activity of AM females was affected much more than that of AM males during our early studies (Lyon and McClure, 1994), but in the second series of experiments, this difference appeared also during the extinction phase and in UN animals. UN males tended to show some behavioral changes that have been closely tied to schizophrenia (increased switching; perseveration in holepoking).

These findings are particularly important with respect to the time of prenatal treatment used, and its relationship to stages of brain development in the rat. It could be argued that the GD 11-14 or 12-15 period in the rat is closer to the end of the first trimester than to the late second trimester which has been emphasized by Mednick et al. (1988) and Barr et al. (1990) with respect to exposure to influenza epidemics. The findings of the effects of undernutrition in the UN animals also fits with the report of increased DA activity in adult animals following both prenatal undernutrition (Marichich et al., 1979) and prenatal (GD 12- 15) treatment with d-amphetamines (Holson et al., 1985). It should be noted that undernutrition effects may be somewhat greater in females than in males, in agreement with the greater risk for schizophrenia in female children of mothers exposed to late first trimester starvation as reported by Susser and Lin (1992).

In their work on the Dutch Hunger Winter, and its apparent effect on the outcome of pregnancies during that period, Susser and Lin reported an increased tendency for female offspring to become schizophrenic following a late *first* trimester exposure to starvation in the mother. There was also a trend for the males in the same direction, but it was not statistically significant. It remains possible that some aspects of schizophrenia may be mimicked or elicited by the effects of prenatal undernutrition. The animal evidence is being examined in detail at this time and will be reported elsewhere (Lyon and Bracha, 1994).

In relation to rat experiments, it may be worthwhile to point out that Carlson et al. (1987) showed that 24 hour food deprivation in the rat resulted in increased DA activity in the medial prefrontal cortex, but not in the substantia nigra or nucleus accumbens.

Comments on Right/Left Turning and Lateral Preference. There is evidence that schizophrenic patients, even those never medicated, rotate bodily more often to the left side than to the right (Bracha, 1987; 1989). This finding has been supported by Nancy Lyon's demonstration of increased turning to the left side in a choice-response situation in both schizophrenic and manic patients (see Lyon and Satz, 1991; Lyon et al., 1992). The demonstration of turning preference should be differentiated from that of handedness, which due to learning and modification postnatally may not reflect the natural tendency. For instance, the choice of pressing a right or left button in a two-choice task is more likely to reveal increased switching between sides than a distinct bias toward only one side (Lyon et al., 1986; Frith and Done, 1983).

Turning in the rat does not have the strong right-side bias of humans, but it has been shown to be at least partially dependent on the dopaminergic balance between the right and left striatum (Glick and Shapiro, 1985). Thus when we are able to demonstrate a doubling of lateral preference strength to either the right or the left in the rat (see above), it suggests that the striatal DA balance has been altered. Additional measures of lateral preference in the rat would be desirable.

Bracha's measures of bodily rotation in humans used a rotometer apparatus that recorded all turns in the right or left direction taken during the day by schizophrenic patients or by control subjects (Bracha, 1987). In collaboration with Dr. Bracha we have run overnight measures of bodily rotation in a rotometer apparatus designed for use with rats. During their nocturnal high activity period, the rotometer evidence indicated, as in other measures of activity, that UN animals were generally more active than AM animals. However, we also found that AM rats showed significantly increased right/left switching on one-third turn measures, although they did not show a significant preference for either the right or left side. The presence of increased switching in direction appears similar to the right/left switching increase noted in schizophrenics and manics on a two-choice button-operated task (Lyon and Gerlach, 1988; Lyon et al., 1992). It is also similar to the increased holepoke switching ratio mentioned above in AM animals.

In summary, although we do not have evidence of a distinct lateral bias, as in human schizophrenic and manic patients, we did find evidence of significantly increased switching from side-to-side. The older adult rats used in these single overnight bodily rotation experiments sometimes provided too few rotation counts to give a reliable measure of performance, but practical problems did not allow increasing the session length in these experiments. Further experiments are underway, including experiments with rotation under the effects of amphetamine stimulation.

Preliminary Evidence for Alcohol/Water Intoxication. Both alcohol and water intoxication are well-known problems among schizophrenic patients, and in each case they may be so extreme as to lead to the death of the patient if unchecked (Cuffel et al., 1993; Illowsky and Kirch, 1988). It is therefore important to ask whether an animal model of schizophrenia can produce evidence of either type of over-drinking. For that reason, studies were made using a two-bottle preference task with a cage containing an activity wheel. These experiments were done in collaboration with Drs. D. E. McMillan and T. Hudzik, of the Department of Pharmacology and Toxicology, and Dr. W. B. Lawson of the Department of Psychiatry and Behavioral Sciences, at the University of Arkansas for Medical Sciences.

The results (Lyon et al., 1993) indicated that AM animals drank significantly more 5% alcohol when only that was offered, and tended to show over-drinking of either alcohol or water under different experimental conditions involving presence or absence of access to an activity wheel.

In the first experimental series, the sequence was: presentation of water only with activity wheel, activity wheel with alcohol only, closing access to the activity wheel with alcohol present, and then with both water and alcohol present, and finally allowing wheel activity with both fluids present. In the second experiment, access to the wheel was not prevented under any conditions, so only the first conditions, wheel + water only and wheel + alcohol only, were similar. There was no prevention of wheel access in the presence of alcohol and water together as there was in the first experiment.

The results showed some interesting similarities and differences. In both experiments, AM animals showed greater intake of 5% alcohol than did UN animals when only alcohol was presented. Furthermore, in the first experiment, when both water and alcohol had been present without wheel access and the wheel was again made available, at this point the AM animals began a significant and long-lasting (>10 days) increase in alcohol intake in preference to water. In the second experiment, when both alcohol and water were present and wheel activity was *not* prevented the AM animals tended to show significantly increased *water* intake compared with that of the UN animals. In both experiments, the UN animals tended to show increased activity in the wheel as compared to AM animals, but they did not show evidence of overdrinking alcohol.

In both experiments, the number of subjects is small (N=6) and further study is needed. However, the preliminary results suggest that the AM treatment model may also provide a useful parallel to alcohol and water intoxication problems in schizophrenia.

NEUROANATOMICAL RESULTS

The above evidence confirmed significant behavioral changes in animals exposed to prenatal treatment with d-amphetamine. It also demonstrated that there were significant behavioral similarities and also some significant differences between the AM animals and the UN animals with respect to schizophrenia-like behaviors. However, the demonstration of behavioral similarities to schizophrenia raises the important question of whether there are neuroanatomical changes in the brains of AM animals that have some similarity to the abnormalities found in schizophrenia.

Most previous animal models (Lyon, 1991a,b) rely on lesion techniques or upon generalized toxic drug effects. Most recently, postnatal lesions of the hippocampus have been suggested as potential models for schizophrenia (Schmajuk, 1987; Lipska et al., 1993; Mittleman et al., 1993). Except for postnatal lesion models, it has been difficult to show any significant behavioral correlations with demonstrated changes in brain anatomy.

Therefore, it was thought necessary, in parallel with the fetal developmental changes that must have taken place in schizophrenia, to demonstrate changes in the neuroanatomy of animals following treatments given only during fetal development. Such prenatal treatments should not produce massive losses of brain tissue such as those typically following intracerebral injection of neurotoxins, fetal brain lesions, or brain lesions made shortly after birth, since in all of these cases, there would be residual structural and/or glial alterations that are not found in the brain tissue of most schizophrenic individuals (Gilles et al., 1983; Lyon and Barr, 1991). The following analysis therefore concentrates on regions of the brain found to be disorganized or disturbed in cell number in postmortem schizophrenic brain tissue.

Mediodorsal Thalamic Nucleus (MD)

Initial results with the GD 11-14 prenatal treatment with amphetamine indicated that offspring had a significant decrease (-24.3%; $p < 0.02$; t-test) in the number of neurons in the mid-region of the MD. This decrease was not found in the lateral portion of the nucleus, nor was it found with any "window" of treatment within the GD 15-20 range. This finding appears to agree with the loss of neurons in the MD in schizophrenia (Pakkenberg, 1990; 1992).

The functional significance of this finding is that the MD sends heavy projections to the medial prefrontal cortex. Lesions involving these projections have been demonstrated to result in deficiencies in reversal learning in non-human primates by Zola-Morgan and Squire (1985), and in the rat by Robinson and Mair (1992). In the rat, damage to the MD is also associated with a loss of response in the delayed non-matching to sample (DNMTS) paradigm. This paradigm requires the animal to retain the memory of the location of a particular stimulus in order to respond after the delay to a different location. It will be seen that this is highly similar to the reversal learning that we used in our experiments and in which we found deficits in the speed of learning for AM animals. As noted earlier, the change in cognitive "set" required by the reversal test and in the DNMTS is similar to the demands of the Wisconsin Card Sort Test, with which schizophrenic patients frequently have difficulty. In the card sort test, "set" is related to a request that the subject change from identifying the card forms by color to identifying them by shape and vice versa. Inability to switch between these two cognitive "sets" is a relatively stable symptom in schizophrenic subjects (Daniel et al., 1991; Berman and Weinberger, 1990). In relation to the present findings, these considerations suggest that loss of neurons in the MD may be directly related to the deficits in reversal learning which we have observed in AM rats.

Entorhinal Cortex (EC)

The EC is a significant region with respect to the hippocampal formation, since it provides major input from all of the sensory pathways in the brain to the hippocampus through the perforant pathway. Furthermore, it has been reported that there are significant changes in the cellular distribution within the EC in brain tissue from schizophrenics (Jakob and Beckmann, 1986; Arnold et al., 1991). It was therefore natural for us to consider looking at EC as a region that might be involved if the present animal model did indeed mimic schizophrenia. To test this, pregnant mothers were treated with amphetamine using three different treatment windows: GD 11-14; 15-17; and 18-20. It may be seen from the developmental table regarding cell birth (Fig. 1) that these three windows will affect widely different stages of brain growth, and should yield very different neuroanatomical consequences.

Horizontal sections taken at various levels in the ventral to dorsal dimension show an increase of cells in the EC. The increase is seen only in the GD 11-14 window, and does not vary significantly with ventral to dorsal location (Lawrence et al., 1993). Although the increase is small ($+21\%$; $p < 0.05$ by t-test), both its statistical significance and the lack of an effect in two later windows of gestation indicate that it is real. Treatment with *in utero* amphetamine alters the structure of the rat's EC.

Functionally, changes in the location of cells in EC may lead to an abnormal input to the hippocampus with resulting effects upon the ability to use spatial "cognitive maps" to solve location problems (O'Keefe and Nadel, 1978). Such a defect could also result in some difficulty in learning and remembering the location of baits in the holeboard task. More specific tests of spatial location under the pressure of time delay, as in the delayed non-matching to sample task, would be useful in determining the accuracy of this suggestion.

Nucleus Accumbens (NAC)

The nucleus accumbens is an important region in the brain with respect to dopaminergic systems, but its study has been complicated by the finding that it consists of both a shell and a core region which have different neurotransmitters and may be related to different behavioral functions (Voorn et al., 1988; Berendse et al., 1992).

The present findings are that following the GD 11-14 prenatal treatment there was a mean 19% decrease in the number of neurons in the core region of NAC itself in the AM animals. However, the variance was large and the difference did not quite reach statistical significance (P < 0.06). These counts are difficult and further investigations are needed, particularly also in the shell region of NAC where the majority of ventral tegmental projections arrive.

Significant cell losses have been reported in NAC in schizophrenia by Pakkenberg (1990), but the exact relationship to sub-divisions of the nucleus in the rat is not known at this time. Further investigations will also be necessary to establish the relevance of these connections. The NAC is known to be involved in many of the behavioral changes dependent on dopaminergic systems, as documented above (see also Willner and Scheel-Kruger, 1991). Functionally, the NAC appears to be related to the initiation of behavior (Koob and Swerdlow, 1988), in particular regarding changes in the frequency of repetitive responses, as well as to the temporal sequence of responses in general. It has been theorized that the actual form of the response is decided in other parts of the striatum with a close relationship to cortical interactions. (Alexander et al., 1990).

Pedunculopontine (PPTg)/Laterodorsal (LDTg) Tegmental Nuclei

These nuclei contain a population of cells which contain both choline acetyl transferase and nitric oxide synthase (NOS; Vincent et al., 1983; Vincent and Kimura, 1992). Significant increases in the number of these cells have been reported by Karson et al. (1991) in postmortem schizophrenic brain tissue. We have also found increases in the number of cells in the LDTg of the AM animals (Nielsen et al., 1992; Nielsen et al., 1994) and preliminary evidence supports a similar finding in the PPTg (unpublished).

Nitric oxide may have general neuromodulatory functions within the nervous system. Release of nitric oxide is necessary for penile erection (Burnett et al., 1992) and has been associated with dilation of the perivascular musculature (Bredt et al., 1990). Most recently, it has been demonstrated that nitric oxide, as a free radical, can have both neurotoxic and neuroprotective effects in the brain depending upon the redox milieu in which the NO release occurs (Lipton et al. 1993; Coyle and Puttfarcken, 1993).

It is possible that the NOS-positive, cholinergic cells of the PPTg/LDTg may be involved in the etiology of schizophrenia. The PPTg/LDTg system is thought to affect the temporal sequence of behavior by means of oscillatory functions that involve both nigrostriatal and thalamocortical systems (Skinner and Garcia-Rill, 1990). The NOS-positive, cholinergic cells of the PPTg and LDTg are appropriately located to perform such a function, as well as to modify the activity of many other areas of the brain. Some important aspects of the anatomy of these connections are shown in Figure 5, where two roughly parallel, upward-reaching systems, connected to the LDTg and PPTg respectively, are illustrated. The PPTg has important projections to the substantia nigra and corpus striatum and indirectly to the NAC (Gould et al., 1989; Blaha and Winn, 1993). The LDTg has prominent projections to rostral thalamic nuclei, including the mediodorsal and anterior nuclei. These projections, including those to MD, could be closely related to sleep-waking and oscillatory functions (Pape and Mager, 1992; Steriade et al., 1987a,b; 1993; Kayama et al., 1992). Projections to the nigra may also be important in evaluating the possibility that the PPTg acts as a driving force for the nigrostriatal DA system, which may be abnormally active in schizophrenia (Garcia-Rill et al., 1991; Blaha and Winn, 1993). There are also some descending projections, from about 10% of the cholinergic NOS-containing cells of the PPTg and LDTg, to the medioventral medullary "motor region". However, the majority of projections to the medioventral medulla from the PPTg and LDTg are from the non-cholinergic (i.e. non- NOS-containing) cells (Skinner et al., 1990). These ventrally projecting, NOS-containing, cells do not appear to provide more than a small number of connections to caudal medullary regions. It would appear that the major influence of the nitric oxide system in the brainstem is directed toward the more rostral aspects of the cerebral hemispheres.

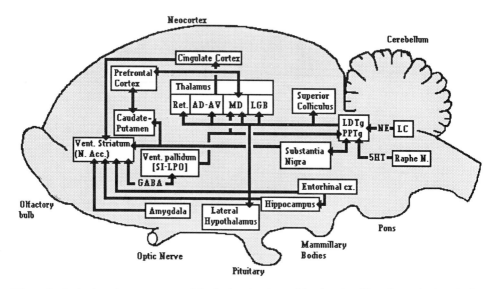

Figure 5. Projections between areas of the brain related to schizophrenia. Note the projections both rostral and caudal from the pedunculopontine tegmental nucleus (PPTg) and the laterodorsal tegmental nucleus (LDTg). LC, locus coeruleus; Raphe N., raphe nuclei; N. Acc., nucleus accumbens; SI-LPO, substantia innominata - lateral preoptic area; AD-AV, anterior dorsal and anterior ventral nuclei of the thalamus; Ret, reticular nucleus of the thalamus; LGB, lateral geniculate body of the thalamus.

It may be concluded that the PPTg/LDTg complex has projections specifically affecting both the nigrostriatal and the mesocorticolimbic systems, both of which have been implicated in schizophrenia. The increased number of NOS-containing cells in the PPTg/LDTg in schizophrenia may also be related to the finding that there are many partially migrated, or improperly oriented, NOS-containing cells in the frontal and temporal cortex of schizophrenic patients (Akbarian et al., 1993a,b). Exactly how these systems exert their effects upon behavior is not yet clear.

SUMMARY

Behavioral Parallels to Schizophrenia

The following points indicate a significant series of behavioral parallels between human schizophrenics and rats treated *in utero* with amphetamine.   Since we cannot reliably measure in the rat certain types of cognitive experience commonly reported by human schizophrenics (i.e. hallucinations, delusions) it is necessary to look at the basic structure of behavior to find other similarities. The following list of behavioral alterations found in the present animal model is highly consistent with behavioral abnormalities that have been described in many schizophrenic patients. As with other potentially diagnostic systems for schizophrenia, no single item on this list is exclusively found in that disorder, but in concert they suggest a strong correlation.   References are given to selected supporting literature from the study of human schizophrenic patients.

1. Perseverative responding (Lyon et al., 1986; Armitage et al., 1964; Lyon and Gerlach, 1988; Frith and Done, 1983)
2. Increased response switching (Lyon et al., 1986; Lyon and Gerlach, 1988)
3. Lateral preference strength altered and/or increased (Lyon and Satz, 1991; Lyon et al., 1992; Bracha, 1987; Bracha, 1989)
4. Difficulty in reversal learning (changing "set"; Daniel et al., 1991; Armitage et al., 1964; Berman and Weinberger, 1990)
5. Hyperactivity of increasingly stereotyped nature developing at the young adult stage (Bleuler, 1950)
6. Evidence of tendency toward alcohol/water intoxication (Cuffel et al., 1993; Illowsky and Kirch, 1988)
7. Increased response to cholinergic stimulation (Tandon and Greden, 1989; Tandon et al., 1993)
8. Increased sensitivity to dopaminergic stimulation (Angrist, 1983; Lieberman et al., 1985; Levy et al., 1993).

So far, purely stereotyped behavior has not been demonstrated in AM animals, nor has complete behavioral "breakdown" been observed, as might be expected when animals reach a stage similar to that of severe onset of schizophrenic symptoms. However, AM animals have not yet been thoroughly tested under stress, which might provoke increased signs of abnormality.   The general evidence presented does support a model of incipient schizophrenia, prior to the full-blown symptomatology, with male/female differences similar to those found in schizophrenia.

Neuroanatomical Parallels to Schizophrenia

Neuroanatomical measures also support the similarity of amphetamine-treated rats and human schizophrenics. Four of these are relevant:

1. Reduced neuronal number in mediodorsal thalamic nucleus (Pakkenberg, 1990)
2. Reduced neuronal number in nucleus accumbens (Pakkenberg, 1990)
3. Alterations in structure of the entorhinal cortex (Jakob and Beckmann, 1986)
4. Increased neuronal number in LDTg and PPTg (Karson et al., 1991).

In conclusion, this fetal development system appears to be the first animal model of schizophrenia with both strong behavioral and neuroanatomical parallels to the human disease. We are continuing to examine the affected animals and relevant controls. Even at this stage, however, the fetal amphetamine model of schizophrenia appears to be worth examining in other studies related to the etiology, treatment, or prevention of human schizophrenia.

ACKNOWLEDGMENTS

The authors also wish to acknowledge the excellent technical assistance of Joshua Layne and Bobby Freeman. M. Lyon was supported in part by a UAMS Medical Research Endowment grant and by the Marie Wilson Howells Fund from the UAMS Department of Psychiatry (Chairman: Frederick G. Guggenheim). W.O. McClure was supported in part by the Hedco Foundation and the NIH.

REFERENCES

Akbarian, S., Bunney, W.E. Jr., Potkin, S.G., Wigal, S.B., Hagman, J.O., Sandman, C.A., and Jones, E.G., 1993a, Altered distribution of nicotinamide-adenine dinucleotide phosphate-diaphorase cells in frontal lobe of schizophrenics implies disturbances of cortical development, *Arch. Gen. Psychiatry* 50: 169-177.

Akbarian, S., Vinuela, A., Kim, J.J., Potkin, S.G., Bunney, W.E., Jr., and Jones, E.G., 1993b, Distorted distribution of nicotinamide-adenine dinucleotide phosphate-diaphorase neurons in temporal lobe of schizophrenics implies anomalous cortical development, *Arch. Gen. Psychiatry* 50: 178-187.

Alexander, G.E., Crutcher, M.D., and DeLong, M.R., 1990, Basal ganglia-thalamocortical circuits: Parallel substrates for motor, oculomotor, "prefrontal" and "limbic" functions. *in* "Progress in Brain Research. 85th edition," Uylings, H.B.M., VanEden, C.G., DeBruin, J.P.C., Corner, M.A., Feenstra, M.G.P., eds. Elsevier Science Publishers.

Angrist, B., 1983, Psychoses induced by central nervous system stimulants and related drugs, *in* "Stimulants: Neurochemical, Behavioral, and Clinical Perspectives," Creese, I., ed., Raven Press, New York.

Armitage, S.G., Brown, C.R., and Denny, M.R., 1964, Stereotypy of response in schizophrenics, *J. Clin. Psychol.* 20: 225-230.

Arnold, S.E., Hyman, B.T., Hoesen Van, G.W., and Damasio, A.R., 1991, Some cytoarchitectural abnormalities of the entorhinal cortex in schizophrenia, *Arch. Gen. Psychiatry* 48: 625-632.

Ayllon, T., and Azrin, N., 1968, "The Token Economy: A Motivation System for Therapy and Rehabilitation," Appleton-Century-Crofts, NY.

Barr, C.E., Mednick, S.A., and Munk-Jorgensen, P., 1990, Exposure to influenza epidemics during gestation and adult schizophrenia: A 40 year study. *Arch. Gen. Psychiatry* 47:869-874.

Bayer, S.A., and Altman, J., 1991, "Neocortical Development," Raven Press, NY.

Bellack, A.S., and Hersen, M., 1993, "Handbook of Behavior Therapy in the Psychiatric Setting," Plenum Press, NY.

Berendse, H.W., Groenewegen, H.J., and Lohman, A.H.M., 1992, Compartmental distribution of ventral striatal neurons projecting to the mesencephalon in the rat, *J. Neurosci.* 12:2079-2103.

Blaha, C.D., and Winn, P., 1993, Modulation of dopamine efflux in the striatum following cholinergic stimulation of the substantia nigra in intact and pedunculopontine tegmental nucleus-lesioned rats, *J. Neurosci.*, 3: 1035-1044.

Bleuler, E., 1950, "Dementia Praecox," International University Press, New York.

Blundell, J.E., and Latham, C.J., 1978, Pharmacological manipulation of feeding behaviour: possible influences of serotonin and dopamine on food intake, *in* "Central Mechanism of Anorectic Drugs," Garratini, S., and Samanin, R., eds. Raven Press, NY.

Berman, K.F., and Weinberger, D.R., 1990, The prefrontal cortex in schizophrenia and other neuropsychiatric diseases: *in vivo* physiological correlates of cognitive deficits. *in:* "Progress in Brain Research. 85th edition," Uylings, H.B.M., VanEden, C.G., DeBruin, J.P.C., Corner, M.A., Feenstra, M.G.P., eds. Elsevier Science Publishers.

Bogerts, B., 1993, Recent advances in the neuropathology of schizophrenia, *Schiz. Bull.* 19: 431-445.

Bogerts, B., Meertz, E., and Schonfeldt-Bausch R., 1985, Basal ganglia and limbic system pathology in schizophrenia. *Arch. Gen. Psychiatry* 42: 784-791.

Bracha, H.S., 1987, Asymmetric rotational (circling) behavior, a dopamine-related asymmetry: Preliminary findings in unmedicated and never-medicated schizophrenic patients, *Biol. Psychiatry* 22:995-1003.

Bracha, H.S., 1989, Is there a right hemi-hyper-dopaminergic psychosis? *Schiz. Res.* 2:317-324.

Bredt, D.S., Hwang, P.M., and Snyder, S.H., 1990, Localization of nitric oxide synthase indicating a neural role for nitric oxide, *Nature* 347:768-770.

Brown, V.J., and Robbins, T.W., 1989, Deficits in response space following unilateral striatal dopamine depletion in the rat, J. Neurosci., 9:983-989.

Burnett, A.L., Lowenstein, C.J., Bredt, D.S., Chang, T.S.K., and Snyder, S.H., 1992, Nitric oxide: A physiologic mediator of penile erection. *Science* 257:401-403.

Carlsson, A., 1988, The current status of the dopamine hypothesis of schizophrenia, *Neuropsychopharmacol.* 13:179-186.

Carlson, J.N, Herrick, K.F, Baird, J.I., and Glick, S.D., 1987, Selective enhancement of dopamine utilization in the rat prefrontal cortex by food deprivation, *Brain Research* 400:200-203.

Clarke, P.B.S., Reuben, M., and Eli-Bizri, H., 1993, Eserine (physostigmine) blocks nicotinic responses in the rat CNS, *Soc. Neurosci. Abs.* 19:1535.

Coyle, J.T., and Campochiaro, P., 1976, Ontogenesis of dopaminergic-cholinergic interactions in the rat striatum: A neurochemical study. *J. Neurochem.* 27:673-678.

Coyle, J.T., and Puttfarcken, P., 1993, Oxidative stress, glutamate, and neurodegenerative disorders, *Science* 262: 689-695.

Cuffel, B.J., Heithoff, K., and Lawson, W.B., 1993, Correlates of patterns of substance abuse among patients with schizophrenia, *Hosp. Comm. Psychiat.* 44: 247-251.

Daniel, D.G., Weinberger, D.R., Jones, D.W., Zigun, J.R., Coppola, R., Handel, S., Bigelow, L.B., Goldberg, T.E., Berman, K.F., and Kleinman, J.E., 1991, The effect of amphetamine on regional cerebral blood flow during cognitive activation in schizophrenia, *J. Neurosci.* 11: 1907-1917.

Frith, C.D., and Done, D.J., 1983, Stereotyped responding by schizophrenic patients on a two-choice guessing task, *Psychol. Med.* 13: 779-786.

Garcia-Rill, E., Karson, C., Gray, T., Husain, M., Mrak, R., and Skinner, R.D., 1991, The pedunculopontine nucleus. I. Increased cell number in schizophrenia. *Anat. Rec.* 229:29A.

Gilles, F.H., Leviton, A., and Dooling, E.C., 1983, "The Developing Human Brain. Growth and Epidemiologic Neuropathology," John Wright/PSG Inc., Boston.

Glick, S.D., and Shapiro, R.M., 1985, Functional and neurochemical mechanisms of cerebral lateralization in rats. *in:* "Cerebral Lateralization in Nonhuman Species," Glick, S.D., ed., Academic Press, New York.

Gould, E., Woolf, N.J., and Butcher, L.L., 1989, Cholinergic projections to the substantia nigra from the pedunculopontine and laterodorsal tegmental nuclei, *Neuroscience* 28:611-623.

Holson, R.R., Adams, J., Buelke-Sam, J., Gough, R., and Kimmel, C.A., 1985, d-Amphetamine as a behavioral teratogen: Effects depend on dose, sex, age and task, *Neurobehav. Toxicol. Teratol.* 7:753-758.

Holson, R.R., and Pearce, B., 1992, Principles and pitfalls in the analysis of prenatal treatment effects in multiparous species *Neurotoxicol. and Teratol.* 14:221-228.

Huttunen, M.O. and Niskanen, P., 1978, Prenatal loss of father and psychiatric disorders, *Arch. Gen. Psychiat.* 35: 429-431.

Illowsky, B.P., and Kirch, D.G., 1988, Polydipsia and hyponatremia in psychiatric patients. *Am. J. Psychiatry* 145:675-683.

Jakob, H., and Beckmann, H., 1986, Prenatal developmental disturbances in the limbic allocortex in schizophrenia, *J. Neurotrans.* 65:303-326.

Karson, C.N., Garcia-Rill, E., Biedermann, J., Mrak, R.E., Husain, M.M., and Skinner, R.D., 1991, The brain stem reticular formation in schizophrenia, *Psychiatry Res.: Neuroimaging* 40:31-48.

Karson, C.N., Casanova, M., Kleinman, J., and Griffin, W.S.T., 1993, Choline acetyltransferase in schizophrenia, *Am. J. Psychiatry* 150:454-459.

Kayama, Y., Ohta, M., and Jodo, E., 1992, Firing of 'possibly' cholinergic neurons in the rat laterodorsal tegmental nucleus during sleep and wakefulness, *Brain Res.* 569:210-220.

Koob, G.F., and Swerdlow, N.R., 1988, The functional output of the mesolimbic dopamine system. *in:* "The Mesocorticolimbic Dopamine System," Kalivas, P.W., and Nemeroff, C.B., eds. Annals New York Academy of Sciences, New York.

Kovelman, J.A., and Scheibel, A.B., 1984, A neurohistological correlate of schizophrenia, *Biol. Psychiatry* 19:1601-1621.

Levy, D.L., Smith, M., Robinson, D., Jody, D., Lerner, G., Alvir, J., Geisler, S.H., Szymanski, S.R., Gonzalez, A., Mayerhoff, D.I., Lieberman, J.A., and Mendell, N.R., 1993, Methylphenidate increases thought disorder in recent onset schizophrenics, but not in normal controls, *Biol. Psychiatry* 34:507-514.

Lieberman, J.A., Kane, J.M., Gadaletta, D., Ramos-Lorenzi, J., Bergmann, K., Wegner, J., and Novacenko, H., 1985, Methylphenidate challenge tests course of schizophrenia, *Psychopharmac. Bull.* 21:123-129.

Lipska, B.K., Jaskiw, G.E., and Weinberger, D.R., 1993, Postpubertal emergence of hyperresponsiveness to stress and to amphetamine after neonatal excitotoxic hippocampal damage: a potential animal model of schizophrenia, *Neuropsychopharmacology* (in press).

Lipton, S.A., Choi, Y-B., Pan, Z-H., Lei, S.Z., Chen, H-SV., Sucher, N.J., Loscalzo, J., Singel, D.J., and Stamler, J.S., 1993, A redox-based mechanism for the neuroprotective and neurodestructive effects of nitric oxide and related nitroso-compounds, *Nature* 364:626-632.

Lyon, M., 1991a, Animal models of mania and schizophrenia. *in:* "Behavioral Models in Psychopharmacology: Theoretical, Industrial, and Clinical Perspectives," Paul, W., ed. Cambridge University Press, Cambridge, England.

Lyon, M., 1991b, Animal models with parallels to schizophrenia, *in:* "Neuromethods Volume 18: Animal Models in Psychiatry I," Boulton, A., Baker, G., and Martin- Iverson, M., ed. Humana Press, Clifton, NJ.

Lyon, M., and Barr, C.E., 1991, Possible interactions of obstetrical complications and abnormal fetal brain development in schizophrenia, *in:* Fetal Neural Development and Adult Schizophrenia, Mednick, S.A., Cannon, T.D., Barr, C.E., and Lyon, M., eds. Cambridge University Press, Cambridge pp.134-149

Lyon, M., and Bracha, H.S., 1994, Fetal amphetamine/undernutrition and schizophrenia, *Proc. Am. Psych. Assoc., Ann. Meet.*, Philadelphia, PA.

Lyon, M., and McClure, W.O. 1994, Investigations of fetal development models for substance abuse and schizophrenia. I. Prenatal d-amphetamine effects upon early and late juvenile behavior in the rat, *Psychopharmacology*, in press.

Lyon, M., and Robbins, T., 1975, The action of central nervous system stimulant drugs: A general theory concerning amphetamine effects, *in:* "Current Developments in Psychopharmacology, 2nd ed.," Essman, W., and Valzelli, L., eds. Spectrum Publications, Inc., New York.

Lyon, M., Hudzik, T., Lawson, W.B., and McMillan, D.E., 1993, Potential animal model of increased ETOH intake in schizophrenia: Prenatal d-amphetamine exposure vs. pair- feeding control conditions, *Schiz. Res.* 9:243-244.

Lyon, N., and Gerlach, J., 1988, Perseverative structuring of responses by schizophrenic and affective disorder patients, *J. Psych. Res.* 22:261-277.

Lyon, N., and Satz, P., 1991, Left turning (swivel) in medicated chronic schizophrenic patients, *Schiz. Res.* 4: 53-58.

Lyon, N., Mejsholm, B., and Lyon, M., 1986, Stereotyped responding by schizophrenic outpatients: Cross-cultural confirmation of perseverative switching on a two-choice task, *J. Psych. Res.* 20:137-150.

Lyon, N., Satz ,P,. Fleming, K., Green, M.F., and Bracha, H.S., 1992, Left turning (swivel) in manic patients, *Schiz. Res.* 7:71-76.

Mair, R.G., Robinson, J.K., Koger, S.M., Fox, G.D., and Zhang, Y.P., 1992, Delayed-nonmatching-to-sample performance is impaired by extensive, but not by limited, lesions of the thalamus in the rat, *Behav. Neurosci.* 106:646-656.

Marichich, E.S., Molina, V.A., and Orsingher, O.A., 1979, Persistent changes in central catecholaminergic system after recovery of perinatally undernourished rats, *J. Nutr.* 109:1045-1050.

Mednick, S.A., Machon, R.A., Huttunen, M.O., and Bonett, D., 1988, Adult schizophrenia following prenatal exposure to an influenza epidemic, *Arch. Gen. Psychiatry* 45:189-192.

Mednick, S.A., and Schulsinger, F., 1968, Some premorbid characteristics related to breakdown in children with schizophrenic mothers, *J. Psychiat. Res.* 6:267-291.

Mittleman, G., LeDuc, P.A., and Whishaw, I.Q., 1993, The role of D1 and D2 receptors in the heightened locomotion induced by direct and indirect dopamine agonists in rats with hippocampal damage: an animal analogue of schizophrenia, *Behav. Brain. Res.* 55:253-267.

Muller, E.E., Liuzzi, A., Cocchi, D., Panerai, A.E., Oppizzi, G., Locatelli, V., Mantegazza, P., Silvestrini, F., and Chiodini, P.G., 1977, Role of dopaminergic receptors in the regulation of growth hormone secretion, *in:* "Advances in Biochemical Psychopharmacology, Vol. 16: Nonstriatal dopaminergic neurons," Costa, E., and Gessa, G.L., eds., Raven Press, New York.

Nielsen, M., Lyon, M., Tanimura, S., and McClure, W.O., 1994, Prenatal exposure to amphetamine increases the number of neurons positive for nitric oxide synthase in the laterodorsal tegmental nucleus of the brain. *Brain Res.*, submitted.

Nielsen, M., Lyon, M., and McClure, W.O., 1992, Prenatal amphetamine exposure increases the number of neurons positive for nitric oxide synthase (NOS) in the laterodorsal tegmental nucleus of the rat, *Soc. Neurosci. Abst.* 18:1596.

Oades, R.D., 1982, Search strategies on a hole-board are impaired in rats with ventral tegmental damage: Animal model for tests of thought disorder, *Biol. Psychiatry* 17:xx

O'Keefe, J., and Nadel, L., 1978, "The Hippocampus as a Cognitive Map, First Ed.," Oxford University Press, Oxford.

Otake, M., and Shull, W.J., 1984, *In utero* exposure to A-bomb radiation and mental retardation: A reassessment, *Br. J. Radiol.*, 57:409-414.

Pakkenberg, B., 1990, Pronounced reduction of total neuron number in mediodorsal thalamic nucleus and nucleus accumbens in schizophrenics, *Arch. Gen. Psychiatry* 47:1023-1028.

Pakkenberg, B., 1992, The volume of the mediodorsal thalamic nucleus in treated and untreated schizophrenics, *Schiz. Res.* 7:95-100.

Pape, H.C., and Mager, R., 1992, Nitric oxide controls oscillatory activity in thalamocortical neurons, *Neuron* 9:441-448.

Robbins, T.W., Mittleman, G., O'Brien, J., and Winn, P., 1990, The neuropsychological significance of stereotypy induced by stimulant drugs. *in:* "Neurobiology of Stereotyped Behaviour," Cooper, S.J., and Dourish, C.T., eds. Clarendon Press, Oxford.

Roberts, G.W., 1990, Schizophrenia: the cellular biology of a functional psychosis, *Trends Neurosci.* 13:207-211.

Robinson, J.K., and Mair, R.G., 1992, MK-801 prevents brain lesions and delayed- nonmatching-to-sample deficits produced by pyrithiamine-induced encephalopathy in rats, *Behav. Neurosci.* 106:623-633.

Schiørring, E., 1971, Amphetamine induced selective stimulation of certain behaviour items with concurrent inhibition of others in an open-field test with rats, *Behaviour* 39:1-17.

Schmajuk, N. A., 1987, Animal models for schizophrenia: The hippocampally lesioned animal. *Schiz. Bull.* 13:317-327.

Skinner, R.D. and Garcia-Rill, E., 1990, Brainstem modulation of rhythmic functions and behaviors. *in:* "Brainstem Mechanisms of Behavior," Klemm, W.R., and Vertes, R.P., eds. John Wiley, New York.

Skinner, R.D., Kinjo, N., Ishikawa, Y., Biedermann, J.A., and Garcia-Rill, E., 1990, Locomotor projections from the pedunculopontine nucleus to the medioventral medulla, *NeuroReport* 1:207-210.

Steriade, M., Domich, L., Oakson, G., and Deschenes, M., 1987a, The deafferented reticular thalamic nucleus generates spindle rhythmicity, *J. Neurophysiol.* 57:260-273.

Steriade, M., Parent, A., Pare, D., and Smith, Y., 1987b, Cholinergic and non-cholinergic neurons of cat basal forebrain project to reticular and mediodorsal thalamic nuclei, *Brain Research* 408:372-376.

Steriade, M., McCormick, D.A., and Sejnowski, T.J., 1993, Thalamocortical oscillations in the sleeping and aroused brain, *Science* 262:679-685.

Susser, E.S., and Lin, S.P., 1992, Schizophrenia after prenatal exposure to the Dutch Hunger Winter of 1944-45, *Arch. Gen. Psychiatry,* in press.

Tandon, R., and Greden, J.F., 1989, Cholinergic hyperactivity and negative schizophrenic symptoms. A model of cholinergic/dopaminergic interactions in schizophrenia, *Arch. Gen. Psychiatry* 46:745-753.

Tandon, R., Greden, J.F., and Haskett, R.F., 1993, Cholinergic hyperactivity and negative symptoms: behavioral effects of physostigmine in normal controls, *Schiz. Res.* 9:19-23.

Ushijima, I., Yamada, K., Inoue, T., Tokunaga, T., and Furukawa, T., 1984,: Muscarinic and nicotinic effects on yawning and tongue protruding in the rat, *Pharm. Biochem. Behav.* 21:297-300.

Ushijima, I., Mizuki, Y., Imaizumi, J., Yamada, M., Noda, Y., Yamada, K., and Furukawa, T., 1985, Characteristics of yawning behavior induced by apomorphine, physostigmine and pilocarpine *Arch. Int. Pharmacodyn.* 273:196-201.

Van Eden, C.G., 1986, Development of connections between the mediodorsal nucleus of the thalamus and the prefrontal cortex in the rat, *J. Comp. Neurol.* 244:349-359.

Vincent, S.R., and Kimura, H., 1992, Histochemical mapping of nitric oxide synthase in the rat brain, *Neuroscience* 46:755-784.

Vincent, S.R., Satoh, K., Armstrong, D.M., and Fibiger, H.C., 1983, NADPH-diaphorase: a selective histochemical marker for the cholinergic neurons of the pontine reticular formation, *Neurosci. Lett.* 43:31-36.

Voorn, P., Kalsbeek, A., Jorritsma-Byham, B., and Groenewegen, H.J., 1988, The pre- and postnatal development of the dopaminergic cell groups in the ventral mesencephalon and the dopaminergic innervation of the striatum of the rat, *Neuroscience* 25:857-887.

Willner, P., and Scheel-Kruger, J., 1991, "The Mesolimbic Dopamine System: From Motivation to Action," John Wiley, New York.

Zola-Morgan, S., and Squire, L.R., 1985, Amnesia in monkeys after lesions of the mediodorsal nucleus of the thalamus, *Ann. Neurol.* 17:558-564.

METAL EXPOSURE OF THE SQUIRREL MONKEY FETUS AS A MODEL OF HUMAN NEUROPSYCHIATRIC DISORDERS

Bengt Lögdberg[1,2] and Karin Warfvinge[2]

Department of Neuropathology[1]
and Institute of Environmental Medicine[2],
Lund University, Lund, Sweden

THE NEUROPSYCHIATRIC SPECTRUM

Figure 1 gives a tentative overview of the spectrum of chronic neuropsychiatric disorders, i.e., cognitive and emotive disturbances leading to long-term continuous or repeated need of help from the health care system, and an indication of the change of their prevalence over age. In total, these disorders may affect in the order of 10-20% or more of a population, and are responsible for a large part of human suffering and economic costs in any society. For the sake of prevention, research into the causes of these entities is important. Little is known even of the specific time of the etiology/pathogenesis. There is, obviously, more evidence for a prenatal etiology/pathogenesis, as to specific agents and times of origin, for those disorders which are diagnosed at an early postnatal age, e.g., mental retardation, than for those which are diagnosed later, such as dementia (see Figure 1). However, the high prevalence, in mental retardation, of other neuropsychiatric disorders (see, e.g., Dosen, 1989) suggests the possibility that it is not uncommon that also these disorders have a prenatal etiology/pathogenesis. In the case of schizophrenia, there are indications of both prenatal ("developmental") and late ("degenerative") pathogeneses. An example of an established link between fetal disturbances and a much later development of a neuropsychiatric disturbance is the high incidence of Alzheimer's dementia in Down's syndrome.

All of these neuropsychiatric disorders can be described as syndromes encompassing a combination of cognitive and emotive - and often motor and social - disturbances. Extensive research in the field of environmental medicine has focused on the influence of specific environmental factors on the development of defined cognitive functions. For instance, indications have been found that exposure during early brain development to the heavy metals lead and methylmercury may decrease the psychometrically measured cognitive level in a population, apparently displacing the normal distribution to the left, thus implying an increased incidence of mental retardation (see below). Whether this is also true for the cognitive and emotive functions disturbed in the other neuropsychiatric disorders is not known, partly due to the less precise definition of those functions and their disturbances and to the lack of

Neural Development and Schizophrenia, Edited by S.A. Mednick
and J.M. Hollister, Plenum Press, New York, 1995

valid and reliable tests to measure them. Thus, with the possible exception of mental retardation, it remains to be investigated whether the great global increase of human lead exposure over the last 150 years, or the particularly high lead- and methylmercury-exposure of certain populations, may have influenced the incidence or prevalence of various neuropsychiatric disorders.

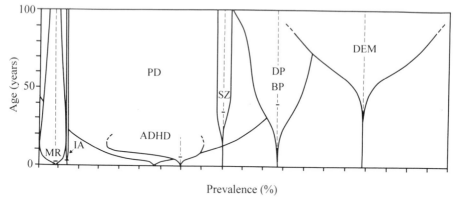

Figure 1. The neuropsychiatric spectrum. The chronic neuropsychiatric disorders included in this tentative and approximative sketch are arranged from left to right according to the mean age at which they are diagnosed (indicated by short, thick horizontal lines): mental retardation (MR), infantile autism (IA), personality disorder (PD), attention-deficit hyperactivity disorder (ADHD), schizophrenia (SZ), depressive and bipolar psychoses (DP, BP), and dementia (DEM). Prevalences are given as functions of age (each mark on the x-axis represents one %). Dashed vertical lines divide the incidences between the sexes: left side - males, right side - females. Epidemiological data on the prevalence of ADHD-like syndromes in later life, and of various personality disorders throughout life, are very limited.

The effects of lead and methylmercury will be described here as possible models for other environmental factors, as well as genetic factors, causing neuropsychiatric disorders by their influence on fetal brain development. Due to the simple metabolism and to good analytical techniques, lead and methylmercury offer the advantage of an accurate, precise and relatively simple characterization of exposure, externally as well as internally in individual organs or even individual cells. In contrast, it is for instance more difficult to control the internal fetal dose of influenza A viruses, and to analyze effects on the fetal brain of the virus itself, in relation to secondary effects due to, e.g., hyperthermia, anorexia, or an immune response.

DETERMINANTS OF THE VARIATIONS IN HUMAN BRAIN FUNCTIONS

Considering that neuropsychiatric disorders consist of disturbances in various cognitive and emotive functions, what in turn is the overall impact of variations of environmental factors on such human neurobehavioral functions? Studies on monozygotic twins reared apart indicate that genetic factors may explain about 50–70% of the variance of neurobehavioral traits in adult human populations on repeated testing (see, e.g., Bouchard et al., 1990). In allegedly hereditary neurological and psychiatric diseases, genetic factors may explain between 27% (multiple sclerosis) and 100% (Huntington's chorea) of the incidence (see, e.g., Torrey, 1992). Among the specific neurobehavioral functions studied, about 70% of the variance of results in traditional cognitive tests has relatively consistently been shown to be explained by genetic factors, and only about 10% by measurement error, probably partly due to the good psychometric properties of these tests. This leaves about 20% of the variance in these neurobehavioral functions to be explained by environmental factors, at least as far as the investigated populations in Western Europe and North America are concerned.

In view of the relative stability of individual neurobehavioral traits during adulthood, it may be hypothesized that a large part of the variation due to environmental factors should be traced back to influences during brain development, whether pre- or postnatal. Based on epidemiological, clinical and experimental results, a tentative list of the most important environmental factors interfering with brain development – ranked in a descending series according to their estimated influence on the variance in these populations – would include: psychosocial stress and understimulation, ethanol, viruses, malnutrition, narcotics and pharmaceuticals, lead, smoking, methylmercury, and ionizing radiation. With a modification of the ranking and a reduction of the overall variance figure, this tentative list may apply to environmental factors interfering with the neurobehavioral functions of the brain during its adult period. With modifications of the ranking and perhaps the overall variance figure, it might also apply to various environments globally, although this has not been much investigated.

The analysis of the influence of each individual environmental factor, in epidemiological studies, is confounded by the interaction of different combinations of environmental and genetic factors. The relative influence of the environment, and its individual factors, on emotive and social neurobehavioral states and traits is much less known and more difficult to study than cognitive traits, due to the poorer psychometric properties of tests used to measure them. This is an important limitation in risk assessment.

The unborn child was until quite recently considered to be relatively unaffected by environmental factors, embedded behind barriers (abdominal wall, uterus, placenta, and fetal membranes). About 50 years ago, however, it was realized clinically that ambient microbiological factors (rubella; Gregg, 1942) can cause severe and irreversible prenatal brain damage, and it has been shown that rubella could be an important cause of infantile autism (Desmond et al., 1967). Later it was shown that chemical factors released in the general environment (methylmercury; Matsumoto et al., 1965) or used individually to obtain psychopharmacological effects (ethanol; Jones et al., 1973) could cause similar damage at doses which seem to cause no changes, or only small and reversible changes in postnatal human brains. A concern arose that environmental factors apparently not interfering much with adults, or even children, might cause serious disturbances in the prenatal development of the human brain (see, e.g., Schardein, 1985).

In general, however, it has proved difficult to evaluate the overall as well as the specific influence of such environmental factors on the human prenatal brain development, probably due to their lower potency. Such influence, and its implications for neuropsychiatric disorders, has not been scientifically evaluated at all for most factors.

EFFECTS OF LOW LEAD LEVELS ON THE DEVELOPING BRAIN: EPIDEMIOLOGICAL, CLINICAL, AND EXPERIMENTAL EVIDENCE

More than 3000 publications exist from epidemiological, clinical, and experimental studies relevant to the question of whether pre- or early postnatal low-level lead exposure (i.e. lead concentrations in blood below 20–40 μg/dl (about 1–2 μmol/l) or equivalent) may cause neurobehavioral disturbances in children (Kazantis, 1989). As with many other environmental factors, this hypothesis has proved difficult to test adequately. There are large differences in the lead dose in various studies. Generally, the epidemiological studies are "low-exposure" studies (defined here as blood lead levels below 25 μg/dl (below about 1.2 μmol/l)), the clinical and experimental nonhuman primate studies "medium-" to "high-exposure" studies (i.e., blood lead around 40–60 μg/dl (about 2–3 μmol/l)), the rodent experimental studies "high-" to "very high-exposure" studies (i.e., blood lead from over 60 up to several hundred μg/dl (about 3 up to 10 μmol/l and more)) and the chicken experimental studies probably "very high-" to "extremely high-exposure" studies (i.e., involving tissue concentrations equivalent to blood lead levels in mammals of several hundred to several thousand μg/dl (about 10 to more than 100 μmol/l)). Table 1 lists some of the important limitations, on the basis of existing data, in the evaluation of effects and risks of lead exposure of the developing brain, particularly the fetal brain; and thus the limitations for the testing of the hypothesis that low lead levels may permanently damage the developing brain.

Table 1. Summary of some important methodological problems in human (epidemiological and clinical) and experimental studies of relevance to the evaluation of effects and risks of lead exposure of the developing human brain.

Epidemiological and clinical studies	Experimental studies
Genetic and environmental confounders	High-dose models
Uncertain direction of causality	Cognitively inadequate models
Only recent prospective studies	"Malnutrition" as confounder
Limited prenatal exposure documentation	Cerebellum more sensitive than cerebrum
Few prenatal clinical case studies	No corresponding late fetal period
No neuropathological examinations	Few fetal models

Epidemiological studies published over the last 30 years, most of them retrospective or cross-sectional, have important methodological limitations, particularly in the control of confounding factors and the analysis of causality. These limitations have precluded firm conclusions on the basis of such data only. Over the years, the number of confounding factors analyzed in the studies has grown, and increasingly sophisticated statistical techniques have been elaborated for controlling them. However, not even the most ambitious prospective studies ongoing (Bellinger et al., 1987, 1991; Diedrich et al., 1991, 1993; Ernhart et al., 1986, 1989; McMichael et al., 1988; Baghurst et al., 1992; Cooney et al., 1989; see, e.g., Davis and Svendsgaard, 1987) have been able to establish a firm causal relationship between low lead levels and disturbed brain functions.

The following illustrates the problem of direction of causality: During the postnatal development, a neurobehaviorally deviant child, both a "hyperactive" disturbed child and a "supernormal" highly explorative child, may ingest more lead from the environment than other children. In the first case, it would result in a positive correlation with an underlying direction of causation opposite to the one hypothesized, and in the other case it would result in the absence of a correlation ("masking" of possible adverse effects of lead on the brain) or a negative correlation. During prenatal development, fetal stress may be the cause of, as well as the result of, lead accumulation (high lead concentrations in the fetus and placenta have been observed following experimental growth retardation in rats; to be published). Such mechanisms do not seem to have been addressed in postnatal studies.

To reach firmer conclusions regarding the direction of causality during prenatal development, experimental data are essential. The few recent epidemiological studies will not provide data relating to the hypothesis of neurobehavioral disturbances at adult age for another 5-10 years, and there are indications that the influence of postnatal confounders will make it difficult to test this hypothesis adequately. Furthermore, in most prospective epidemiological studies, the documentation of prenatal lead exposure has been limited to the determination of lead concentration in blood at birth.

There are only a few clinical case reports with well-documented prenatal lead exposure (Palmisano et al., 1969; Singh et al., 1978; Ghafour et al., 1984). These studies do not provide firm evidence for prenatal brain damage caused by lead, in view of the few indications of neurobehavioral disturbances, and the absence of neuropathological examinations. An early study indicated the possibility of congenital neuropathological effects, but early postnatal exposure did not seem to have been excluded as a cause (Rennert, 1881). This is in contrast to the convincing clinical and pathological evidence linking methylmercury exposure to prenatal brain damage (Matsumoto et al., 1965; Choi et al., 1978).

Experiments with lead exposure of chickens during early embryonic development have produced clear effects on the development of the embryo and its brain (Hammet and Wallace, 1928; Catizone and Gray, 1941; Karnofsky and Ridgeway, 1952; Butt et al., 1952; Gilani, 1973; Hirano and Kochen, 1973; de Gennaro, 1978). These data, however, are difficult to apply in human risk assessment, since lead salts were administered *in ovo* and can be estimated to have resulted in tissue concentrations of probably several hundred $\mu g/g$, i.e., several thousand times the concentrations relevant to humans. Most experimental studies in the recent literature have used rodents. However, rodents also have several limitations as animal models of the effects of lead on the developing brain. First of all, like chickens, they obviously do not develop the cerebral structures necessary for more sophisticated sensorimotor, cognitive, and social neurobehavioral functions found in humans, and small lead-induced disturbances of these functions might not arise in such an experimental model. Furthermore, they seem to be relatively insensitive to lead compared to humans, in that much higher lead concentrations in blood and other tissues are required to produce morphological damage in the developing brain (for details, see Lögdberg, 1993a). These high doses often cause a condition similar to malnutrition, which in itself has been shown to adversely influence brain development (see, e.g., Balázs et al., 1979), thus confounding the cause–effect analysis. Furthermore, the morphological brain damage is mainly found in the cerebellum (Pentschew and Garro, 1966), which does not conform to the cognitive and sensorimotor, predominantly cerebral, disturbances of lead suspected from the human low-dose studies. Finally, rodents have a short gestation, and seem to be lacking the corresponding latter part of gestation found in primates, including some cell populations of importance for normal cerebrogenesis, e.g., the subpial granular layer (unpublished observations), and do not seem to reproduce the lead-induced prematurity found or suspected in human studies. The much fewer studies using nonprimates from other mammalian orders have similar limitations and have, together with the very few studies on nonhuman primates, contributed relatively little data pertaining to the question of lead effects on the prenatal brain.

For psychometric methodological reasons, it is the correlation between lead and minor cognitive disturbances that has been best characterized. Some data suggest that the negative influence of lead occurs evenly in the population, thus displacing the whole normal distribution of cognitive functions to the left. In the case of an average decrease by 5 IQ-points this would cause a fourfold increase in the prevalence of individuals with an IQ below 80, i.e., with borderline or more severe mental retardation (from 4% to 16%), and there would be a similar decrease at the other end of the normal distribution (Needleman and Bellinger, 1991). Similar influences on other neurobehavioral traits and states, such as empathy, emotions, or reliable and sensitive measures of attentional capacity, should be further investigated. Such neurobehavioral functions are, however, difficult to study in most experimental models. Moreover, for psychometric methodological reasons, reference values for such functions in general human populations are not well known or easily obtained. Early, less well controlled studies have shown positive correlations between lead exposure and disturbances in attention and activity (e.g., clinical syndromes such as attention-deficit hyperactivity disorder (ADHD), etc.) (e.g., David et al., 1972). Mental retardation and infantile autism have been linked to lead in some studies (David et al., 1976; Moore et al., 1977; Moore, 1980; Accardo et al., 1988), although a causal relationship is far from established for these disorders.

PATHOGENETIC MECHANISMS OF LEAD

There are several possible biochemical toxic mechanisms for the effects of lead on the developing brain, including the binding of lead to SH- and other groups of proteins, particularly of enzymes important for cell growth such as protein kinase C (Markovac and Goldstein, 1988) or -aminolevulinic acid dehydratase (ALAD) (Hernberg and Nikkanen, 1970), the catalysis of tRNA by lead (Brown et al., 1983), and the competition of lead with other trace elements such as calcium, zinc, iron and copper (see Miller et al., 1990, for a review). There seem to be no data indicating that lead is an essential element for any biochemical system. Rather, several of the biochemical studies above, as well as neurophysiological data (e.g., Schwartz and Otto, 1987) suggest the absence of a threshold for toxic effects of lead on the developing nervous system within the range of lead levels currently found in humans.

Which developmental processes may be influenced through these and other mechanisms, to produce the minor cognitive and visuomotor disturbances suspected to occur following low-level lead exposure? These processes, like the processes of neurhomogeny (see below), may in principle be found throughout our phylo-ontogenetic developmental history, from the nucleotide biochemistry in our ancestors' gametes to social behavior in the community. Lead has been shown to be toxic to the genome, also in utero, in some studies (see, e.g., Gerber, 1980; Qazi et al., 1980; Nayak et al., 1989), to the ovum (Vermande-Van Eck and Meigs, 1960), to the spermatogenesis (see, e.g., Lancranjan et al., 1975; Uzych, 1985; Brady et al., 1975), to the blastocyst at implantation (Wide and Nilsson, 1977), to the embryo during organogenesis (see, e.g., Ferm and Carpenter, 1967), to the postnatal developing brain (Gibson, 1904), and to the adult brain (see, e.g., Yokoyama et al., 1988; Stollery et al., 1991). The effects of lead on the fetal brain have been relatively little studied in mammals.

The disturbances in the genome, gametes, blastocyst, and early embryo, referred to above, seem to occur only at relatively high tissue concentrations of lead, which produce clinical toxicity in the parental organisms and often early death or gross malformations of the conceptus. Towards the other end of the phylo-ontogenetic developmental history, i.e., the adult brain, disturbances of cognitive functions by lead may occur already at lead concentrations in blood above 40-60 μg/dl (about 2-3 μmol/l), in the absence of overt clinical toxic symptoms; however, these effects appear to be essentially reversible.

It is hypothesized that small and irreversible effects on the brain and its functions, which are suspected in epidemiological studies to follow lead exposure below this level, may occur during the fetal, as well as the early postnatal human development. The fetal period may be of particular importance for the pathogenesis of small disturbances, as well as for the mechanisms responsible for neurhomogenesis (see below), since graded dose–effect relationships might exist for effects of lead on various developmental processes during this period, such as mitosis, migration, differentiation, and selective death of cells.

NEURHOMOGENY

The gap between the extensive epidemiological and experimental literature -- with a few clinical case reports in-between -- is maintained by fundamental problems inherent in the scientific study of the mechanisms and risks of minor disturbances in human cognitive, emotive, and social neurobehavioral development, using experimental animal models. Research into the possibilities and ways of extrapolating such experimental results to humans can be seen as progressing along two lines of inquiry: (1) What are *homologous* neurodevelopmental mechanisms (i.e., *the same* ontogenetically, and possibly phylo-genetically), across various combinations of species which include *Homo sapiens*? (2) What are *homospecific* neurodevelopmental cell populations and mechanisms (i.e., more or less *unique* to *Homo sapiens*)? The first question can be said to represent the major line or strategy in basic neurodevelopmental research; while the second represents a much smaller research area, mainly due to methodological and ethical limitations and constraints. However, the information collected in both these complementary research areas is essential for the possibility of extrapolating results from animal experiments to humans, and the combination of them will be referred to in this text as the study of "neural homogeny" or "neurhomogeny". Thus, the study of the effects of lead from a perspective of neurhomogeny would concern the effects of lead on the development of the human nervous system, combining information which can be extrapolated from studies on other more or less closely related species, with information shown to be specific to humans. The neurhomogeny of behavioral disturbances would be the information on the development of neurobehavioral disturbances, and thus neurobehavior, which is specific to humans, and that which is shared with one or more other species. To help bridge the gap between the epidemiological and experimental studies, so that they can compensate for each other's limitations and thus more adequately support human risk assessment, it is important to obtain data from animal models which are neurhomogenetically well characterized and found to be similar to humans. In order to elaborate logically coherent risk management on the basis of risk assessment obtained as above, it is furthermore necessary to relate the risks to an assessment of human ethical values concerning various types and degrees of neurobehavioral disturbances ("neuroethics" - see Lögdberg, 1993a).

From the perspective of neurhomogeny, the squirrel monkey has several advantages as an experimental model: its adult neurohistology, neurophysiology (including neuro-pharmacology), and neurobehavior, and its reproduction, have been well characterized (see, e.g.,Rosenblum and Coe, 1985); it has a visual, manual-motor, cognitive and social behavior similar to that of other primates, including man, some aspects of which are only seldom found in other mammalian orders; it has a brain/body size ratio and a biparietal/pelvic outlet diameter ratio more similar to humans than those of larger primates (Napier and Napier, 1967; Schultz, 1949; own observations); and it has a relatively highly differentiated and well characterized emotive behavior compared to other primates, as interpreted through vocalization (Ploog, 1979). Its relatively small size makes housing in social groups feasible, with the possibility of studying social behavior *per se* as well as a sensitive indicator of cognitive (Cheney et al., 1986) and emotive (Ploog, 1979) disturbances.

LEAD, METHYLMERCURY, AND THE SQUIRREL MONKEY FETAL BRAIN

Relationships between fetal brain disturbances and later development of schizophrenia and other neuropsychiatric disorders have been much investigated and discussed in recent years. Such investigations are difficult, since the influence of environmental factors on the human fetal brain during development and on subsequent neurobehavioral functions is complex and not well characterized. Inorganic lead has been much investigated in this respect, particularly in view of the large global increase of anthropogenic lead in the environment. The apparently greater sensitivity to lead of the developing brain, compared to the adult brain, has been demonstrated. However, due mainly to methodological difficulties, no clear-cut causal relationship between low-level lead exposure of the developing brain (particularly in the prenatal period) and subsequent neurobehavioral disturbances has been shown. The extrapolation of experimental results to humans has been particularly difficult, due to differences in fetal brain development and later neurobehavioral functions in humans and common laboratory animals. To this end, and with the long-term objective of obtaining data helping to bridge the gap between the existing epidemiological and experimental literature, we have developed techniques for studying and characterizing the squirrel monkey as a nonhuman primate model of human brain development (e.g., Lögdberg, 1988; Lögdberg 1994a). The model has been used to test the hypothesis that lead may cause fetal brain damage with subsequent permanent neurobehavioral disturbances. Thirty-five squirrel monkey pregnancies were exposed to lead during various parts of the fetal development and to various blood lead concentrations (about 20-80 μg/dl; i.e., about 1-4 μmol/l). Fourteen pregnancies were exposed to methylmercury as comparative controls.

Brain growth and histology

The gestational age was reduced and the pre- and perinatal mortality increased (Lögdberg et al., 1987). Examination of the central nervous systems was performed in twelve offspring before or at birth (Lögdberg et al., 1988). The mean cerebral weight was significantly reduced for the fetal age (about 10%). A similar reduction of placental weight was seen. A few cerebra were paradoxically overweight for the fetal age and the body weight, possibly due to white matter edema. Histological examination of the CNS revealed large numbers of characteristic perivascular, petechial hemorrhages in the white matter in six of the twelve cerebra (see Figure 2). In two of these cases, such hemorrhages were also found in the white matter of the cerebellum, brain stem, and spinal cord. No signs of disturbed cell migration could be detected.

The reduction of gestational length is consistent with the results in two prospective epidemiological studies (McMichael et al., 1986; Dietrich et al., 1986), and with preliminary results from a third prospective study (Rothenberg et al., 1989), as well as with earlier cross-sectional studies (e.g., Moore et al., 1982). No experimental data linking reduced gestational length to lead exposure seem to have been reported previously. There seems to be a lack of human data concerning placental effects such as reduced growth and histopathology, and such effects appear to have been experimentally confirmed only recently (e.g., Nayak et al., 1989). The pre- and perinatal mortality rate is comparable with that in previous studies of women exposed occupationally, directly, or via their husbands (Oliver, 1911, Pindborg, 1945; see Rom, 1976 for a review of early studies). This effect is also in accordance with a few more recent case reports (Wilson, 1966; Valentino et al., 1984) and with studies showing increased lead concentrations in fetal and placental tissues from human stillbirths and neonatal deaths (Bryce-Smith et al., 1977; Wibberley et al., 1977).

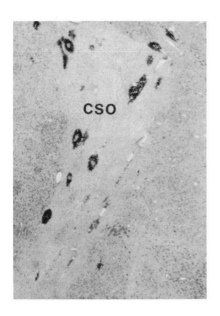

Figure 2. CSO = centrum semiovale in the basal region of the cerebrum, with petechial perivascular hemorrhages. Newborn squirrel monkey exposed to lead during the fetal development. HE, × 35.

Although lead concentrations in blood below 60 μg/dl (about 3 μmol/l) have long been suspected to cause damage to the prenatal human nervous system, no neuropathological study has confirmed this hypothesis. In the experimental literature, no brain damage has been described as a consequence of prenatal lead exposure via the mother, intoxicated either perorally or by air, i.e., the routes relevant to humans. Only very high doses of lead, given parenterally, have produced such damage (see, e.g., Singh et al., 1976; and Miller et al., 1982). Previous experimental studies have demonstrated increased pre- and perinatal mortality, or neuropathological effects in neonates, but at blood lead levels above 500 µg/dl (about 24 µmol/l) – an exposure level which has been associated with clinical signs reminiscent of severe malnutrition here probably acting as a confounder (see, e.g.,Winder et al., 1983; and Lögdberg, 1993a). The appearance of some toxic signs in the adult male squirrel monkeys at lead concentrations above about 120 µg/dl (about 5 µmol/l) is consistent with the dose-effect relationship found in adult humans, and the absence of such or other signs of lead toxicity in the pregnant females suggest the absence of the above confounder in the present study. The results of the present study support the hypothesis that there is a causal relationship between prenatal lead exposure and permanent brain damage in humans.

The indications of a fetal cerebral growth retardation are consistent with the reduction of neonatal head circumference in an epidemiological study (McMichael et al., 1986), and with the brain growth retardation following intraperitoneal lead injections in pregnant guinea pigs (Edwards and Beatson, 1984). It may be related to disturbances in cell proliferation (Lögdberg, 1994b) or cell differentiation.

The hemorrhagic encephalopathy found in the present study has not been reported previously as a result of human prenatal lead exposure, but clinical evidence suggests such an effect (Rennert, 1881; Ghafour et al.,1984). However, similar hemorrhagic lesions have previously been produced in fetal rodents and chicken, using very high lead levels. However, the cerebral hemorrhagic lesions reported here are similar to those seen in the infant "lead encephalopathy" following peroral lead exposure of humans (Blackman, 1937; Okazaki et al., 1963; Popoff et al., 1963; Niklowitz and Mandybur, 1975) and squirrel monkeys (Zook et al., 1980). In these cases of human lead encephalopathy, and in early postnatal lead encephalopathy in experimental animals (Thomas et al., 1971; Goldstein et al., 1974), the brain lead concentrations were 1.5-25 µg/g (about 70–500 nmol/g), compared to 0.1–0.7µg/g (about 5–35 nmol/g) in the present study. Early postnatal lead exposure of rats, with resulting brain lead concentrations, Pb-B values, and brain/blood lead concentration ratios within or slightly above the ranges in the present study, has not produced any morphological effects (Mykkanen et al., 1979; Grant et al., 1980; Collins et al., 1982). These results suggest that the fetal brain may be more sensitive to lead than the infant brain, and that primates (including humans) may be more sensitive to lead than rodents.

The hemorrhagic lesions are reminiscent of those found in neonatal sepsis with endotoxic endothelial damage and those found in coagulation dyscrasias. The normal megakaryocyte density in the offspring, the maternal blood indices, and the absence of hemorrhages in other organs does not, however, indicate severely reduced clotting ability. Besides probable toxic effects of lead on the cerebrum directly, or via the placenta, a few other factors could be of crucial importance in the pathogenesis, for example reduced gestational length. Prematurity in humans (defined as a 7.5% reduction in gestational length, i.e.,3/40 weeks, or more) is known to predispose to brain hemorrhages, especially after a difficult birth. Similarly, prematurity could partly explain the higher frequency of cerebral petechial hemorrhages in the offspring exposed to lead from about 6 weeks gestational age, compared to those exposed from about 9 weeks, in spite of relatively lower Pb-B values. However, a large numbers of hemorrhages was also found in lead-exposed fetuses born at about full-term. In addition, several facts point to the importance of parturition in the pathogenesis of the hemorrhages. A large number of brain hemorrhages was found only after vaginal birth. By analogy, the supernormal cerebral weights, probably due to edema, occurred only postnatally. Furthermore, signs of old hemorrhages (iron-containing macrophages) were found only weeks after birth, thus probably not arising in utero. Part of the explanation of the role of parturition could be that the squirrel monkey, like humans, but unlike ordinary laboratory animals, has a small pelvic size compared to the head size of the newborn. This may result in mechanical stress on the fetal head at birth and to birth complications (to be published). Perinatal asphyxia may be another factor which might have contributed to the development of the hemorrhages. It has been shown in subhuman primates that perinatal asphyxia superimposed on prenatal brain retardation (due to placental insufficiency), may result in acute neurological damage and perinatal death (Brann and Myers, 1975). The vascular congestion and necrobiotic neurons found in some of the present cases could be the result of asphyxia, although a direct toxic effect of lead on the neurons cannot be excluded.

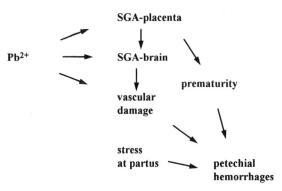

Figure 3. A tentative pathogenesis of lead-induced fetal brain disturbances. SGA = small for gestational age.

In conclusion, placental insufficiency and a direct effect of lead on the fetal brain may have caused a cerebral parenchymal and endothelial growth retardation. These factors, combined with prematurity, birth-associated mechanical stress, and asphyxia, may have precipitated the cerebral edema and extensive hemorrhages seen *post partum* (see Figure 3). It is noteworthy that such lesions were virtually absent in the fetuses delivered by caesarean section. This suggests that caesarean section may be indicated in cases of prenatal lead exposure, by analogy with other conditions predisposing to perinatal brain hemorrhages, e.g., neonatal thrombocytopenia (Miller et al., 1987).

Neurobehavior

In a group of offspring with mean prenatal maternal blood lead values of about 50 μg/dl, the "clinical" neurobehavioral examination at about 2 years of age revealed signs of decreased aggressiveness, lower position in the social hierarchy, impaired performance in testing of spatial reversal, and small visuomotor neurological disturbances (Lögdberg, 1993a; Lögdberg, 1994f). Individual monkeys showed short attention span and possible somatosensory disturbances.

In this group, effects on social behavior were the most frequent findings. A reduction of aggressive behavior has been reported previously as a consequence of early postnatal lead exposure of rodents (Hastings et al., 1977; Drew et al., 1979), and indirect indications of this were also found in an epidemiological study (reduced "minor antisocial behavior"; Needleman et al., 1990). The lower position in the social hierarchy found for the lead-exposed group is also consistent with findings in this epidemiological study ("reduced class standing"). In the present study, it could be related to the reduced aggressiveness or to impaired attentional or visuomotor performance, but it could also be due to a reduced cognitive capacity (Cheney et al., 1986) or to other disturbances (see, e.g., Talmage-Riggs and Anschel, 1973).

Various signs of visuomotor disturbances were also found. A lower degree of lateralization in hand preference for grabbing was found in the lead-exposed group, and may be a sign of cerebral functional retardation. The head and upper-limb movements appeared slower or disturbed in the lead-exposed group. Furthermore, in contrast to the controls, the upper-limb speed of the lead-group seemed highly correlated with and perhaps dependent on visual guidance, possibly due to sensorimotor disturbances. Neurological signs were found in the form of Babinski's sign and muscular hypotonus. These visuomotor results show some similarity to those of epidemiological studies in which a positive correlation was found between the neonatal Pb-B level and early postnatal disturbances in reflexes, muscle tonus, and soft neurological signs (Ernhart et al., 1986), as well as disturbances in bilateral coordination, upper-limb speed and dexterity, and a composite index of fine-motor coordination at 6 years of age (Dietrich et al., 1993).

At adult age, monkeys were tested in concurrent schedules of reinforcement in an "operant chamber" where they had to press two different levers in different and changing proportions in order to obtain reinforcers in the form of sucrose pellets, as programmed by a minicomputer (Lögdberg et al., 1994d; Newland et al., 1994). For instance, the maximum number of reinforcers would be given if the monkey made 80% of the presses on the right lever and 20% on the left lever, and this would then be reversed so that the maximum number of reinforcers would be given if the monkey pressed 80% of the times on the left lever. The behavioral adaption following reversals of this type - a measure of learning ability - was studied in a group of eight adult prenatally lead-exposed offspring and eight unexposed age-matched controls. The change in proportion responses to the two levers over time after the reversal of the type described above was fitted to an asymptotic function, using nonlinear regression analysis with least-square technique. Statistical analyses of the main resulting parameters (i.e., which described how well the behavior changed towards the proportions producing most sucrose pellets) – rate and relative magnitude – suggested a dose-effect relationship between the mean maternal blood lead concentration during pregnancy and the relative magnitude of change following a reversal, with a significant reduction of the magnitude already at maternal Pb-B about 20 μg/dl (about 1 μmol/l; see Figure 4, and Lögdberg et al., 1994d).

This finding of a permanently impaired learning capability in concurrent schedules of reinforcements following fetal lead-exposure with maternal blood lead levels as low as about 20 μg/dl (about 1 μmol/l) seems to be consistent with results in a number of epidemiological studies (see, e.g., Davis and Svendsgaard, 1987; Lögdberg, 1993a). Most of the prospective epidemiological studies have shown consistent correlations between prenatal lead exposure and disturbances in cognitive functions during the first 1–2 years of postnatal development. Such consistent correlations have not been found during later development. Whether this is a consequence of difficulties in detecting the role of prenatal lead exposure, considering the addition of other environmental factors over time (e.g., postnatal lead exposure, social factors, etc.), or of a reduction of an early brain damage over time, or a combination of both, is difficult to determine with epidemiological methods. The experimental results presented here support the first interpretation.

Several of these neurobehavioral effects found in the squirrel monkeys may be of relevance to human neuropsychiatric disorders, e.g., the social disturbances, impaired motor coordination and perseveration. One male monkey showed, in addition to the above symptoms, a clinically characteristic "syndrome", most obvious during adolescence, consisting of motor hyperactivity, stereotype movements, and short attentional span with a high degree of distractibility. This combination can be found in humans with attention-deficit hyperactivity disorder, and it is of interest that such symptoms have been described in human children with high lead exposure (e.g., David et al., 1972).

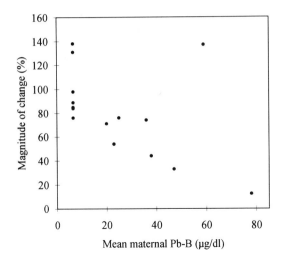

Figure 4. The relationship between maternal Pb-B and relative magnitude of change following a reversal in concurrent schedules of reinforcements. The relative magnitude of change was defined as $b / (0.8 - (a - b)$, according to the best fit of the asymptotic regression function $y = a - be^{-cx}$ (a = the asymptote, b = the absolute magnitude of change, c = the rate of change).

In the absence of postmortem analyses or neuroimaging of the animals here studied, the neuroanatomical localization of the disturbances can only be speculated upon. For instance, the indications of positive Babinski's sign and hypotonus, without apparent muscular weakness or atrophy, suggest some degree of damage to the pyramidal tract, possibly part of the cerebrum. The decreased aggressiveness could be related to damage of the amygdala or its connections (see, e.g., Klüver and Bucy, 1939). It is also of interest that prefrontal cortical lesions may lead to a combination of decreased aggressiveness, lower hierarchical position and cognitive disturbances (Peters and Ploog, 1976). These and other signs might be caused by the petechial hemorrhages in the cerebral white matter. Impairments of learning following reversals in concurrent schedules of reinforcements may neuroanatomically relate to disturbances in the hippocampus or prefrontal cortex, and neurobehaviorally to disturbances in central inhibition of responses ("perserveration"), attention, or spacial memory.

Methylmercury-exposed comparative controls

Examination of the central nervous systems was performed in six methylmercury-exposed offspring (Lögdberg et al., 1994c). Histological examination revealed signs of disturbed cell migration from the subpial granular layer (Brun, 1965) and the periventricular matrix, i.e., a persistence of cells subpially (see Figure 5) and subcortically, and signs of small disturbances in sulcus formation in the cerebrum, as well as a reduction of the external granular layer of the cerebellum. Similar changes have been found following mercury vapor exposure (Lögdberg et al., 1994e).

The effects of prenatal methylmercury exposure were similar to those of lead in many respects. There were, however, no significant effects on the gestational length or the pregnancy outcome, no extensive hemorrhages in the brain, and there were some differences in neurobehavioral effects (e.g., no reflex disturbances, but pathological manual motor behavior; unpublished observations). Furthermore, there were signs of disturbed cell migration, and of a body size growth retardation throughout the postnatal development (unpublished observations). The signs of disturbed cell migration, i.e., a persistence of cells subpially and subcortically and signs of small disturbances in sulcus

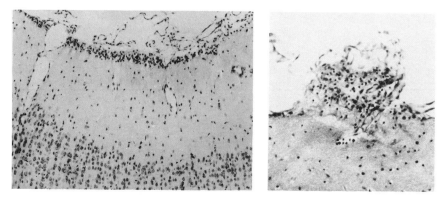

Figure 5. Cerebral neocortex with persistence of cells subpially, in the molecular layer (*left*; HE, x 100), and in the form of a leptomeningeal heterotopia (*right*; HE, x 110). Newborn squirrel monkey exposed to methylmercury during fetal development.

formation in the cerebrum, as well as a reduction of the external granular layer of the cerebellum, were reminiscent of those found in human cases of prenatal methylmercury exposure. This points to the similarity of this developmental process between the squirrel monkey and humans, and indirectly speaks against a significant effect of lead on cell migration in the human fetal brain. An experimentally induced persistence of cells in the subpial granular layer has not been reported previously. The tentative pathogenesis of the methylmercury-induced brain disturbances is shown in Figure 6, and should be compared with that of lead (Figure 3).

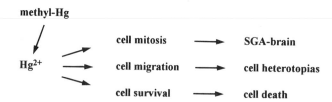

Figure 6. A tentative pathogenesis of methylmercury-induced fetal brain disturbances. SGA = small for gestational age.

PATHOGENETIC RELEVANCE TO NEUROPSYCHIATRIC DISORDERS

The hemorrhages, disturbances in cell migration and tissue growth, caused by prenatal exposure to metals, may be pathogenetically comparable with some of the various signs of neuropathology found postmortem in adult cases of schizophrenia. Thus, the lead-induced white matter hemorrhages at partus might relate to the ventriculomegaly, and to the signs of mild gliosis periventricularly and elsewhere, found as a more or less stable disturbance in many cases of adult schizophrenia (see, e.g., Fisman, 1975; Stevens, 1982; Nasrallah et al., 1983; Pakkenberg, 1987; Crow et al., 1989; Bruton et al., 1990; Bogerts and Falkai, 1991).

The methylmercury-induced sulci abnormalities and increase in the number of heterotopic cells subcortically and in lamina I (from the subpial granular layer), may correspond to similar signs of disturbed cell migration intra- and subcortically found in some cases of schizophrenia (disorientation of hippocampal pyramidal cells; heterotopic cells in the entorhinal cortex; cytoarchitectural disturbances in the prefrontal, anterior cingulate, entorhinal and primary motor cortex; surplus of neurons subcortically in the prefrontal and temporal cortex; wide and shallow cortical sulci of the cerebrum; and abnormal pattern of temporal cortical sulci; see, e.g., McLardy, 1974; Scheibel and Kovelman, 1981; Kovelman and Scheibel, 1984; Bogerts, 1984, 1985; Jacob and Beckmann, 1986; Falkai and Bogerts, 1986; Benes et al., 1986; Benes, 1987; Altschuler et al., 1987; Falkai et al., 1988; Falkai and Bogerts, 1989; Arnold et al., 1991; Conrad et al., 1991; Akbarian et al., 1993a, 1993b).

Finally, the methylmercury- and lead-induced growth retardation, possibly partly due to disturbed mitosis, might correspond to the signs of hypo-/"hetero"plasia of the cerebrum and its lobes, nuclei, and cortices with their various subpopulations of cells (i.e. reduced volumes of the cerebral hemispheres, hippocampus, parahippocampal gyrus including entorhinal cortex, amygdala, mediodorsal thalamic nucleus, and nucleus accumbens; reduction of the number of hippocampal pyramidal cells; reduction of microneuron density in the pulvinar; and abnormal morphology of the corpus callosum; see, e.g., Rosenthal and Bigelow, 1972; Dom et al., 1981; Bogerts et al., 1983; Brown et al., 1986; Pakkenberg, 1987, 1990; Crow et al., 1989; Jeste and Lohr, 1989; Altschuler et al., 1990; Benes et al., 1991)

Within the lead-exposed group, there was a markedly and statistically significant higher perinatal mortality (stillbirths and neonatal deaths) among the male offspring compared to the female offspring, with similar gestational age and lead dose, presumably due to a higher incidence of perinatal white matter hemorrhages. The neurobehavioral status up to adult age was also more impaired in male, compared to female, offspring following similar prenatal lead doses. A similar sex-difference in the incidence of periventricular hemorrhages has been found in a general population of humans (see, e.g., Amato et al., 1987), and might relate to indications of a higher frequency of perinatal complications in the history of male schizophrenics. Such a sex-difference was not obvious among the methylmercury-exposed monkeys.

The developmental neuropathological findings which have been reported in neuropsychiatric disorders other than schizophrenia also include signs of disturbances in cell mitosis and migration in the fetal brain, and hypoxic-ischemic/hemorrhagic lesions in the perinatal brain, although the latter lesions may only remain as discrete histopathological disturbances at adult age which could be difficult to differentiate from postnatal lesions. In the case of mental retardation, there is an abundance of postmortem cases with clear disturbances of the above types (see, e.g., Crome and Stern, 1967). However, a subgroup of 10-50% of cases of mental retardation has no obvious signs of structural brain disturbances at routine analysis. In these, as in most cases of schizophrenia, only a detailed morphometric analysis may reveal neuropathological disturbances (Lögdberg, 1993b). In the case of neuropsychiatric disorders other than schizophrenia and mental retardation, postmortem or magnetic resonance imaging studies of the brain are much fewer, and clear signs of disturbances of cell migration seem only to have been reported in a few cases of bipolar disorder (Bourgeois et al., 1992; Beckman and Jacob, 1993) and infantile autism (Gaffney and Tsai, 1987; Priven et al., 1993). There appears to be a lack of postmortem studies of the neuropathology of attention-deficit hyperactivity disorder and of personality disorders.

CONCLUSIONS

Recent research on the influence of environmental and genetic factors during fetal brain development on the later development of schizophrenia and other neuropsychiatric disturbances may benefit from experiences accumulated in earlier studies of the influence of specific environmental factors, such as lead and methylmercury, on the development of cognitive functions. An overview is given of the research into the influence of inorganic lead on the development of the brain and its cognitive functions, with emphasis on the problems of causality in human studies, and of the validity for humans of experimental studies.

To help bridge the gap between the existing epidemiological and experimental literature, the squirrel monkey was characterized as a nonhuman primate model of the human brain development. Lead and methylmercury exposure of squirrel monkeys during prenatal development produce neuropathological changes, as well as postnatal neurobehavioral disturbances which remained until adult age. These effects appeared to vary with the type of metal, the metal dose, and the developmental stage of metal exposure. The neuropathological effects - subtle disturbances in cell migration, and in tissue growth, and petechial white matter hemorrhages - may be pathogenetically comparable to findings reported in human cases of schizophrenia and other neuropsychiatric disorders. Some of the neurobehavioral effects - e.g., perseveration and social effects - may also relate to disturbances in human neuropsychiatric disorders.

In view of these results and the concept of neurhomogeny (see above) the squirrel monkey may offer advantages as an experimental model for the study of factors regulating the normal and abnormal human fetal brain development, compared to models used earlier, and particularly for the analysis of the multiple and interlinked disturbances in brain development hypothesized for many cases of schizophrenia and other neuropsychiatric disorders.

ACKNOWLEDGEMENT

These investigations were supported by the Swedish Work Health Fund, Svenska Läkarsällskapet and the Lund University Medical Faculty.

REFERENCES

Accardo P, Whitman B, Caul J, Rolfe U (1988) Autism and plumbism. A possible association. *Clin. Pediatr. Phila.* 27: 41–44.

Akbarian S, Bunney WE Jr, Potkin SG, Wigal SG, Hagman JO, Sandman CA, Jones EG (1993a) Altered distribution of nicotinamide-adenine-dinucleotide-phosphate-diaphorase cells in frontal lobe of schizophrenics implies disturbances in cortical development. *Arch. Gen. Psychiat.* 50:169-177.

Akbarian S, Viñuela A, Kim JJ, Potkin SG, Bunney WE Jr, Jones EG (1993b) Distorted distribution of nicotinamide-adenine-dinucleotide-phosphate-diaphorase neurons in temporal lobe of schizophrenics implies anomalous cortical development. *Arch. Gen. Psychiat.* 50:178-187.

Altschuler LL, Conrad A, Kovelman JA, Scheibel A (1987) Hippocampal pyramidal cell orientation in schizophrenia. *Arch. Gen. Psychiatr.* 44: 1094-1098.

Altschuler LL, Casanova MF, Goldberg TE, Kleinman JE (1990) The hippocampus and parahippocampus in schizophrenic, suicide and control brains. *Arch. Gen. Psychiat.* 47: 1029-1034.

Amato M, Howald H, von Muralt G (1987) Fetal sex distribution of peri- and intraventricular hemorrhage in preterm infants. *Eur. Neurol.* 27: 20-23.

Arnold SE, Hyman BT, van Hoesen GW, Damasio AR (1991 Some cytoarchitectural abnormalities of the entorhinal cortex in schizophrenia. *Arch. Gen. Psychiat.* 48: 625-632.

Baghurst PA, McMichael AJ, Wigg NR, Vimpuni G., Robertson E., Roberts RJ, Tong S-L (1992) Environmental exposure to lead and children's intelligence at the age of seven years: The Port-Pirie cohort study. *N. Engl. J. Med.* 327: 1279-1284.

Balázs R, Lewis PD, Patel AJ. Nutritional deficiencies and brain development, *in*: "Human growth", F Falkner, JM Tanner, eds., Bailliere Tindall, London, Vol. 3, pp 415-480, 1979.

Beckmann H, Jakob H (1991) Prenatal disturbances of nerve cell migration in the entorhinal region: a common vulnerability factor in functional psychoses? *J. Neural. Transm. Gen. Sect.* 84: 155-164.

Bellinger DA, Leviton C, Waternaux H, Needleman, Rabinowitz M (1987) Longitudinal analyses of prenatal and postnatal lead exposure and early cognitive development. *New Engl. J. Med.* 316: 1037-1043.

Bellinger D, Sloman J, Leviton A, Rabinowitz, M, Needleman HL, Waternaux C (1991) Low-level lead exposure and children's cognitive function in the preschool years. *Pediatrics* 87: 219-227.

Benes FM (1987) An analysis of the arrangement of neurons in the cingulate cortex of schizophrenic patients. *Arch. Gen. Psychiat.* 44: 608-616.

Benes FM, Davidson B, Bird ED (1986) Quantitative cytoarchitectural studies of the cerebral cortex of schizophrenics. *Arch. Gen. Psychiat.* 43: 31-35.

Benes FM, McSparren J, Bird ED, SanGiovanni JP, Vincent SL (1991) Deficits in small interneurons in prefrontal and cingulate cortices in schizophrenic and schizoaffective patients. *Arch. Gen. Psychiat.* 48: 996-1001.

Blackman Jr SS (1937) The lesions of lead encephalitis in children. *Bull. Johns Hopkins Hosp.* 61: 1-61.

Bogerts B (1984) Zur Neuropathologie der Schizophrenien. *Fortschr. Neurol. Psychiat.* 52: 428-437.

Bogerts B, Lesch A, Lange H, Zech M, Tutsch J (1983) Hypotrophy of the corpus callosum in schizophrenia. *Neurosci. Lett.*, suppl. 14: 413.

Bogerts B, Falkai P, 1992, Clinical and neurodevelopmental aspects of brain pathology in schizophrenia, *in*: "Developmental Neuropathology of Schizophrenia", SA Mednick, TD Cannon, CE Barr, JM LaFosse, eds., Plenum Press, New York, NY: pp 93-120.

Bouchard Jr TJ, Lykken DT, McGue M, Segal NL, Tellegen A (1990) Sources of human psychological differences: The Minnesota study of twins reared apart. *Science* 250: 223-228.

Bourgeois JA, Nisenbaum J, Drexler KG, Dobbins KM, Hall MJ (1992) A case of subcortical grey matter heterotopia presenting as bipolar disorder. *Compr. Psychiatr.* 33:407-410.

Brady K, Herrera Y, Zenick H (1975) Influence of parental lead exposure on subsequent learning ability of offspring. *Pharmacol. Biochem. Behav* 3: 561-565.

Brann Jr AW, Myers RE (1975) Central nervous system findings in the newborn monkey following severe in utero partial asphyxia. *Neurology* 25: 327-338.

Brown RS, Hingerty BE, Dewan JC, Klug A (1983) Pb(II)-catalyzed cleavage of the sugar-phosphate backbone of yeast tRNA(Phe) – implications for lead toxicity and self-splicing RNA. *Nature* 303: 543-546.

Brown R, Colter N, Corsellis JAN, Crow TJ, Frith CD, Jagoe R, Johnstone EC, Marsh L (1986) Postmortem evidence of structural brain changes in schizophrenia. Differences in brain weight, temporal horn area and parahippocampal gyrus compared with affective disorder. *Arch. Gen. Psychiat.* 43: 36-42.

Brun A. The subpial granular layer of the fetal cerebral cortex in man. *Acta Pathol. Microbiol. Scand.*, Suppl. 179, 1965.

Bruton CJ, Crow TJ, Frith CD, Johnstone EC, Owens DGC, Roberts GW (1990) Schizophrenia and the brain: a prospective clinico-neuropathological study. *Psychol. Med.* 20: 285-304.

Bryce-Smith D, Deshpande RR, Hughes J, Waldron HA (1977) Lead and cadmium levels in stillbirths. *Lancet* 1: 1159.

Butt EM, Pearson HE, Simonsen DE (1952) Production of meningoceles and cranioschisis in chick embryos with lead nitrate. *Proc. Soc. Exp. Biol. Med.* 79: 247-249.

Catizone O, Gray P (1941) Experiments on chemical interference with the early morphogenesis of the chick. II. The effects of lead on the central nervous system. *J. Exp. Zool.* 87: 71–83.

Cheney D, Seyfarth, R, Smuts B (1986) Social relationships and social cognition in nonhuman primates. *Science* 234: 1361–1366.

Choi BEH, Lapham LOW, Amin-Zaki L, Saleem T (1978) Abnormal neuronal migration, deranged cerebral cortical organization, and diffuse white matter astrocytosis in the human fetal brain: A major effect of methylmercury poisoning in utero. *J. Neuropath. Exp. Neurol.* 37: 719–733.

Collins MF, Hrdina PD, Whittle E, Singhal RL (1982) Lead in blood and brain regions of rats chronically exposed to low doses of the metal. *Toxicol. Appl. Pharmacol.* 65: 314–322.

Conrad AJ, Abebe T, Austin R, Forsythe S, Scheibel AB. Hippocampal pyramidal cell disarray in schizophrenia as a bilateral phenomenon. *Arch. Gen. Psychiat.* 48: 413–417.

Cooney GH, Bell A, McBride W, Carter C (1989) Neurobehavioral consequences of prenatal low lead exposure to lead. *Neurotoxicol. Teratol.* 11: 95–104.

Crome L, Stern J, 1967, "The Pathology of Mental Retardation", Little, Brown and Company, Boston.

Crow TJ, Ball J, Bloom SR, Brown R, Bruton CJ, Colter N, Frith CD, Johnstone EC, Owens DC, Roberts GW (1989) Schizophrenia as an anomaly of development of cerebral asymmetry: a postmortem study and a proposal concerning the genetic basis of the disease. *Arch. Gen. Psychiatr.* 46: 1145–1150.

David O, Clark J, Voeller K (1972) Lead and hyperactivity. *Lancet* 2: 900–903.

David OJ, McGann B, Hoffman S, Sverd J, Clark J (1976) Low lead levels and mental retardation. *Lancet* 6: 1376–1379.

Davis JM, Svendsgaard DJ (1987) Lead and child development (Commentary). *Nature* 329: 297–300.

de Gennaro LO (1978) The effects of lead nitrate on the central nervous system of the chick embryo. I. Observations of light and electron microscopy. *Growth* 42: 141–155.

Dietrich KN, Krafft KM, Bier M, Succop PA, Berger O, Bornschein RL (1986) Early effects of fetal lead exposure: Neurobehavioral findings at 6 months. *Int. J. Biosoc. Res.* 8: 151–168.

Dietrich KN, Berger OG, Succop PA (1993) Lead exposure and the motor developmental status of urban six-year-old children in the Cincinnati prospective study. *Pediatrics* 91: 301–307.

Dom R, de Saedeler J, Bogerts B, Hopf A (1981) Left globus pallidus abnormality in never-medicated patients with schizophrenia. *Proc. Nat. Acad. Sci. USA* 84: 561–563.

Dosen A (1989) Diagnosis and treatment of mental illness in mentally retarded children: A developmental model. *Child Psychiat. Hum. Dev.* 20: 73-84.

Drew WG, Kostas J, McFarland DJ, De Rossett SE (1979) Effects of neonatal lead exposure on apomorphine-induced aggression and stereotypies in the rat. *Pharmacol.* 18: 257–262.

Edwards MJ, Beatson J (1984) Effects of lead and hyperthermia on prenatal brain growth of guinea pigs. *Teratology* 30: 413–421.

Ernhart CB, Wolf AW, Kennard MJ, Erhard P, Filipovich HF, Sokol RJ (1986) Intrauterine exposure to low levels of lead: The status of the neonate. *Arch. Environ. Health* 41: 287–291.

Ernhart CB, Morrow-Tlucak M, Wolf AW, Super D, Drotar D (1989) Low level lead exposure in the prenatal and early preschool periods: intelligence prior to school entry. *Neurotoxicol. Teratol.* 11: 161–170.

Falkai P, Bogerts B (1986) Cell loss in the hippocampus of schizophrenics. *Eur. Arch. Psychiat. Neurol. Sci.* 236: 154-161.

Falkai P, Bogerts B, Rozumek M (1988) Cell loss and volume reduction in the entorhinal cortex of schizophrenics. *Biol. Psychiat.* 24: 515-521.

Falkai P, Bogerts B (1989) Morphometric evidence for developmental disturbances in brains of some schizophrenics. *Schizophrenia Res.* 2: 99.

Ferm VH, Carpenter SJ (1967) Developmental malformations resulting from the administration of lead salts. *Exp. Mol. Pathol* 7: 208-213.

Fisman M (1975) The brain stem in psychosis. *Brit. J. Psychiat.* 126: 414-422.

Gaffney GR, Tsai LY (1987) Magnetic resonance imaging of high level autism. *J. Autism Dev. Disord.* 17: 433-438.

Gerber GB, Léonard A, Jacquet P (1980) Toxicity, mutagenicity and teratogenicity of lead. *Mutat. Res.* 76: 115-141.

Ghafour SY, Khuffash FA, Ibrahim HS, Reavey PC (1984) Congenital lead intoxication with seizures due to prenatal exposure. *Clin. Ped.* 23: 282-283.

Gibson JL (1904) A plea for painted railings and painted walls of rooms as the source of lead poisoning among Queensland children. *Australasian Med. Gaz.* 23: 149-153.

Gilani SH (1973) Congenital anomalies in lead poisoning. *Obstet. Gynekol.* 41: 265-268.

Goldstein GW, Ashbury AK, Diamond I (1974) Pathogenesis of lead encephalopathy: Uptake of lead and reaction of brain capillaries. *Arch. Neurol.* 31: 382–389,

Grant LD, Kimmel CA, West Gl, Martinez-Vargas CM, Howard JL (1980) Chronic low-level lead toxity in the rat: II. Effects on postnatal physical and behavioral development. *Toxicol. Appl. Pharmacol.* 56: 42–58.

Gregg NM (1942) Congenital cataract following German measles in the mother. *Trans. Ophthal. Soc. Austral.* 3: 35–46.

Hammett FS (1928) Studies in the biology of metals. VII. The influence of lead on the development of the chick embryo. *J. Exp. Med.* 48: 659–665.

Hastings L, Cooper GP, Bornschein RL, Michaelson IA (1977) Behavioral effects of low level neonatal lead exposure. *Pharmacol. Biochem. Behav.* 7: 37–42.

Hernberg S, Nikkanen J (1970) Enzyme inhibition by lead under normal urban conditions. *Lancet* 1: 63–64.

Hirano A, Kochen JA (1973) Neurotoxic effects of lead in the chick embryo. *Morphologic studies* 29: 659–668.

Howard JD, Mottet NK (1986). Effects of methylmercury on the morphogenesis of the rat cerebellum. *Teratology* 34: 89–95.

Jacob H, Beckmann H (1986) Prenatal developmental disturbances in the limbic allocortex in schizophrenics. *J. Neural Transm.* 65: 303-326.

Jeste DV, Lohr JB (1989) Hippocampal pathological findings in schizophrenia. *Arch. Gen. Psychiat.* 46: 1019-1024.

Jones KL, Smith DW. Recognition of the fetal alcohol syndrome in early infancy. *Lancet* 2: 999–1001, 1973.

Karnofsky DA, Ridgway LP (1952) Production of injury to the central nervous system of the chick embryos by lead salts. *J. Pharmacol. Exp. Ther.* 104: 176–186.

Kazantis G, 1989, Lead: ancient metal – modern menace, *in*: "Lead Exposure and Child Development; an International Assessment", MA Smith, LD Grant, AI Sors, eds., Kluwer Academic Publishers, Lancaster, pp 119–128.

Klüver H, Bucy P (1939) Preliminary analysis of functions of the temporal lobe in monkeys. *Arch. Neurol. Psychol.* 42: 979–1000.

Kovelman JA, Scheibel AS (1984) A neurohistological correlate of schizophrenia. *Biol. Psychiat.* 16: 1601-1621.

Lancranjan I, Popescu HI, Gavanescu O, Klepsch I, Serbanescu M (1975) Reproductive ability of workmen occupationally exposed to lead. *Arch. Environ. Health* 30: 396–400.

Lögdberg B, Berlin M, Schütz A (1987) Effects of lead exposure on pregnancy outcome and the fetal brain of squirrel monkeys. *Scand. J. Work Environ. Health* 13: 135-145.

Lögdberg B, Brun A, Berlin M, Schütz A (1988) Congenital lead encephalopathy in monkeys. *Acta Neuropathol. (Berl.)* 77: 120-127.

Lögdberg B (1988) Alphaxolone-alphadolone acetate for anesthesia of squirrel monkeys of different ages. *J. Med. Primatol.* 17: 163–167.

Lögdberg B, 1993a, "Fetal Lead and Brain Development. Studies in a Nonhuman Primate", Thesis, Lund.

Lögdberg B (1993b) Prefrontal neocortical disturbances in mental retardation. *J. Intell. Disabil. Res.* 37:459-468.

Lögdberg B (1994a) Methods for timing of pregnancy and monitoring of fetal body and brain growth in squirrel monkeys. *J. Med. Primatol.* In press.

Lögdberg B (1994b) Lead reduces mitosis of cultured fetal cerebral and placental cells from rat, monkey and human. Submitted for publication.

Lögdberg B, Berlin M, Brun A (1994c) Effects of methylmercury on the fetal brain of the squirrel monkey. Submitted for publication.

Lögdberg B, Newland C, Sheng Y, Berlin M (1994d) Effects of fetal lead exposure on learning in squirrel monkeys. Submitted for publication.

Lögdberg B, Warfvinge K, Hua J, Berlin M. (1994e) Fetal brain disturbances by mercury vapor in monkeys. Submitted for publication.

Lögdberg B (1994f) Effects of fetal lead exposure on the postnatal neurobehavioral status in monkeys. To be published.

Markovac J, Goldstein GW (1988) Picomolar concentrations of lead stimulate brain protein kinase C. Nature 334: 71–73.

Matsumoto HI, Koya GO, Takeuchi T (1965) Fetal Minamata disease – A neuropathological study of two cases of intrauterine intoxication by a methylmercury compound. J. Neuropath. Exp. *Neurol.* 24: 563–574.

135

McLardy T (1974) Hippocampal zink and structural deficits in brains from chronic alcoholics and some schizophrenics. *J. Orthomol. Psychiatry* 4:32-36.

McMichael AJ, Vimpani GV, Robertson EF, Baghurst PA, Clark PD. (1986) The Port Pirie cohort study: maternal blood lead and pregnancy outcome. *J. Epidemiol. Community Health* 40: 18-25.

McMichael AJ, Baghurst PA, Wigg NR, Vimpani GV, Robertson EF, Roberts RJ (1988) Port Pirie cohort study: environmental exposure to lead and children's abilities at the age of four years. *N. Engl. J. Med.* 319: 468-475.

Miller CD, Buck WB, Hembrough FB, Cunningham WL (1982) Fetal rat development as influenced by maternal lead exposure. *Vet. Hum. Toxicol.* 24: 163-166.

Miller DT, Etzel RA, McFarland JG, Aster RH, White GC. (1987) Prolonged neonatal autoimmune atrombocytopenic purpura associated with anti-Bak(a). Two cases in siblings. *Am. J. Perinatol.* 4: 55-58.

Miller GD, Massaro TF, Massaro EJ (1990) Interactions between lead and essential elements: a review. *Neurotoxicology* 11: 99-120.

Moore MR, 1980, Prenatal exposure to lead and mental retardation, *in*: "Low Level Lead Exposure: the Clinical Implications of Current Research", HL Needleman, ed., Raven Press, New York, NY, pp 53-65.

Moore MR, Meredith PA, Goldberg A (1977) A retrospective analysis of blood-lead in mentally retarded children. *Lancet* 1: 717-719.

Moore MR, Goldberg A, Pocock SJ, Meredith A, Stewart IM, MacAnespie H, Lees R, Low A (1982) Some studies of maternal and infant lead exposure in Glasgow. *Scot. Med. J.* 27: 133-122.

Mykkanen HM, Dickerson JWT, Lancaster MC (1979) Effect of age on the tissue distribution of lead in the rat. *Toxicol. Appl. Pharmacol.* 51: 447-454.

Napier JR, Napier PH, 1967, "A Handbook of Living Primates", Academic Press, London-New York, NY.

Nasrallah HA, McCalley-Whitters M, Rauscher FP et al. (1983) A histological study of the corpus callosum in chronic schizophrenia. *Psych. Res.* 8: 151-160.

Nayak BN, Ray M, Persaud TV, Nigli M (1989). Relationship of embryotoxicity to genotoxicity of lead nitrate in mice. *Exp. Pathol.* 36: 65-73.

Needleman HL, Schell A, Bellinger D, Leviton A, Allred E (1990) The long-term effects of exposure to low doses of lead in childhood: An 11 year follow-up. *N. Engl. J. Med.* 322: 83-88.

Needleman, H.L., and Bellinger, D (1991) The health effects of low level exposure to lead. *Annu. Rev. Public Health* 12:111-140.

Newland C, Sheng Y, Lögdberg B, Berlin M (1994) Prenatal exposure to lead or methylmercury impairs aquisition and maintenance of concurrent schedule performance in squirrel monkeys. To be published.

Niklowitz WJ, Mandybur TI (1975) Neurofibrillary changes following childhood lead encephalopathy: Case report. *J. Neuropathol. Exp. Neurol.* 34: 445-455.

Okazaki H, Aronson SM, DiMaio DJ, Olvera JE (1963) Acute lead encephalopathy of childhood. *Trans. Am. Neurol. Assoc.* 88: 248-250.

Oliver T (1911) A lecture on lead poisoning and the race. *Brit. Med. J.* 1: 1096-1098.

Pakkenberg B (1987) Postmortem study of chronic schizophrenic brains. *Brit. J. Psychiat.* 151:744-752.

Pakkenberg B (1990) Pronounced reduction of total neuron numbers in mediodorsal thalamic nucleus and nucleus accumbens in schizophrenics. *Arch. Gen. Psychiat.* 47: 1023-1028.

Palmisano PA, Sneed RC, Cassady G (1969) Untaxed whiskey and fetal lead exposure. *J. Pediatr.* 75: 869-872.

Pentschew A, Garro F (1966) Lead encephalo-myelopathy of the suckling rat and its implications on the porphyrinopathic nervous diseases. *Acta. Neuropath. (Berl.)* 6: 266-278.

Peters M, Ploog D (1976) Frontal lobe lesions and social behavior in the squirrel monkey: A pilot study. *Acta Biol. Med. Germ.* 35: 1317-1326.

Pindborg S (1945) Om sølverglødsforgiftning i Danmark. *Ugeskr. Læg.* 107: 1-6.

Ploog D (1979) Phonation, Emotion, Cognition, with Reference to the Brain Mechanisms involved. *Brain and Mind, Ciba Found. Series* 69, Excerpta Medica, Amsterdam, pp 79-98.

Popoff N, Weinberg S, Feigin I (1963) Pathologic observations in lead encephalopathy with special reference to the vascular changes. *Neurology* 13: 101-112.

Qazi QH, Medahar C, Yuceoglu AM (1980) Temporary increase in chromosome breakage in an infant prenatally exposed to lead. *Hum. Genet.* 53: 201-203.

Rennert O (1881) Über eine hereditäre Folge der chronischen Bleivergiftung. *Arch. Gynäkol.* 18: 109-131.

Rom WN (1976) Effects of lead on the female and reproduction: A review. *Mt. Sinai. J. Med.* 43: 542-552.

Rosenblum LA, Coe CL, eds., 1985, "Handbook of Squirrel Monkey Research", Plenum Press, New York and London.

Rosenthal R, Bigelow LB (1972) Quantitative brain measurements in chronic schizophrenia. *Brit. J. Psychiat.* 121: 259-264.

Rothenberg SJ, Schnaas L, Cansino-Ortiz S, Perroni-Hernándes E, de la Torre P, Neri-Mendéz C, Ortega P, Hidalgo-Loperena H, Svendsgaard D. (1989) Neurobehavioral deficits after low level lead exposure in neonates: the Mexico City pilot study. *Neurotoxicol. Teratol.* 11: 85-93.

Schardein JL, 1985, "Drug and chemical toxicology, Vol 2: Chemically induced birth defects", Marcel Dekker Inc., New York and Basel.

Scheibel AB, Kovelman JA (1981) Disorientation of the hippocampal pyramidal cells and its processes in the schizophrenic patient. *Biol. Psychiat.* 16: 101-102.

Schultz AH (1949) Sex differences in the pelves of primates. *Amer. J. Phys. Anthropol.* 7: 401-423.

Schwartz J, Otto D (1987) Blood-lead, hearing threshold, and neurobehavioral development in children and youth. *Arch. Environ. Health* 42: 153-160.

Singh NP, Thind IS, Vitale LF, Pawlow M (1976) Lead content of tissues of baby rats born of, and nourished by, lead-poisoned mothers. *J. Clin. Med.* 87: 273-280.

Singh N, Donovan CM, Hanshaw JB (1978) Neontal lead intoxication in a prenatally exposed infant. *J. Pediatr.* 93: 1019-1021.

Stevens JR (1982) Neuropathology of schizophrenia. *Arch. Gen. Psychiat.* 39: 1131-1139.

Stollery BT, Broadbent DE, Banks HA, Lee WR (1991) Short term prospective study of cognitive functioning in lead workers. *Brit. J. Ind. Med.* 48: 739-749.

Talmage-Riggs G, Anschel S (1973) Homosexual behavior and dominance hierarchy in a group of captive female squirrel monkeys. *Folia Primat.* 19: 61-72.

Thomas JA, Dallenbach FD, Manaroma T (1971) Considerations on the development of experimental lead encephalopathy. *Virchows Arch. A. Path. Anat.* 352: 61-74.

Torrey EF (1992) Are we overestimating the genetic contribution to schizophrenia? *Schizophrenia Bull.* 18: 159-170.

Uzych L (1985) Teratogenesis and mutagenesis associated with the exposure of human males to lead: a review. *Yale J. Biol. Med.* 58: 9-17.

Valentino M, Coppa G, Ruschioni A (1984) Gradidanza in un'operaia esposta al piombo. *Med. Lav.* 75: 296-299.

Vermande-Van Eck GJ, Meigs JW (1960) Changes in the ovary of the rhesus monkey after chronic lead intoxication. *Fertil. Steril.* 11: 223-234.

Wibberley DG, Khera AK, Edwards JH, Rushton DI (1977) Lead levels in human placentae from normal and malformed births. *J. Med. Genet.* 14: 339-345.

Wide M, Nilsson O (1977) Differential susceptibility of the embryo to inorganic lead during preimplantation in the mouse. *Teratology* 16: 273-276.

Wilson AI (1966) Effects of abnormal lead content of water supplies on maternity patients. The use of a simple industrial screening test in antenatal care in general practice. *Scot. Med. J.* 11: 73-82.

Winder C, Garten LL, Lewis PD (1983) The morphological effects of lead on the developing central nervous system. *Neuropathol. Appl. Neurobiol.* 9: 87-108.

Yokoyama K, Araki S, Aono H (1988) Reversability of psychological performance in subclinical lead absorption. *Neurotoxicology* 9: 405-410.

Zook BC, London WT, Wilpizeski CR, Sever JL (1980) Experimental lead paint poisoning in nonhuman primates. *J. Med. Primatol.* 9: 343-360.

AMPA RECEPTOR-INDUCED DOPAMINERGIC CELL DEATH: A MODEL FOR THE PATHOGENESIS OF HYPOFRONTALITY AND NEGATIVE SYMPTOMS IN SCHIZOPHRENIA

Gabriel A. de Erausquin[1] and Ingeborg Hanbauer[2]

[1]Psychiatry Department, Yale University School of Medicine
New Haven, Connecticut
[2]National Heart and Lung Institute, National Institutes of Health
Bethesda, Maryland

INTRODUCTION

In the conclusion of their article on the role of glutamate in schizophrenia, Wachtel and Turski (1990) stated that *"because of the uncertainties surrounding the aetiology of schizophrenia, studies should be initiated with the goal of determining what role...excitatory amino acids play in this disorder."* Indeed, a wealth of information has been acquired about the interrelations between the dopaminergic and the glutamatergic systems, and several hypotheses about the physiopathology of schizophrenia have arisen. The dopaminergic and glutamatergic systems have been found to interact with each other at the biochemical, synaptic, and neural network levels.

Voltage-clamp intracellular recordings in slices of rat mesencephalon showed that agonists of the excitatory aminoacids receptors (a-Amino-3-hydroxy-5-methylisoxazole-4-propionic acid (AMPA), kainate, and quisqualate) increased the input conductance of dopaminergic neurons, whereas the antagonist N-methyl-D-Aspartate (NMDA) was associated with a decrease in input conductance (Mercuri et al., 1992). Biochemical (Girault et al., 1990) and behavioral (Schmidt et al., 1990) data indicate that NMDA stimulates a biochemical pathway that antagonizes indirectly a dopamine regulated biochemical pathway in the neostriatum. In striatonigral neurons dopamine D_1 receptor activation leads to an increase in levels of cAMP, followed by activation of cAMP-dependent protein kinase. One of the substrates of the cAMP-dependent protein kinase is DARPP-32, a dopamine and cAMP regulated phosphoprotein (Girault et al., 1990). DARPP-32 is highly enriched in striatonigral neurons, and its phosphorylation turns it into a potent inhibitor of phosphatase-1, an enzyme with broad range substrate specificity (Girault et al., 1990). Thus, it seems likely that one of the actions of DARPP-32 is to prevent dephosphorylation of other substrates phosphorylated by cAMP-dependent protein kinase, therefore enhancing other effects of dopamine. The residue of DARPP-32 phosphorylated by cAMP-dependent kinase is dephosphorylated by calcineurin, a very specific calcium-dependent phosphatase that is activated by NMDA stimulation (Girault et al., 1990). Hence,

Neural Development and Schizophrenia, Edited by S.A. Mednick
and J.M. Hollister, Plenum Press, New York, 1995

NMDA blockage would result in a facilitation of dopamine action by preventing the glutamate induced dephosphorylation of DARPP-32 in the nigrostriatal neurons (Girault et al., 1990).

In fact, in rats dizolcipine restores motility in animals treated with haloperidol (a dopaminergic D_2 antagonist) but not with reserpine (which depletes monoamines), indicating that some remaining dopaminergic activity appears to be necessary for NMDA antagonists to exert anticataleptic effects (Schmidt et al., 1990). Moreover, rats trained to discriminate a selective D_2 antagonist, cross generalize to dizolcipine administration (Greenamyre and O'Brien, 1991).

Whole cell recording in dopaminergic neurons of rat mesencephalon slices show that excitatory post-synaptic potentials have a fast component induced by non-NMDA currents and a slow component contributed by NMDA channels (Mereu et al., 1991). Injection of kainic acid, but not NMDA, into the SNc induced seizures in rats, which were prevented by a specific kainic receptor antagonist (Maggio et al., 1990). These observations suggest that nigral dopaminergic neurons may express mainly non-NMDA type glutamate receptors.

In striatal slices (Bouger et al., 1991) and in striatal synaptosomes (Araneda and Bustos, 1981; Llinas et al., 1984; Krebs et al., 1991) NMDA induced [3H]dopamine release, suggesting that dopaminergic terminals may express NMDA receptors. In contrast, NMDA induced activation of tyrosin hydroxylase (TH) in striatum was not blocked by tetrodotoxin (which abolishes nerve action potential), suggesting that the receptors may not be located in the dopaminergic terminal (Arias Montana et al., 1992). One possible explanation for these contradictory data has been proposed by Hanbauer et al. (1992), who showed that NMDA-mediated [3H]dopamine release in mesencephalic culture neurons was prevented by inhibiting the synthesis of nitrate oxide (NO), a highly diffusible gas. NO appears to convey a signal from the post-synaptic to the pre-synaptic cell, suggesting that NMDA may indirectly regulate dopamine release.

Direct evidence for the presence of AMPA receptors subunits in the rat SNc and Ventral Tegmental Area (VTA) (Petralia and Wenthold, 1992) and in particular in TH-immunoreactive neurons (Martin et al., 1993), has been provided by immunocytochemistry. However, information regarding NMDA receptor subunits is not yet available.

At the network level, glutamate and dopamine operate independently of each other on GABAergic inhibition of the excitatory thalamocortical pathway, which forms an important part of a cortico-striatal-thalamo-cortical feedback loop that protects the cortex from an informational overload and hyperarousal (Wachtel and Turski, 1990). Similarly, direct injection of AMPA into the SNc induces prolonged rotatory behavior contralateral to the injection site (Mascó, de Erausquin, Hanbauer & Gale, unpublished observation). Clearly, interactions between the dopaminergic and glutamatergic systems occur at multiple loci in the adult brain, and dysfunctional interactions leading to a decrease in glutamatergic function and secondary increase in dopaminergic output have been suggested to underlie the so called *positive symptoms* of schizophrenia and other psychosis (v.g., Wachtel and Turski, 1990; Kornhuber, 1990; Reynolds, 1992). This hypothesis is supported by the psychotomimetic action of drugs like phencyclidine (Reynolds et al., 1992), and ketamine (Krystal et al., 1993), which have NMDA receptor blocking properties.

On the other hand, *negative symptoms* of schizophrenia seem to correlate best with a decrease in dopaminergic function as well as with a relative lack of activation in the frontal lobes, a phenomenon usually described as *hypofrontality* (Andreasen, 1989; Weinberger, 1987). Interestingly, it has been shown that in developing rats, a lesion of the dopaminergic projection fibers to the prefrontal cortex results in mesocortical dopaminergic underactivity and compensatory **mesolimbic overactivity**

(Weinberger, 1987). Such a lesion during development in humans would manifest itself clinically as *negative* and *positive* symptoms of schizophrenia, respectively (Weinberger, 1987). However, there is no information yet about the neurodevelopmental aspects of this interaction.

Two possible explanations for the initial loss of dopaminergic neurons have been suggested. They include the presence of serum antibodies against a mitochondrial protein (Kilindreas et al., 1992); and a deficiency in Ca^{++}-ATPase, which has been shown in erythrocytes of schizophrenic patients (Kluge and Kuhne, 1985). Both of these defects should affect all subpopulations of neurons equally, and hence the question of the specificity of the dopaminergic neuronal death is left unanswered (de Erausquin et al., 1993).

One alternative of more direct interest for the experiments described here is that the neuronal phenotype (and its relative sensitivity to excitotoxic injury) should be defined by subcellular properties linked to calcium homeostasis, including the presence of soluble calcium binding proteins (Mattson et al., 1991). The best studied among these proteins are calbindin-D28K (CB), calretinin (CR) and parvalbumin (PV); they are found within specific subpopulations of neurons, are present throughout the cell, and exhibit a high degree of affinity for calcium (Celio, 1990; Resibois and Rogers, 1992).

Unusual calcium buffering, specific translocation requirements, and/or specific coupling mechanisms are among the functions that have been claimed for CB, CR and PV, but very little proof is available for any of them. In peripheral tissues, PV was associated with the termination of fast contractions in muscle (Celio and Heizmann 1982), where PV was found to transiently bind Ca^{++} and return it quickly to the endoplasmic reticulum thus allowing prompt relaxation (Celio, 1990).

Stable transfection of CB into a cell line reduced Ca^{++} entry through VDCCs and improved the ability of the cells to reduce $[Ca^{++}]_i$ transients evoked by depolarization (Lledo et al., 1992). GABAergic and glutamatergic neurons are believed to contain higher levels of calcium binding proteins, perhaps in order to provide resistance to the neurotoxic effects of the excitatory aminoacids (Iacopino and Christakos, 1990b; Jacobowitz and Winsky, 1991). Very little is known about the function of CR, whose sequence is 60 % homologous to CB, and is highly expressed in sensory cells in the retina, organ of Corti and sensory ganglia (Ichikawa et al., 1991; Rogers, 1987).

In summary, these proteins seem good candidates to explain the relative differences in the ability of subgroups of otherwise identical neurons to handle $[Ca^{++}]_i$ loads. In fact, some evidence seems to suggest that their developmental expression in dopaminergic neurons may follow a timetable such that a vulnerable window exists (Liu and Graybiel, 1992; Abbott and Jacobowitz, 1993). In rats, TH expression (a marker of dopaminergic function) appears by embryonic day 14, whereas CB begins to appear at day 20, and thereafter increases in waves until postnatal day 3 (Liu and Graybiel, 1992). Again, CR seems to be expressed earlier in some regions, but it is unclear to what extent is expressed in dopaminergic neurons (Abbot and Jacobowitz, 1993). During this window the dopaminergic phenotype would be already expressed but the protective action of calcium binding proteins would be lacking, therefore exposing dopaminergic neurons to excitotoxic damage.

We here present a series of experiments aimed at establishing some form of evidence for the participation of $[Ca^{++}]_i$ dependent mechanisms (de Erausquin et al., 1993) in the selective *"pruning"* of subpopulations of dopaminergic neurons during a specific sensitive neurodevelopmental window (namely the equivalent of the human second trimester; Nasrallah, 1993), which would lead to a mesocortical dopaminergic deficit in the adult.

MATERIAL AND METHODS

E14 Mesencephalic Cultures

The mesencephalic region of embryonic day 14 (E14) rat pups was dissected into PBS containing 6mg/ml glucose and mechanically dissociated. Cells were plated onto 8-well slides coated with poly-D-lysine and laminin in culture media containing equal volumes of MEM and HAM-F12 with 15% equine serum, 2mM glutamine, 6mg/ml glucose and antibiotics. Cells were grown for 5 days at which point 10uM ARA-C (cytosine ß-D-arabino furanoside) was added to stop glial growth.

Imaging

Dopaminergic neurons (3-5 % of the total cells plated) were identified by 5,7-dihydroxytryptamine (5,7-DHT) uptake. The methods are described in detail elsewhere (de Erausquin et al., 1994). Briefly: The fluorescence of 5,7-DHT as well as of Ca^{++} chelator Fura-2 were monitored using an Attofluor Digital Fluorescence Microscopy System (Atto Instruments, Inc., Rockville, MD) based on a Zeiss Axiovert 35 inverted epifluorescence microscope. Rapid bleaching of 5,7-DHT prevented further interference with the Fura-2 signal. Paired time sequence (334 nm/390 nm) images of Fura-2 fluorescence were captured and stored. A computer controlled CDD camera allowed alternative capture at high and low gain (sensitivity) for the image emission detector in those experiments in which the dimmer fluorescence coming from dendrites was monitored. $Ca^{2+}]_i$ was calculated according to external standards.

Identification of Dopaminergic Neurons and FURA-2 Loading

Cultures dishes were incubated 30-45 min in 25 μM 5,7-DHT in the presence of 50 μM ascorbic acid at 37°C under regular culture conditions, and dopaminergic neurons were identified under the microscope by intravital fluorescence elicited by uptake of the dye. After identification of 5,7-DHT positive dopaminergic cells, cultures were incubated on the microscope stage with Fura-2 AM (20 min at 22°C) and washed with PBS solution (1 mM Ca^{2+}; 5 mM Mg^{2+}, 6 mg/ml glucose). Cells were kept after washing for 15 to 20 min at room temperature in the same buffer.

Quantification and Statistics

In the Calcium fluorescence experiments two way ANOVA (for unbalanced designs) for between treatment comparisons, followed by post-hoc Mann-Whitney multiple means comparisons was used. For differences between time points under the same treatment, one way ANOVA was used.

RESULTS

[CA^{++}]$_i$ Modulation in Mesencephalic Neurons "In Vitro" by EAA Receptor Agonists

In primary cultures of ventral tegmental mesencephalon grown for 5 to 9 days *in vitro*, each microscopic field selected contained usually two or three dopaminergic cells among as many other neurons. Exposure of these cultures to NMDA in Mg^{++}-free buffer caused at most a very transient and small increase of [Ca^{++}]$_i$ in neurons. Indeed, in these cultures, NMDA failed to induce any significant increase in somatic cytosolic $[Ca^{++}]_i$ over a wide range of concentrations (up to 500 μM) in the absence of magnesium (de Erausquin et al., 1992). However, in adult rat striatum NMDA receptor activation induces TH expression (Arias Montaño et al., 1992). On the other hand, preliminary data from our laboratory indicated that cultures exposed to 500 μM NMDA for 24 hr showed a trend towards increased number and length of primary and higher order dendrites in dopaminergic neurons (data not shown).

In contrast, a short exposure to glutamate or other non-NMDA agonists caused a dose dependent increase in $[Ca^{++}]_i$ in both neuronal subpopulations (de Erausquin et al., 1994). This $[Ca^{++}]_i$ rise was blocked by the L-type voltage dependent calcium channel blocker nifedipine but not by the N-type blocker w-conotoxin (Table 1). On the other hand, we have previously shown that N-type, but not L-type, blockers prevent depolarization-induced $[Ca^{++}]_i$ increase in the dopaminergic neurites, as well as dopamine release from dopaminergic neurons (de Erausquin et al., 1992), suggesting that functional specificity in different subcellular calcium pools in dopaminergic neurons may depend at least partly upon localization of clusters of voltage dependent calcium channels (de Erausquin et al., 1992). In dopaminergic neurons, the non-NMDA receptor antagonist NBQX shifted the dose response curve for AMPA to the right without altering the resting $[Ca^{++}]_i$, whereas NMDA antagonists had no effect (de Erausquin et al., 1994).

Table 1. Effect of voltage dependent calcium channel blockers on Fura-2 measured intracellular calcium in dopaminergic neurons *"in vitro"*.

TREATMENT	BASAL $[Ca^{++}]_i$	10 μM AMPA	50 μM AMPA
NONE	50+/-4.0	137+/-15	172+/-25
w-conotoxin (15 μg/ml)	67+/-8.0	n.m.	167+/-22
nifedipine	50+/-8.0	55+/-10 **	119+/-11 **

Mesencephalic cultures from E14 rat embryos were grown "in vitro" for 5 to 9 days. Dopaminergic cells were identified by uptake of autofluorescent 5.7-dihydroxytryptamine and then loaded with Fura-2.
**: p < 0.05 when compared to controls (NONE).

Non-NMDA Receptor Agonists Selectively Disrupt $[CA^{++}]_i$ in Embryonic Dopaminergic Neurons

Exposure to low doses of AMPA-receptor agonists was followed by a recovery of $[Ca^{++}]_i$ to resting values occurred within 5 min in all neurons (de Erausquin et al., 1994). In contrast, when cells were exposed higher doses, resting $[Ca^{++}]_i$ levels were recovered only in non-dopaminergic neurons, with just a slight decrease detected in dopaminergic neurons (Figure 1). Loss of $[Ca^{++}]_i$ homeostasis in dopaminergic neurons was prevented by pretreatment with a blocker of calcium-induced calcium release, indicating a role for intracellular Ca^{++}-sensitive Ca^{++} stores (de Erausquin et al., 1994).

Non-NMDA receptor-mediated excitotoxicity occurred when dopaminergic neurons where exposed to an agonist (v.g.,kainic acid) for a relatively short period of time (5 min), and involved protracted increases in $[Ca^{++}]_i$ long after the withdrawal of the stimulus. In contrast, other neurons in the same culture responded with an increase in $[Ca^{++}]_i$ which was reversible after removal of the excitatory aminoacids. Pretreatment with the ryanodine receptor antagonist dantrolene prevented both the protracted elevation in $[Ca^{++}]_i$ and cell death, suggesting that calcium-induced calcium release from intracellular stores was a necessary step for the toxic mechanism to occur (de Erausquin et al., 1994). It is presently not understood why calcium-sensitive calcium stores are regulated differently in embryonic dopaminergic neurons and in other neurons at the same developmental stage. Indeed, functional evidence for the

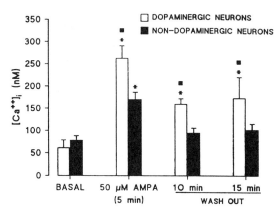

Figure 1. Destabilization of $[Ca^{++}]_i$ homeostasis by 50 μM AMPA is selective to dopaminergic neurons in culture.

Mesencephalic cultures from E14 rat embryos were grown *"in vitro"* for 5 to 9 days. Dopaminergic cells were identified by uptake of 5,7,Dihydroxitryptamine and then loaded with Fura-2. Each column represents the average value from three experiments.

■: $p < 0.01$ compared to non-dopaminergic neurons in the same point
*: $p < 0.01$ compared to basal.

presence of these stores in the central nervous system has been hard to find and most neurons either do not express them, or do so under very particular circumstances such as $[Ca^{++}]_i$ overload during membrane depolarization (Kostyuk and Tepikin, 1991; Fohrman et al., 1993).

DISCUSSION

Neural Development and Schizophrenia

Schizophrenics have a higher rate of perinatal and obstetric complications, as well as more congenital and minor physical abnormalities than the general population (Nasrallah, 1993), indicating a disrupted developmental process. In addition, structural brain abnormalities suggestive of developmental deviation have been repeatedly shown by *in vivo* imaging in schizophrenic patients (Shelton & Weinberger, 1986; Nasrallah, 1993), and children at risk for schizophrenia manifest early neurointegrative deficits, which also suggest a defect in maturation of the central nervous system (Fish et al., 1992). Because the lesions listed in schizophrenics affect developmental steps that span throughout the fetal life, there is a high degree of controversy as to the timing of the that would cause the clinical symptoms of the disease (Nasrallah, 1993). Evidence that exposure to the influenza virus during *the second trimester* of pregnancy significantly increases the risk for schizophrenia in the offspring (Mednick et al., 1988; Barr et al., 1990; O'Callaghan et al., 1992) is the only instance in which a critical period has been identified that could explain the appearance of the clinical syndrome of schizophrenia.

As pointed out by Nasrallah (1993): *"Despite the abundance of evidence for a disruption of neurodevelopment in schizophrenia, the nature of this perturbation remains a mystery."* The data presented here can be best discussed in the context of their relevance for the stated problem, since they may shed some light precisely on *"the nature of the perturbation"* leading to decreased dopaminergic activity in the mesocortical system.

Expression of calcium binding proteins CR and CB follows that of TH hydroxylase in the VTA in rat embryos with a delay, so that by E14 no dopaminergic neurons seem to express CR or CB, whereas by E20 most of them do (Liu and Graybiel, 1992; Abbott and Jacobowitz, 1993). Since stimulation of AMPA subtype glutamatergic receptors appears to be toxic for dopaminergic neurons at a time when they do not express calcium binding proteins (Figure 1), the presence of such a timeshift between the expression of the two proteins can be viewed as a vulnerable window for this neuronal subpopulation. Most interestingly, this window corresponds to the human second trimester of pregnancy, which has been shown to be linked to a liability to acquire schizophrenia (Mednick et al., 1988; Barr et al., 1990).

As mentioned before, AMPA receptor-mediated induction of calcium binding proteins has been reported in Purkinje neurons in the cerebellum (Batini et al., 1993). Protective effects of CB have also been repeatedly reported in adult dopaminergic neurons in the substantia nigra, particularly in the context of parkinsonism (v.g., Iacopino & Christakos, 1990). However, a direct relationship between developmental expression of TH and CR with sensitivity to excitatory aminoacid-induced toxicity, at a time corresponding to the human susceptible period (to influenza) is not yet available.

Neuropathology of Schizophrenia: Primary Versus Secondary Neurodevelopmental Lesions

Histopathological changes have been identified in the prefrontal cortex (Benes et al., 1986; Akbarian et al., 1993a), entorhinal cortex (Arnold et al., 1991; Falkai & Bogerts, 1991; Akbarian et al., 1993b), hippocampus and parahippocampus (Conrad et al., 1991; Jeste & Lohr, 1989; Akbarian et al., 1993b) of post-mortem schizophrenic brains. Altogether, these findings consistently suggest disruptions in at least one neurodevelopmental process, possibly including neuronal proliferation and elimination, migration, sprouting and elongation, and pruning (Nasrallah, 1993).

However, given the intense interconnection among all the structures where structural abnormalities have been found, it is extremely difficult to establish what is the effect of the primary etiologic process, and what is the transformation of related structures secondary to neural plasticity (Weinberger, 1987; Carlsson & Carlsson, 1990; Nasrallah, 1993). Thus, although several theoretical models have been proposed, there is a paucity of experimental data which could provide information on the possible pathogenetic mechanisms involved in the primary lesion(s) (Nasrallah, 1993).

Pathogenesis of Schizophrenia: Calcium-Binding proteins, Apoptosis and the Ventral Tegmental Area

At least *in vitro*, stimulation of AMPA-sensitive glutamate receptor activation can trigger a calcium dependent process leading to selective death of dopaminergic neurons (de Erausquin et al., 1993). This process depends upon activation of Ca^{++}-induced Ca^{++}-release from intracellular stores by extracellular Ca^{++} entering the neurons through L-type voltage dependent calcium channels (de Erausquin et al., 1993). Unpublished data from our laboratory suggest that AMPA receptor agonists induce a series of morphological changes in TH-immunoreactive neurons that are suggestive of pruning of the dendritic tree followed by possibly cell death (manuscript in preparation). However, although the developmental expression of CR and TH in rat embryos at a later time (Liu and Graybiel, 1992) suggests that this effect should be protected by the expression of CR in the same neurons, direct evidence for such an event is lacking. Indeed, mesencephalic dopaminergic neurons do not survive well in culture if plated after E14, making these experiments unattainable at the present time.

Selective dopaminergic neuronal death in mesencephalic cultures differs from other models of excitotoxicity in several important ways. Indeed, the time course of cell death (present only after 6 to 24 hours) does not coincide with delayed excitotoxicity in other neuronal *in vitro* systems (v.g.,de Erausquin & al, 1990), but may represent programmed cell death (Gerschenson and Rotello, 1992). AMPA or Kainate receptor-induced cell death in most other systems requires very prolonged exposures (Koh et al., 1990; Weiss & al, 1990), in the range of hours, whereas it has been shown that a brief exposure to AMPA may determine the fate of dopaminergic neurons at least under certain experimental conditions (de Erausquin et al., 1993).

So, is it possible that programmed cell death could be involved in selective dopaminergic cell death? Several pieces of indirect evidence seem to support this hypothesis. Apoptosis is in many cell systems, including neurons, a $[Ca^{++}]_i$ dependent process (Lee et al., 1993).

In prostate cell lines expression of a hybrid calbindin gene is specifically associated with protection against apoptosis in the absence of hormone (Lee et al., 1993), and overexpression of CB protects lymphocytes against glucocorticoid, cAMP and calcium ionophore-induced apoptosis (Lee et al., 1993). Protection against apoptosis has been demonstrated also in PC12 cells (a rat pheochromocytoma cell line which may express a well characterized dopaminergic neuronal phenotype) by treatment with Nerve Growth Factor (NGF) (Mesner et al., 1992), which induces the expression of two calcium-binding proteins with some homology to the ones discussed here (Altman, 1992).

In neurons with a dopaminergic phenotype, there is also some indirect evidence that oxidative stress can induce programmed cell death. Brain Derived Neurotrophic Factor protects against 6-OH-dopamine toxicity in a human dopaminergic neuroblastoma cell line by induction of glutathione reductase (Spina et al., 1992). Expression of *c-jun* and *c-fos* proto-oncogenes is rapidly induced in cell lines undergoing apoptosis (Lee et al., 1993), and in rat SNc dopaminergic neurons, 6-OH-dopamine lesions induced a substantial increase in *c-jun* (but not *c-fos*) proto-oncogene expression (Jenkins et al., 1993). However, AMPA induced neurotoxicity does not seem to involve production of free radicals, since cotreatment with superoxide dismutase (SOD) did not protect TH-immunoreactive neurons in preliminary experiments (unpublished data).

Overexpression of the proto-oncogene *bcl-2* prevents apoptosis in sympathetic neurons (García et al., 1992), as well as in neuronal PC12 (Mah et al., 1993). Interestingly, the *bcl-2* protein is membrane bound, and is associated with the nuclear envelope, the endoplasmic reticulum, and the inner mitochondrial membrane (Jacobson et al., 1993). However, human mutant cell lines that lack mitochondrial DNA, and therefore do not have a functional respiratory chain, can still be induced to die by apoptosis, and they can be protected by overexpression of *bcl-2*, suggesting that neither apoptosis nor the protective effect of *bcl-2* depend on mitochondrial respiration (Jacobson et al., 1993). On the other hand, they also suggest that the protective effect of *bcl-2* can not be mediated by an alteration in mitochondrial function (Jacobson et al., 1993).

In summary, the data presented demonstrate the existence of a susceptible period during rat neural development, in the course of which dopaminergic neurons in rat mesencephalon have not yet started to express CR or CB. Based on the known data on expression of calcium binding proteins, it can be predicted that dopaminergic neurons will loose their sensitivity to AMPA receptor agonists after E20, and into adulthood. We submit that these data represent a model for the human susceptible period during the second trimester of pregnancy. If the mother is exposed to influenza (or a similar environmental injury), increased glutamatergic stimulation of the dopaminergic neurons in the VTA would result excessive pruning of their dendritic tree and possibly in neuronal death, thus accounting for the presence of *negative symptoms* in the schizophrenic subject. Over time, *positive symptoms* would develop as a consequence of compensatory increases in the activity of the mesolimbic dopaminergic system, as suggested by Weinberger (1987).

REFERENCES

Akbarian S., Bunney W.E., Potkin S.G., Wigal S.B., Hagman J.O, Sandman C.A. and Jones E.G.: Altered distribution of NADPH-diaphorase cells in frontal lobe of schizophrenics implies disturbances of cortical development. Arch. Gen. Psych., **50**: 169-177 (1993).

Akbarian S., Vinuela A., Kim J.J., Potkin S.G., Bunney W.E. and Jones E.G.: Distorted distribution of NADPH-diaphorase neurons in temporal lobe of schizophrenics implies anomalous cortical development. Arch. Gen. Psych., **50**: 178-187 (1993).

Altman J.: Programmed cell death: the paths to suicide. TiNS, **15**: 278-281 (1992).

Andreasen N.C.: Neural mechanisms of negative symptoms. Brit. J. Psych. **155**, Supp. 7: 93-98 (1989).

Araneda R. and Bustos G.: Modulation of dendritic release of dopamine by NMDA receptors in substantia nigra. J. Neurochem., **52**: 962-997 (1989).

Arias Montano J.A., Martinez-Fong D. and Aceves J.: Glutamatic stimulation of tyrosine hydroxylase is mediated by NMDA receptors in the rat striatum. Brain Res. **569**: 317-322 (1992).

Arnold S.E., Hyman B.T., Van Hoesen G.W. and Damasio A.R.: Some cytoarchitectural abnormalities of the entorhinal cortex in schizophrenia. Arch. Gen. Psych., **47**: 625-632 (1991).

Barr C.E., Mednick S.A. and Munk-Jorgensen P.: Exposure to influenza epidemics during gestation and adult schizophrenia. A 40 year study. Arch. Gen. Psych., **47**: 869-874 (1990).

Benes F.M., Davidson J. and Bird E.D.: Quantitative cytoarchitectural studies of the cerebral cortex of schizophrenics. Arch. Gen. Psych., **43**: 31-35 (1986).

Bowyer J.F., Scallet A.C., Holson R.R., Lipe G.W., Slikker W. Jr., and Ali S.F.: Interactions of MK-801 with glutamate, glutamine and methamphetamine evoked release of [3H]dopamine from striatal slices. J. Pharmacol. Exp. Ther. **257**: 262-270 (1991).

Carlsson M. and Carlsson A.: Schizophrenia: A subcortical neurotransmitter imbalance syndrome? Schizophrenia Bull., **16**: 425-432 (1990).

Celio M.R.: Calbindin-D28K and parvalbumin in the rat nervous system. Neuroscience, **35**: 375-475 (1990).

Conrad A.J., Abebe T., Austin R., Forsythe S. and Scheibel A.B.: Hippocampal pyramidal cell disarray in schizophrenia as a bilateral phenomenon. Arch. Gen. Psych., **48**: 413-417 (1991).

de Erausquin G.A., Manev H., Guidotti A., Costa E, and Brooker G.: Gangliosides normalize distorted single cell $[Ca^{++}]_i$ dynamics after toxic doses of glutamate in cerebellar granule cells. Proc. Natl. Acad. Sci., **87**: 8017-8021 (1990).

de Erausquin, G.A., Brooker G., and Hanbauer I.: K+-evoked dopamine release depends on a cytosolic Ca++ pool regulated by N-type calcium channels. Neurosci. Lett. **145**: 121-125 (1992).

de Erausquin, G.A., Brooker G., Costa E. and Hanbauer I.: Persistent AMPA stimulation alters $[Ca^{++}]_i$ homeostasis in cultures of embryonic dopaminergic neurons. Mol. Brain Res., (1994, in press).

Falkai P. and Bogerts B.: Qualitative and quantitative assessment of pre-alpha cell clusters in the entorrhinal cortex of schizophrenics. A neurodevelopmental model of schizophrenia? Schizophrenia Res., **4**: 357-358 (1991).

Fish B., Marcus J., Hans S.L., Auerbach J.G. and Perdue S.: Infants at risk for schizophrenia: Sequelae of a genetic-neurointegrative defect. Arch. Gen. Psych., **46**: 221-235 (1992).

Fohrman E.B., de Erausquin G.A., Costa E. and Wojcik W.: Muscarinic m3 receptors and dynamics of intracellular calcium in cerebellar granule neurons. Eur. J. Pharmacol. (Mol. Pharmacol. Section), **245**: 263-271 (1993).

García I., Martinou I., Tsujimoto Y. and Martinou J.C.: Prevention of programmed cell death of sympathetic neurons by the bcl-2 proto-oncogene. Science, **258**: 302-304 (1992).

Girault J.A., Halpain S. and Greengard P.: Excitatory aminoacids antagonists and Parkinson's Disease. TiNS, **13**: 325-326 (1990).

Greenamyre J.T. and O'Brien C.F.: NMDA antagonists in the treatment of Parkinson's Disease. Arch. Neurol. **48**: 977-981 (1991).

Hanbauer I., Wink D., Osawa Y, Edelman G.M. and Gally J.A.: Role of nitric oxide in NMDA evoked release of [3H] dopamine from striatal slices. NeuroReport, **3**: 409-412 (1992).

Iacopino A.M. and Christakos S.: Specific reduction of calcium binding protein (28KD calbinidin-D) gene expression in aging and neurodegenerative diseases. Proc. Natl. Acad. Sci., **87**: 4078-4082 (1990).

Jacobowitz D. & Winsky L.: Immunocytochemical localization of calretinin in the forebrain of the rat. J. Comp. Neurol., **304**: 198-218 (1991).

Jacobson M.D., Burne J.F., King M.P., Miyashita T., Reed J.C. and Raff M.C.: bcl-2 blocks apoptosis in cells lacking mitochondrial DNA. Nature, **361**: 365-369 (1993).

Jenkins R., O'Shea R., Thomas K.L. and Hunt S.P.: c-jun Expression in substantia nigra neurons following 6-OH dopamine lesions in the rat. Neurosci. **53**: 447-455 (1993).

Jeste S.D. and Lohr J.B.: Hippocampal pathologic findings in schizophrenia: a morphometric study. Arch. Gen. Psych., **46**: 1019-1024 (1989).

Kilindreas K., Latov N., Strauss D.H., Gorig A.D., Hashim G.A., Gorman J.M. and Sadig S.A.: Antibodies to the human 60 kDa heat-shock protein in patients with schizophrenia. Lancet, **340**: 569-572 (1992).

Kluge H. and Kuhne G.E.: Preliminary findings on calmodulin stimulated Ca++-ATPase of erythrocytic ghosts on psychotic patients. Eur. Arch. Psych. Neurol. Sci., **235**: 57-59 (1985)..

Koh J.-Y., Goldberg M.P., Hartley D.M. and Choi D.W.: Non-NMDA receptor mediated neurotoxicity in cortical culture. J/ Neurosci., **10**: 693-705 (1990)

Kornhuber J.: Glutamate and schizophrenia (letter). TiPS, **11**: 357 (1990).

Kostyuk P.G. & Tepikin A.V.: Calcium signals in nerve cells. NIPS, **6**: 6-10 (1991).

Krebs M.O., Desce J.M, Kemel M.L., Gauchy C., Godeheu G., Cheramy A and Glowinsky J.: Glutamatergic control of dopamine release in the rat striatum: evidence presynaptic NMDA receptors in dopaminergic nerve terminals. J. Neurochem., **56**: 81-85 (1991).

Krystal J.H., et al.: Subanesthetic effects of the non-competitive NMDA antagonist ketamine in humans. Arch. Gen. Psych., (1992, in press).

Lee S., Christakos S. and Small M.B.: Apoptosis and signal transduction: clues to a molecular mechanism. Curr. Opin. in Cell Biol., **5**: 266-291 (1993).

Liu F.C. and Graybiel A.M.: Heterogeneous development of calbindin-D28K expression in the striatal matrix. J. Comp. Neurol., **320**: 304-322 (1992).

Lledo P.M., Somasundaram B., Norton A.J., Emson P.C. and Mason W.T.: Stable transfection of calbinin-D28K into the GH3 cell line alters calcium currents and intracellular calcium homeostasis. Neuron **9**: 943-954 (1992).

Llinas R., Greenfield S.A. and Jahnsen H.: Electrophysiology of pars compacta cells in the in vitro substantia nigra - a possible mechanism of dendritic release. Brain Res., **294**: 127-132 (1984).

Maggio R., Liminga U. and Gale K.: Selective stimulation of kainate but not quisqualate or NMDA receptors in substantia nigra evokes limbic motor seizures. Brain Res., **258**: 223-230 (1990).

Martin L.J., Blackstone C.D., Levey A.I., Huganir R.L. and Price D.L.: AMPA glutamate receptor subunits are differentially distributed in rat brain. Neurosci., **53**: 327-358 (1993).

Mednick S.A., Máchon R.A., Huttunen M.O., and Bonnett D.: Adult schizophrenia following prenatal exposure to an influenza epidemic. Arch. Gen. Psych., **45**: 189-192 (1988).

Mercuri N.B., Stratta F., Calabresi P. and Bernardi G.: Electrophysiological evidence for the presence of ionotropic and metabotropic EAA receptors on dopaminergic neurons of the rat mesencephalon. An in-vitro study. Funct. Neurol. **7**: 231-234 (1992).

Mereu G., Costa E., Armstrong D.M. and Vicine S.: Glutamate receptors subtypes mediate excitatory synaptic currents of dopamine neurons in mid-brain slices. J. Neurosci. **11**: 1356-1366 (1991).

Mesner P.W., Winters T.R. and Grenn S.H.: Nerve growth factor withdrawal-induced cell death in neuronal PC12 cells resembles that in sympathetic neurons. J. Cell Biol., **119**: 1669-1680 (1992).

Nasrallah H.A.: Neurodevelopmental pathogenesis of Schizophrenia. Psych. Clin. North Am., **16**: 269-280 (1993).

O'Callaghan E., Sham P., Takei N., Glover G. and Murray R.M.: Schizophrenia after prenatal exposure to 1957 Az influenza epidemic. Lancet, **2(337)**: 1248-1250 (1992).

Petralia R.S. and Wenthold R.J.: Light and electron immunocytochemical localization of AMPA-selective glutamate receptors in the ray brain. J. Comp. Neurol., **318**: 329-354 (1992).

Raff M.C., Barres B.A., Burne J.F., Coles H.S., Ishizaki Y. and Jacobson M.D.: Programmed cell death and the control of cell survival: lessons from the nervous system. Science, **262**: 695-700 (1993).

Resibois A., and Rogers J.H.: Calretinin in rat brain: an immunohistochemical study. Neurosci. **46**: 101-134 (1992).

Reynolds G.P.: Developments in the drug treatment of schizophrenia. Trends Pharmacol. Sci. **13**: 116-121 (1992).

Rogers J.H.: Calretinin: a gene for a novel calcium binding protein expressed principally in neurons. J. Cell Biol. **105**: 1343-1353 (1987).

Schmidt W.J., Bubser M., and Hauber W.: Excitatory aminoacids and Parkinson's Disease (reply). Trends Neurosci., **13**: 327 (1990).

Shelton R.C. and Weinberger D.R.: X-ray computerized tomography studies in schizophrenia: a review and synthesis. *in*: Nasrallah HA (*ed*): The Handbook of Schizophrenia, vol. 1. Amsterdam, Elsevier Sci. Pub. (1986). pp: 207-250

Spina M.B., Squinto S.P., Miller J., Lindsay R.M. and Hyman C.: Brain-derived neurotrophic factor protects dopamine neurons against 6-OH-dopamine and N-methyl-4-phenyl-pyridinium ion toxicity: involvement of the glutathione system. J. Neurochem. **59**: 99-106 (1992).

Wachtel H. and Turski L.: Glutamate: A new target in schizophrenia? Trends Pharmacol. Sci. **11**: 219-220 (1990).

Weinberger D.R.: Implications of normal brain development for the pathogenesis of schizophrenia. Arch. Gen Psych., **44**: 660-669 (1987).

Weiss J.H., Hartley D.M., Koh J-Y, and Choi D.W.: The calcium channel blocker nifedipine attenuates slow excitatory amino acid neurotoxicity. Science, **247**: 1474-1477 (1990).

CHILDHOOD RISK FACTORS FOR ADULT SCHIZOPHRENIA IN A GENERAL POPULATION BIRTH COHORT AT AGE 43 YEARS

Peter Jones[1], Robin Murray[1], and Bryan Rodgers[2]

[1]Department of Psychological Medicine, Institute of Psychiatry, De Crespigny Park, London United Kingdom

[2]NH & MRC Social Psychiatry Research Unit, The Australian National University, Canberra, ACT, Australia

INTRODUCTION

The search for risk factors for many chronic, physical illnesses of adult life has begun to concentrate on childhood, and sometimes even fetal life (Barker et al., 1989; Barker et al., 1990; Godfrey et al., 1993; Fine et al., 1985; Barker & Osmond, 1986; Colley et al., 1973; Martyn et al., 1988). Mechanisms which may explain these child-adult continuities include the programming thought to occur following impaired fetal nutrition and growth (Poskitt & Cole, 1977; Lucas, 1991), and infections, both *in utero* (Fine et al., 1985) and in childhood (Pullen & Hay, 1982). Continuities between early factors and adult psychological morbidity have been accepted for considerably longer, and exploration of possible mechanisms for the link has given rise to several explanatory models.

For some psychiatric conditions, such as childhood conduct disorder and adult antisocial personality disorder, continuities are clear between similar symptoms in childhood and adult life; it appears that the adult illness itself is already manifest in childhood, there being no period of discontinuity between early appearance of a risk factor and the adult condition (Robins, 1966; Rutter & Giller, 1983). For others, such as depression and the emotional or neurotic disorders, continuity of symptoms from childhood to adult life is less common. However, it is becoming increasingly recognised, and models of psychosocial risk involving the establishment in childhood of "vulnerability" have been proposed on the basis of empirical data (Rodgers, 1990 a&b; Rutter, 1984).

Neural Development and Schizophrenia, Edited by S.A. Mednick
and J.M. Hollister, Plenum Press, New York, 1995

Schizophrenia has been linked to psychological abnormalities in childhood since the first clear descriptions of the illness (Kraepelin, 1896; 1919). However, these abnormalities, which include social awkwardness and withdrawal (Watt, 1978), are different from those characterising the adult, positive schizophrenic syndrome, such as hallucinations, delusions, and disorders of thought form and structure. It remains unclear whether these childhood abnormalities render an individual vulnerable to a quite separate, schizophrenic illness later in life, or whether they are the earliest manifestations of that illness itself, changing in character as the brain matures and the personality develops.

Neuropathological studies of adults with schizophrenia indicate that developmental processes may have gone awry in some areas, particulary in the formation of hippocampal structures (Roberts, 1990). Pregnancy and delivery complications have been found to be more common in the histories of adults with schizophrenia than controls in many (O'Callaghan et al., 1990; Lewis et al., 1989) although not all studies (Done et al., 1991; Buka et al., 1993). Similarly, there is evidence from population samples of an association of schizophrenia with prenatal exposure to influenza (Mednick et al., 1988; Sham et al., 1992; but see also Crow, 1992; Crow & Done, 1992; Selten & Slaets, 1994), maternal malnutrition (Susser & Lin, 1992)and, possibly, with urban rather than rural upbringing (Lewis et al., 1992).

These strands of evidence in favour of some early abnormality in schizophrenia continue through childhood. Many studies indicate that mean childhood intelligence test scores were lower in adults with schizophrenia than in control groups (Aylward et al., 1984), and subtle differences in neurological development have been demonstrated in both unselected schizophrenic subjects (Walker & Lewine, 1990) and children at high genetic risk of the disorder (Fish, 1977; Erlenmeyer-Kimling et al., 1982; Fish et al., 1992). Evidence of childhood develomental deviance in around one third of adults with schizophrenia has given rise to the notion of a distinct, neurodevelopmental subtype of the disorder.

However, demonstrating associations between early childhood events and adult outcome presents particular methodological problems which may have clouded the true picture. Not only are retrospective designs prone to differential recall bias resulting in spurious associations, but there is also the possibility that subtle effects remain undetected due merely to random inaccuracies in the recall of events occurring long ago. Exposures tend to be classified as either present or absent, and the subsequent consideration of the nature of the risk conferred is similarly dichotomised (Gittleman-Klein & Klein, 1969; Cannon-Spoor et al., 1982; Watt & Lubensky, 1976; Done, et al 1994). Moreover, few studies in this area have had population controls available and most rely on demonstrating differences in group means, leading to further emphasis on 'abnormality' versus 'normality', as well as to lack of comparibility between studies. The notion of the distribution of risk conferred by early factors in the population as a whole has not been investigated.

This investigation aimed to characterise in a general population sample, associations between adult onset schizophrenia and childhood behavioural, social, intellectual and neurodevelopmental factors. We were fortunate in that the data allowed emphasis on the distribution of risks within the population and the investigation of individual development. The aims of this initial study were twofold. We wished to assess, in a general population sample, associations which have been demonstrated in previous studies between adult schizophrenia and childhood characteristics in sociodemographic, neurodevelopmental, behavioural and intellectual domains. Secondly, we wished to examine the longitudinal course of developmental differences between cases and their peers in the cohort.

METHODS

Sample

The study sample was drawn from the Medical Research Council National Survey of Health and Development (NSHD). This is a stratified, random sample (n=5362) of a survey of births in England, Scotland and Wales during the week 3-9th March 1946 (RCOG, 1948). The original survey, comprising 13,687 mothers, was carried out due to concerns over a fall in the birth rate (which proved unfounded) and in order to collect information intended for use in planning for the National Health Service which would be introduced in 1948 (Wadsworth, 1987). Following a decision championed by Dr James Douglas and colleagues, the present sample was followed-up. Data on this cohort, described elsewhere extensively (Atkins et al., 1981; Wadsworth, 1991), were collected on 11 occasions before age 16 years and, so far, on 9 thereafter. The risk set (ie survey members at risk of being identified as schizophrenic in adulthood) used in this investigation comprised all subjects alive and living in the U.K. at age 16 years (n=4746).

Identification of Cases

Cases of schizophrenia with onset between ages 16 and 43 years, when the most recent NSHD interview occurred, were defined using a two stage screen. This aimed at high specificity (low proportion of false positives in the cases), rather than high sensitivity (high proportion of true positives identified as cases), although we believe the latter was, in fact, achieved.

The first stage identified all survey members for whom there was any evidence to suggest schizophrenia, severe unclassified mental illness, unspecified psychiatric hospital admission or use of prescribed neuroleptic drugs, using the following sources:

i) The 9 questionnaire and interview contacts made between 16 and 43 years of age made enquiries into all hospital in- and out-patient contacts, general practice visits, and recorded survey members' own descriptions of their illnesses and prescribed neuroleptic drug use.

ii) Appearances in the Mental Health Enquiry (MHE) for England and Wales which were identified up to age 36 years, and up to age 44 for the Scottish MHE. These data were independent of follow-up by the National Survey.

iii) A short version (Rodgers & Mann, 1986) of the Present State Examination (PSE; Wing et al., 1974) administered at age 36, which included probe questions for psychosis.

In the second stage, DSM-IIIR (APA, 1987) operational criteria for schizophrenia or schizo-affective disorder were applied to all clinical material on survey members thus identified, blind to all information collected between birth and 16 years. Clinical information was available from a variety of sources including abstracted details of mental state during admissions and from complete case notes. The former, and sometimes the latter, were supplied by hospitals in response to routine requests by the NSHD whenever a hospital admission had been identified and for those who responded positively to probes for psychosis in the short PSE. Survey members also described their symptoms during the routine interviews.

In order to investigate the effect of diagnostic misclassification, cases of schizophrenia were divided according to the certainty of diagnosis. Group 1 comprised those who fulfilled DSM-IIIR criteria for schizophrenia or schizo-affective disorder. Group 2 comprised those where positive DSM-IIIR criteria were fulfilled, but where no statement could be found of relevant exclusions. For example, positive schizophrenic phenomena were described, but affective symptoms were not mentioned and so could not be excluded. Age at onset was defined as the age at which a case was first seen by a psychiatrist or, when unavailable, the age at which NSHD records first indicated a psychiatric problem.

Control subjects were defined as the entire risk set, excluding those identified as cases of schizophrenia.

Selection of Variables of Interest Analyzed as Exposures

In order to avoid multiple comparisons, and guided by the existing literature on antecedents of adult schizophrenia, variables referring to the period prior to age 16 were selected for analysis in the following four domains:

socio-demographic, e.g. socio-economic class & sex
physical and neuro-developmental, e.g. sexual maturity & motor milestones
cognitive e.g. educational attainment test scores
socio-behavioural e.g. mothers' and teachers' comments on behaviour.

Where possible, variables were selected where data existed for more than one age enabling assessment of developmental change. Variables examined, together with their derivation, are summarised in the Appendix.

Statistical Analysis

Associations between schizophrenia and the childhood variables were expressed in terms of odds ratios (OR) corrected in logistic regression models for confounding by sex and socioeconomic status (s.e.s.) which was defined on the basis of father's occupation. For variables up to age 8, s.e.s. at birth was used, otherwise that at age 15 was employed. With such a rare outcome as schizophrenia, these odds ratios provide a convenient and accurate estimate of incidence rate ratios, i.e. a comparison of the incidence of schizophrenia in individuals from two groups. Initial analysis of continuous variables was performed using tertiles of normal distributions (Breslow & Day, 1980). Linear trends in risk were assessed and where present, these variables were subsequently modelled in their continuous form. Principal components analysis (Pearson, 1901; Manly, 1986) was used to reduce the complexity of educational test data, where several tests had been administered at each age.

A measure of individual "deviance" from the control mean, measured in units of standard normal deviates, was calculated for variables which had been shown to differentiate cases from controls in univariate analyses. A positive or negative value was assigned according to what constituted a desirable score e.g. late attainment of motor milestones (a value higher than the control mean) was assigned a negative standard normal deviate score whereas for the cognitive tests, a negative score was assigned to values lower than the control mean. Scores for variables at each age were summated to give a score for each individual. Cumulative scores were then calculated and analyzed graphically in order to provide a pictorial representation of different developmental trajectories in the cases and controls.

Table 1. Occupational group of father at birth of survey member. Trend for higher status in cases.

Socio-economic group at birth	Cases	Controls	Odds ratio vs I & II (95% c.i.)
I & II	9	1077	1
III non-manual	9	1149	0.9 (0.3 - 2.6)
III manual	8	1262	0.8 (0.3 - 2.2)
IV & V	4	1214	0.4 (0.1 - 1.4)

χ^2 test for trend 2.5 p=0.1

RESULTS

Four thousand seven hundred and forty six (4746) subjects, alive and living in the U.K. at age 16 years, constituted the risk set. There were 2477 males (52.2%). There were 81 survey members for whom there was evidence, up to age 43 years and eight months, of a diagnosis of schizophrenia, use of regular neuroleptic medication, undefined severe mental illness or a psychiatric admission for unknown cause. Of these, 30 (20 male) were classified as cases of schizophrenia, 22 (73%) fell into group one, as defined above. Controls were the 4716 subjects (2457 men, 52.1%) remaining in the risk set.

Age at onset of schizophrenia. The mean age at onset of schizophrenia in the risk set was 24.3 years (95% c.i. 21.5 - 27; median 21.5 years; range 17 - 43 years). Males had an earlier mean age at onset (23.4 years; 95% c.i. 19.8 - 27.1) than females (25.9 years; 95% c.i. 21.6 - 30.2).

Risk of schizophrenia. Risk of schizophrenia up to age 43 years was 30/4746 = 0.63% (95% c.i. 0.41 - 0.86%). The risk for males (0.81% 95% c.i. 0.45 - 1.2) was greater than that for females (0.44%, 95% c.i. 0.17 - 0.71) but this difference did not reach conventional statistical significance (OR 1.8, 95% c.i. 0.9 - 3.9).

Sociodemographic Characteristics

Social class of survey member at birth is shown in Table 1. There was a trend for higher social class to be associated with cases, but this was small and non-significant (χ^2 trend 2.5, p=0.1). Similarly, there was no evidence of associations between cases and either the administrative characteristics or population size of the place of birth (Tables 2a & 2b). Classification of father's occupation when the survey members were 15 revealed a pattern similar to that at birth.

At age 4, a composite measure of material home circumstances (Table 3) was derived from health visitors' reports of 8 factors concerning the state of housing, crowding therein and a subjective rating of mothering skills (Rodgers, 1978). The impression persisted from the 1946 data of higher risk of schizophrenia in those from more advantaged homes (χ^2 trend 3.0, p=0.08). This small advantage was apparent for all the individual variables except one. Health visitors rated mothers of cases as having worse than average general understanding and management of their child significantly more frequently than controls, independent of social class and sex of their child (OR 5.8, 0.8-31.8, p=0.02). When the children were age 7, 11, 13 and 16, their teachers had been asked to estimate the parental interest in the child's progress at school as "very interested", "average interest" and "low interest". At no age did teachers consider that the parents of the cases had low interest in their child's education.

Table 2a. Administrative classification of birth place.

Administrative area type	Cases (%)	Controls (%)
London	825 (17.5)	2 (6.7)
County urban borough	1507 (32)	7 (23.3)
Municipal borough	725 (15.4)	7 (23.3)
Urban district or small town	703 (14.9)	5 (16.7)
Rural district - villages	2 (0.0)	0
Rural district - parishes	806 (17.1)	7 (23.7)
Towns	116 (2.5)	1 (3.3)
New towns	30 (0.6)	1 (3.3)

Table 2b. Trend for less urban birth place to predict cases.

Recoded administrative area	Cases (%)	Controls (%)	Odds ratio
Cities	16 (53.3)	3057 (64.8)	1
Towns	7 (23.3)	849 (18)	1.6 (0.7-2.1)
Rural communities	7 (23.3)	808 (17.1)	1.7 (0.8-2.1)

χ^2 test for trend 1.5, p=0.2

Table 3. Composite score of home circumstances at age 4 years.

Home circumstances age 4*	Cases (%)	Controls (%)	Odds ratio
Very poor	1 (4.2)	334 (8.5)	1
Poor	4 (16.7)	975 (24.8)	1.4 (0.2 - 12.3)
Reasonable	6 (25)	1186 (30.2)	1.7 (0.2 - 14.1)
Good	13 (54.2)	1438 (36.6)	3.0 (0.4 - 23.3)

Trend $\chi^2 = 3.0, p = 0.08$

Milestones and Physical Development

Early developmental milestones. At age two years health visitors asked mothers the age to the nearest month that the survey members reached the following milestones:- sitting alone, standing alone, walking alone, cutting first tooth, talking - "...other than mumma, dadda or nan".

The mean ages at which speech and gross motor milestones were reached was consistently later for the cases than for controls (Table 4), particularly for walking (cases 1.2 months later, 95% c.i. difference 0.1 - 2.3 months later, p=0.005). The later

156

age at talking of the cases was considerably confounded by sex; in the controls, girls spoke earlier than boys by an average of 1 month (95% c.i. 0.75 - 1.27, p < 0.001). After correction for this effect and for social class, the effect for later talking in the cases remained non-significant and was reduced (OR = 1.1, 95% c.i. 1-1.2, p = 0.2).

Table 4. Age at reaching developmental milestones.

Milestone	Modal value*	Control mean* (s.d.)	Case-control difference* (95% c.i.)
Sitting	6	6.5 (1.5)	0.1 later (0.5 earlier - 0.8 later)
Standing	12	11.4 (2.2)	0.2 later (0.6 earlier - 1.0 later)
Walking	12	13.5 (2.4)	**1.2 later** (0.1 later - 2.3 later)
Teething	6	6.8 (2.2)	0.2 earlier (1.0 earlier - 0.6 later)
Talking	18	14.3 (4.2)	1.2 later (0.4 earlier - 2.8 later)

* months

A variable created following the interview at age 2 years identified survey members who had not yet reached all their milestones. There was an excess of cases over controls in this group, compared with the group where all milestones were seen by the health visitors to have been attained (2/25 cases versus 64/3854 controls; OR = 4.8, χ^2 = 5.4, p = 0.02). Closer examination revealed that, for both those cases, the health visitors had noted that speech had not been attained, whereas for the controls, there was an even spread between motor and language milestones.

Bladder and bowel control. There was no evidence that control of bladder and bowel function differed between cases and controls as children. At age 4 years, 1 case and 73 controls continued to be wet at night regularly (OR adjusted for sex and social class = 1.93; 95% c.i. 0.1 - 13.8) but by age 6 and thereafter, all cases had achieved bladder control at night. By day, all cases were continent at age six and remained so at age 11. The proportions of cases and controls achieving bowel control by ages 12 months, 18 months and six years were virtually identical. No case experienced bowel control problems after 6 years, as opposed to 170 (4%) of the controls.

General physical development and timing of puberty. There was no evidence of differences in general physical development between the cases and controls. This was the case whether odds or means, both adjusted for social class and sex, were examined for the following variables:- birth weight, height at ages 7 and 11, weight at age 7 and 11. No cases fell outside the range of two standard deviations around the control mean. As with general physical development, data recorded during medical examinations revealed no difference in the timing of puberty between cases and controls.

Cognitive Test Scores

Mean, unadjusted scores in the individual educational tests at ages 8, 11 and 13 years are reported elsewhere (Jones et al., 1994c). In essence, cases scored consistently lower than the controls in all tests, at all three ages. Some of these differences reached convential statistical significance, most did not, but the pattern was clear across all sub-scores. In general, this pattern of the differences between the means, together with the confidence limits, suggested that deficits in the scores of the cases were most marked for verbal, non-verbal and mathematical skills, and least for reading and vocabulary. However, these results were confounded by sex and social class (Atkins et al., 1981).

Table 5. Summary of test scores in terms of 1st principal component. Consistent trends for cases to be in the lower tertiles of performance.

AGE 8 - COGNITIVE TESTS - FIRST PRINCIPAL COMPONENT

Tertile	Cases	Controls	Crude OR*	Adjusted OR**
lowest	11	1372	1	1
middle	7	1374	0.6	0.6 (0.2 - 1.6)
highest	6	1376	0.5	0.5 (0.2 - 1.6)

χ^2 test for trend (crude) 1.6, p = 0.2

Summary odds ratio 0.7 χ^2 test for trend (adjusted for sex & social class) 1.9, p = 0.2

AGE 11 - COGNITIVE TESTS - FIRST PRINCIPAL COMPONENT

Tertile	Cases	Controls	Crude OR*	Adjusted OR**
lowest	14	1309	1	1
middle	6	1318	0.4	0.4 (0.1 - 1.1)
highest	6	1316	0.4	0.4 (0.1 - 1.2)

χ^2 test for trend (crude) 3.7, p = 0.05

Summary odds ratio 0.6 χ^2 test for trend (adjusted for sex & social class) 4.0, p = 0.05

AGE 15 - COGNITIVE TESTS - FIRST PRINCIPAL COMPONENT

Tertile	Cases	Controls	Crude OR*	Adjusted OR**
lowest	13	1310	1	1
middle	8	1315	0.6	0.6 (0.2 - 1.5)
highest	4	1317	0.3	0.3 (0.1 - 1.0)

χ^2 test for trend (crude) 4.9, p = 0.03

Summary odds ratio 0.5 χ^2 test for trend (adjusted for sex & social class) 6.2, p = 0.01

* Versus lowest tertile
** Adjusted for sex & social class

Principal components analysis of normalised scores resulted in a single factor, the first principal component (PC 1), explaining some 75% of the variance in scores at each age, and comprised similar (0.72 - 0.91) contributions from each sub-test. Mean values of PC 1, were lower in the cases than controls at age 8 (difference = 0.3, 95% c.i. -0.1 to 0.7), age 11 (difference = 0.2, 95% c.i. -0.1 to 0.5) and at 15 when the gap had widened (difference = 0.48, 95% c.i. 0.1 to 0.9). Division of the distribution of these scores in the controls into tertiles (Table 5) allowed testing of the specific hypothesis of a trend in the inverse association between schizophrenia and test score (i.e. a dose-response relationship between score and risk). The raw data form the body of the tables with the bottom line being a summary odds ratio adjusted for sex and social class, obtained from logistic regression. This represents the increased odds of developing schizophrenia if a score is in the middle tertile versus the highest group, or the lowest versus the middle. Similar results were obtained using quartiles but occasional empty cells hindered analysis. There was no evidence that a non-linear trend gave a better fit to the data, nor was there evidence of an interaction with gender; girls and boys were similar.

The impression gained from the initial investigation of differences in mean values was confirmed but the pattern in the adjusted odds ratios was clearer. Cases were consistently over-represented in the lowest third of the test scores, even at age 8, after which the effect appeared to become more marked. In a similar analysis of individual test scores (not displayed) trend test parameters were highest for non-verbal, verbal and mathematical tests. The tests of vocabulary differentiated least between cases and controls. Reading scores in childhood showed a pattern different from the other tests with the majority of the cases being in the middle tertile at age 15 and a fairly even distribution prior to that time.

The summary measure of IQ was made at three ages, 8, 11 and 15. Logistic regression was used to analyse these repeated measures, taking into account sex, social class, and the effect of previous score. Inclusion of the 1st PC score at age 15 into a model containing sex and social class resulted in a significant improvement in the fit of the model (reduction in deviance; likelihood ratio statistic (LRS) $= 7.7, p = 0.005$). Addition of the score at age 11 resulted in a slight decrease in deviance (LRS $= 1.3$; $p = 0.5$) and change in the odds ratio associated with the 15 year score (OR$=0.59$, p $= 0.03$). Similarly, addition of score at age 8 resulted in a tiny improvement in the fit of the model (LRS$=0.6$; $p = 0.7$) associated with a change in the odds ratio associated with the 15 year score which remained statistically significant (OR $= 0.64; p = 0.04$).

In conclusion, cases tended to score below the controls in all the tests at all three ages - low scores were associated with increased odds of becoming a case, regardless of sex or social class. This was particularly marked for non-verbal, verbal and mathematical tests. General ability was adequately summarised by the PC 1 at each age and this score was lower in cases than controls. The deficit between cases and controls became statistically significant at 15 and remained when regression to the mean in a logistic regression model was taken into account. It appeared that there was a trend for the deficit between cases and controls to become greater with age. Statistical analysis did not confirm this.

Social and Behavioural Characteristics

Play preference. At ages 4 and 6 predicted schizophrenia (Tables 6a & 6b). At both ages, children who displayed a preference for playing alone were more likely to become cases (age 4, OR $= 2.1, p = 0.05$; age 6, OR $= 2.5, p = 0.05$).

Teachers' comments at ages 13 and 15 years. At ages 13 and 15, teachers indicated that the children destined to be cases exhibited several behaviours more commonly than controls. Results are displayed in Table 7 where some items are noted at only one age due to data being unavailable for this analysis. Crude odds ratios refer to the effect in the schizophrenia group as a whole, followed by the effect size (OR) in girls and boys, separately. The final column for each age is the effect size adjusted for confounding by gender. These results need to be interpreted against the finding that, when given the opportunity to single-out individuals as mal-adjusted or problem-children, no teacher identified a child who developed schizophrenia. Thus, all the effects discussed below were likely to have been subtle, even in combination.

Table 6a. Play preference at ages 4.

	Plays alone	Plays with others
Cases	10	20
controls	876	3840
Odds ratio- crude & adjusted*	2.2 (1 - 4.9), p = 0.04; 2.1 (0.9 - 4.7), p = 0.05	

Table 6b. Play preference at ages 6.

	Plays alone	Plays with others
Cases	5	25
controls	355	4361
Odds ratio- crude & adjusted*	2.5 (0.8 - 6.6), p = 0.06; 2.5 (0.8 - 6.9), p = 0.05	

*Adjustment for sex made no difference to the effect size.

There appeared to be strong evidence of a constellation of "anxious", "solitary" behaviours to be noted by teachers when the children were both 13 and 15 years, when different teachers would have rated them. Both girls and boys were *tired and "washed-out"* in class, *avoided rough games and competition* with other children, and appeared *"gloomy"*. They were noted to *"day-dream"* frequently and to be timid in the classroom. At age 13 they were noted to have *problems making friends* and there was some evidence they were *ignored by other children*. At 15 years they were noted *not to be "dare-devils"*. The only behaviour which appeared to change dramatically between 13 and 15 for both boys and girls was *anxiety in class* where girls, particularly, showed a large effect at 13 for which there was little evidence at the later age.

In contrast to the excesses in these rather passive behaviours, neither girls nor boys destined to develop schizophrenia showed evidence of a tendency toward the more anti-social items or those suggesting over-activity and negative attitudes to others. Thus, there was no evidence of *disobedience, resentment of criticism, frequent discipline problems or restlessness during lessons*. There was some evidence at 15 of an association between *truanting* in girls; this may be considered not to be a manifestation of bad behaviour. In general, the majority of the odds ratios are scattered closely around unity, suggesting a truly negative result.

There was evidence that teachers considered that the children who would develop schizophrenia produced *poor or lazy work, not associated with poor concentration*. At 13, they were considered *unduly untidy*, although boys apparently lost this characteristic at the later age. Boys and girls were *poor at games and physical activities*. There were no cases who showed exceptional prowess at an out-of-school activity (Fisher exact test, 2-tailed, p=0.04) and both sexes showed an *excess of twitches and grimaces* at age 15.

Regarding differences between the observed associations for girls and boys, only cautious conclusions can be drawn regarding different odds ratios based on dividing-up

Table 7. Associations between adult onset schizophrenia and behaviour at age 13 and 15 years, as rated by class teachers. (OR = odds ratio)

Teachers' Comments on:-	Age 13 (1959)				Age 15 (1961)			
	Crude OR (95% c.i.)	OR for boys	OR for girls	Adjusted OR (95% c.i.)	Crude OR (95% cl)	OR for boys	OR for girls	Adjusted OR (95% cl)
Tired & Washed Out	3.4 (1-10.7) p=0.02	4.0	2.6	3.5 (1.01-11.7) p=0.02	3.8 (1.2-11.0) p=0.02	2.3**	10.5 p=0.001**	4.3 (1.3-12.4) p=0.002
Marked anxiety in class	3.8 (1.4-10.7)p=0.004	2.3	7.1 p<0.05	3.2 (1.2-9.2) p=0.01	1.1 (0.4-2.5) p=0.9	1.5	0.7	1.1 (0.5-2.8) p=0.9
Truants more than occasionally	Not available				1.6 (0.7-3.5) p=0.3	0.9	3.6 p=0.05	1.51 (0.7-3.4) p=0.7
Ignored by other children	2.3 (0.5-8.2) p=0.2	1.1**	5.6 p=0.02**	2.3 (0.5-8.1) p=0.2				
Shows marked changes in mood	0.8 (0.1-6.0) p=0.8	1.2		0.7 (0.04-5.5) p=0.8				
Avoids rough games	1.8 (0.7-4.6) p=0.2	1.7	2.5	2.0 (0.7-5.1) p=0.1	3.2 (1.3-7.7) p=0.01	2.5	7.9 p=0.004	3.7 (1.4-8.8) p=0.01
Avoids teachers' attention	2.04 (0.7-5.4) p=0.2	1.0**	5.6 p=0.007**	2.2 (0.8-5.9) p=0.08	0.9 (0.3-3.1) p=0.8	1.3	0.9	1.2 (0.3-3.6) p=0.8
Not a dare-devil	Not available				6.6 (1.5-2.4) p=0.001	9.0 p=0.001	5.7 p=0.07	7.6 (1.8-28) p<0.001
Avoids competition	3.4 (1.4-8.1) p=0.002	2.7 p=0.05	5.3 p=0.01	3.4 (1.4-7.8) p=0.002	3.0 (1.2-7.2) p=0.01	1.9**	8.9 p=0.002***	3.1 (1.2-7.4) p=0.006
Poor or lazy worker	2.2 (0.6-7.0) p=0.1	2.0	2.2	2.1 (0.6-6.5) p=0.2	3.4 (1.3-8.8) p=0.01	2.8 p=0.05	4.4 p=0.05	3.1 (1.2-8.1) p=0.008
Poor concentration	1.2 (0.4-3.8) p=0.8	1.2	1.1	1.2 (0.3-3.6) p=1.0	1.1 (3-3.5) p=0.8	1.0	1.2	1.0 (0.4-3.2) p=0.8
Very untidy	3.1 (1.1-8.3) p=0.01	2.8 p=0.05	2.5	2.7 (1.0-2.7) p=0.03	1.7 (0.4-5.9) p=0.4	1.1	3.8	1.4 (0.3-5.2) p=0.5
Work affected by environment (distractibility)	1.7 (0.4-6.2) p=0.3	2.4		1.7 (0.4-5.9) p=0.4				
Exceptional at out-of-school activities	None. Fisher exact test 2-tailed p=0.04							
Poor ability at physical games	3.1 (1.2-7.3) p=0.005	2.5 p=0.01	4.1 p=0.04	2.9 (1.2-7.00) p=0.008	3.8 (1.1-11.9) p=0.03	4.2	3.1	3.8 (1.1-12.1) p=0.03
Appears gloomy	4.02 (1-14.3) p=0.02	3.9	4.3	4.0 (0.9-14.3) p=0.02	3.8 (1.4-9.7) p=0.01	3.6 p=0.02	5.5 p=0.01	4.2 (1.5-11.0) p=0.001
Timid in class and not quarrelsome	2.1 (0.7-5.9) p=0.1	0.7**	6.9 p=0.002**	2.31 (0.7-6.0) p=0.1	2.0 (0.6-5.6) p=0.3	2.0	4.0	2.45 (0.8-7.0) p=0.1
Resentful of criticism	0.8 (0.1-3.5) p=0.8	0.7	1.1	0.9 (0.1-3.8) p=0.9	1.1 (0.4-3.0) p=0.9	1.4	0.6	1.1 (0.4-3) p=1.0
Sometime or frequently disobedient	0.9 (0.3-2.5) p=0.9	1.1	0.5	0.9 (0.3-2.4) p=1.0	1.1 (0.3-3.8) p=0.8	1.0	1.2	1.1 (0.3-3.8) p=0.8
Discipline a problem	0.8 (0.1-3.3) p=0.7	0.5	1.4	0.7 (0.1-3.3) p=0.9	0.9 (0.4-2.1) p=0.8	0.9	0.7	0.8 (0.3-2.0) p=0.8
Restless in class	1.3 (0.6-3.0) p=0.5	1.3	1.1	1.2 (0.5-2.82) p=0.8				
Frequently daydreams in class	2.9 (0.8-9.0) p=0.07	2.7	2.8	2.7 (0.8-8.5) p=0.1	4.6 (1.6-12.3) p=0.002	4.13 p=0.03	5.6 p=0.07	4.5 (1.6-12.2) p=0.002
Problems making friends	4.8 (1.4-15.0) p=0.002	3.1	8.8 p=0.001	4.6 (1.3-14.7) p=0.002				
Noticeable twitches or grimaces					3.1 (0.9-9.6) p=0.03	2.5	3.7	2.8 (0.8-8.7) p=0.06
Thumb sucker					4.8 (0.8-22) p=0.02	8.2 p=0.001		5.05 (0.8-23) p=0.02

(** = interaction term for effect modification by sex, p=0.1)

such a small case group. In the majority of comparisons the confidence limits for girls overlapped those for boys and the differences between the odds ratios may have been due to chance. When testing formally for effect modification by gender, no interaction term was significant at the 5% level, although several approached this. Thus, at 13, girls appeared to avoid teachers attention, to be timid in class (although the effect was present for boys at 15) and to be ignored by other children, whereas boys showed virtually no effects. At 15, girls appeared tired and washed-out and to avoid competition. Truancy was confined to girls at this age. In these items, the odds ratio adjusted for confounding by sex may not be a valid estimation of the true situation. There were other examples where an effect was more marked in girls than boys, but not confined to them, e.g. avoiding rough games at 15 years.

In most instances, given the low statistical power, there was remarkable similarity between the boys and girls, more so in the items related to school work and negative attitudes than those regarding social behaviour. This was the case for situations where an association appeared to exist, and those where the result was resoundingly negative (i.e. odds ratios close to unity). It is interesting that there was convincing evidence of a greater effect for boys than girls in only one out of 25 items. Compared to their peers, this sample of girls who were to develop schizophrenia as adults appeared more abnormal than did the boys. However, this does not necessarily imply that, within this group, the behaviours of girls differed from the boys. The way the questions were phrased (more than average, average, less than average) meant that this question could not be addressed directly.

The multiple items of behavioural information at 13 and 15 years were simplified by the construction of continuous scores based upon principal components analysis of the individual items (see Appendix). These were analysed at both ages in a manner similar to the IQ scores (Jones et al., 1994c).

At 13, the only significant predictor of later schizophrenia was the composite score of sociability. Cases were least likely to be in the tertile containing the most sociable controls (OR $0.3, p = 0.03$) and there was a significant trend ($\chi^2 = 4.0, p = 0.05$) over the tertiles; the less sociable a subject, the more likely they were to develop schizophrenia. Stratification by sex or social class made very little difference to the crude odds ratio, indicating that this trend occurred in both boys and girls and in all socio-economic groups. There was no evidence that emotional stability or negative attitudes to others differentiated cases from controls. The trend for lack of aggression to be associated with cases was not significant, but was in keeping with the findings on anxiety.

At age 15 the scores derived from the teacher ratings gave further evidence of continuity with the results from two years previously. There was a highly significant trend for increasingly anxious behaviour to predict later schizophrenia ($\chi^2 = 9.0, p = 0.003$). Many of the items from which this scale was derived were similar to those making-up the sociability scale which was a significant predictor at age 13. The was no clear pattern for aggressive behaviour at 15.

The continuous data for habit behaviours at 15 were positively skewed (79% of controls had a score of 0, range 0 - 6). These data were re-coded into three categories, no habits, 1 to 3, and 4 to 6 habits reported. There was an excess of cases-to-be in both strata where habits were noticed, the case in the multiple habit stratum representing a highly improbable event (OR $= 17.1, 95\%$ c.i. 0.7 - 159, p=0.01) and the trend was significant at the 0.09 level.

Educational performance and behaviour at 15 years. It was possible that intellectual performance and behaviour each confounded the other's association with the cases; some intellectual deficits, such as reading retardation, are known to be associated with behavioural problems and abnormalities (Rutter & Hersov, 1985). In order to investigate this, the first principal component of the educational test scores at 15 was added to a logistic regression model comprising sex, social class and anxious behaviour, the last modelled as a continuous variable. Addition of PC 1, the "IQ" score, resulted in a significant improvement in the fit of the model (LRS = 12.7, p < 0.001), and both anxiety (OR = 1.3, p < 0.001) and the "IQ" score (OR = 0.5, p = 0.009) remained as significant, seemingly independent predictors of schizophrenia.

General Poor Performance in the Childhoods of Cases of Schizophrenia - A Longitudinal Measure of Deviance

The general pattern of results in all comparisons of cases and controls was for the cases to have performed less well as a group than the controls. The longitudinal data collection allowed this to be investigated further by estimating intra-individual change. A score of "deviance" from the mean value was constructed for each subject. Variables included were those where there had been significant differences between cases and controls, in either direction, and also variables where patterns of differences had been in agreement with the literature but which had failed to reach statistical significance. These scores were treated as cumulative, as at each age subjects could improve their position relative to the mean group score.

Standardized normal deviate scores (Z-scores; difference from the group mean divided by the standard deviation) were calculated for both continuous and categorical variables to arrive at a standardized distance score from the total group (i.e. risk set) mean for each variable of interest. An initial score of 10 was allocated to each subject so as to avoid computational problems associated with processing negative integers. The following 16 variables were selected to contribute to this cumulative deviance score constructed to give eight data points:

Birth	Fathers social class
Age 1	First two principal components of developmental + previous score
Age 4	Play preference + mother's management + previous score
Age 6	Play preference + previous score
Age 8	1st principal component (PC) of educational tests + previous score
Age 11	1st PC of educational tests + previous score
Age 13	Each of the four behavioural self-rating scales + previous score
Age 15	Each of the three behavioural teacher rating scales + 1st PC of educational tests + previous score.

The Z-scores were added in such a way that performance poorer than the mean value (e.g. later milestones, lower educational test score, preference for solo play) was assigned a negative value compared with the mean behaviour of the group, standardized to zero. This strategy yielded a standardised score for each individual which is on an arbitrary "deviance" scale; the values themselves have little meaning and are not displayed.

Between group differences in the cumulative scores were calculated for cases and controls and are displayed in Table 8. A positive difference indicates that cases scored better than the mean tendency, a negative score that they scored worse. The scores demonstrated the relative advantage of the cases at birth in terms of social class. This advantage became eroded by later milestones during the first two years and by age four, the solitary play and poorer mothering of the cases caused a further deterioration of scores. The tendency of a higher proportion of the cases to continue solitary play beyond four years of age lead to continued lowering of scores. The relative improvement at age

163

eight was probably somewhat spurious; the system used to calculate these scores gave greater weight to play alone than to, say, half a standard deviation of educational test score, an arbitrary decision. Deviance was relatively stable until the combination of poor intellectual performance and unusual behaviour at age 15 caused the scores to plummet. Confidence intervals for these differences became wider with age as fewer subjects had complete data necessary to complete the scores. When missing values were modelled using optimum regression or by mean substitution, more cases could be included and narrower confidence limits were obtained. This analysis remains preliminary and is not shown.

Table 8. Difference in culmulative deviance scores between cases and controls. Increasingly negative values indicate cases performing progressively less well than controls.

Age	Difference in accumulated deviances. Cases - Controls	95% c.i. of difference
Birth	+ 0.29	- 0.1 to 0.7
One year	+ 0.14	- 0.53 to 0.8
Four years	- 0.54	-1.4 to 0.3
Six years	- 0.92	- 1.9 to 0.1
Eight years	- 0.72	- 1.9 to - 0.5
Eleven years	- 0.73	- 3.4 to 0.61
Thirteen years	- 0.73	- 2.8 to 1.3
Fifteen years	- 2.68	- 5.6 to 0.3

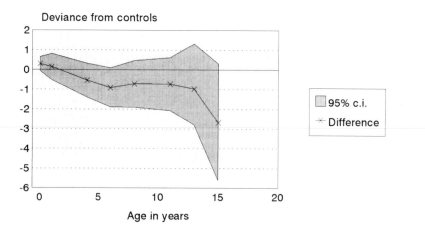

Figure 1. Cumulative developmental deviance from birth to 15 years (Deficit shown by children destined to become cases increases with age. Negative score represents poorer performance by cases - see text.)

These data are shown graphically in Figure 1 which shows the cases becoming increasingly deviant from zero, the null value.

Cases in the two categories of diagnostic certainty did not have a statistically different deviance scores at age 15 (means -7.2 versus -8.7, 95% c.i. difference -9.7 to +6.7). No further statistical analyses of the deviance score are presented.

Missing Data

The characteristics were examined of those survey members who had missing data for the 15 year educational tests. The proportions of cases (n=5, 16.7%) and controls (n=764, 16.2%) were almost identical, as were the proportions of boys and girls in the cases and controls (cases 2 girls missing, 40%; controls 366 girls missing, 47.9%). Parental social class of the cases with missing values showed no significant tendency to cluster (1 social class I, 2 social class II, 2 social class III-N), when compared with the social class distribution of all cases at 15; if anything, those who failed to do the tests came from more advantaged homes. The mean age at onset of those cases with missing values at 15 was 23.4 years versus 24.4 years for the remainder (95% c.i.difference 6.1 years younger to 8.2 years older).

The proportions of cases (11/30, 37%) and controls (2352/4716, 49%), with complete data for the 16 items included in the deviance score, were not significantly different (95% c.i. difference -5% to 29%). However, their deviance scores differ considerably. There is no strong evidence to indicate that the probability of having complete data was related to this score.

DISCUSSION

This investigation of predictors of adult schizophrenia in the NSHD has indicated associations between a variety of childhood characteristics and subsequent schizophrenia in adulthood. Throughout childhood, poor performance in cognitive tests, particularly in non-verbal, verbal and mathematical skills predicted schizophrenia. Those destined to develop the illness rated *themselves* as having low sociability at age 13 and their teachers found them to be anxious at 15 years, regardless of educational performance. Eleven years previously, there was some evidence that mothers noted a preference for the cases-to-be to prefer solitary play and for those mothers to be rated by health visitors as unusual in their mothering skills. Despite normal birth weight and no apparent social disadvantage at birth, age at walking was slightly, but significantly (statistically) delayed.

Low statistical power was a methodological problem. One reason for recruiting as controls the entire risk set other than the cases was to maximise the power of the study (Miettinen, 1969), but the interpretation of negative findings remained a problem. Accordingly, emphasis was placed on patterns of results and confidence limits.

The study had several strengths. The longitudinal nature of the data collection and the use of cross-sectional information, such as educational tests and behavioural ratings, avoided problems with biased recall. Selection of cases proceeded blind to information collected prior to age 16, and several independent sources of information were employed in order to identify the cases. In particular, use of the mental health enquiry meant that survey members who had dropped-out of the NSHD follow-up could still be included as cases. There was only one permanent refusal of follow-up prior to age 16, so the risk set was representative of the immediate post-war generation, alive in the U.K.. Regarding missing data, it appeared that similar proportions of cases and controls had missing exposure data, that such data were not particularly related to sociodemographic characteristics, and that cases with and without missing data had onsets at similar ages.

When effect of possible diagnostic misclassification was assessed, there was no evidence that the results of the cumulative deviance score were related to the quantity of clinical data available for diagnosis. Two differential misclassifications were considered most likely; the classification as schizophrenic of developmentally deviant, "odd" adolescents who would now be classified as having personality disorders, and the misdiagnosis of affective disorder as schizophrenia (Kendell, 1972). These misclassifications would have lead to opposing effects (Foerster et al., 1991; Jones et al., 1993) on the association demonstrated between child development and schizophrenia, and we hope that their net effect has not lead to serious bias.

The control group contained children who had, or later developed, severe illness other than schizophrenia, such as epilepsy and learning difficulties, which are known to be associated with some of the exposures of interest. This retained the population base of the controls, and was the most conservative approach in that it would have reduced associations between exposures and cases. However, this effect was probably very small, given the large size of the control group. Sex and social class confounded many of the associations investigated, and their effects were controlled routinely in the analyses. Definition of these two variables as confounders was largely guided by previous analyses of the NSHD data (Douglas, 1964; Douglas et al., 1968; Rodgers, 1990 a&b; Douglas & Cherry, 1977), together with associations between schizophrenia and social class at birth and male sex demonstrated elsewhere. It was not feasible to divide the cases according to clinical characteristics owing to the small number and lack of fine grained clinical detail. If differences in developmental associations do exist between possible sub-types of the adult clinical syndrome, our estimates of associations will represent *underestimates* of the true effect in which ever sub-group is primarily involved. However, if this were the case, the findings of linear trends in associations for the total case group which we analyzed would have been rather unlikely.

THE FINDINGS

Risk of schizophrenia and sociodemographic characteristics. Case identification was designed to ensure high specificity rather than sensitivity; with such a small number of cases, false positives would have been a serious problem. Nevertheless, the estimated risk of 0.63% by age 43 compares very favourably with the predicted risk of 0.61% by age 40 (Done et al., 1991). No statistically significant predictors of schizophrenia emerged from the measures of social class, although the trend appeared to be for higher social status at birth and perhaps at age four, to predict the illness. Similarly, city birth was not associated with the cases. These findings appear contrary to results from some recent studies of childhood characteristics using routine diagnostic statistics (Lewis et al., 1992). However, effect sizes for associations between social status and place of birth or upbringing are small and probably beyond the resolution of the present study. It is notable, however, that the data from the 1958 U.K. cohort (John Done, personal communication) also indicated that schizophrenia was more common in subjects with fathers in higher status occupations.

The finding that mothers of those destined to develop schizophrenia were rated as less skilled in their management of their children, regardless of the child's sex and the social class of the family, is difficult to explain. It may reflect characteristics solely of the child, the mother, or something unique to the relationship between them. The notion that style of mothering may have a direct causal relationship with schizophrenia has received no empirical support (Hirsch & Leff, 1975; Clare, 1980). In the Danish adoption study (Tienari et al., 1987), quality of rearing environment may have made a contribution to risk of schizophrenia. Robins (1966) found that child guidance clinic attenders who developed schizophrenia were more often removed from their families through neglect, than were attenders healthy as adults, and the former group had generally less favourable family circumstances. The mechanism was unclear. It is known that genetic factors are relevant to schizophrenia (Sham et al., 1994) and it remains possible that what was noticed by the health visitors in our study was a behavioural phenotype manifest in the relationship between infant and mother (Plomin et al., 1994). We plan to examine the exact comments made at the time by the health visitors so as to illuminate the true meaning of this finding. Parental interest in the children's education did not differ between cases and controls indicating that what was noticed was something more subtle than "bad parenting", although the relationship between parent and child is known to be dependent upon developmental stage (Dunn & Plomin, 1994).

Developmental Findings

Within the early, motor milestones, later walking was the only statistically significant predictor of the cases, although there was a pattern for the cases to have reached all motor milestones later than the controls. Reporting bias, leading to terminal digit preference, was evident in these data and may have lead to decreased statistical significance. Given that the control group included children with gross motor disabilities, the findings are likely to be real. Later walking and other perturbations of motor develement have been noted in schizophrenia in studies using a variety of designs (Robins, 1966; Walker & Lewine 1990; Fish et al 1992; Ambelas, 1992). In the present study, these effects were unlikely to be part of a general picture of delayed physical growth as birth weight and both weight and height velocities were similar to controls.

We can only speculate on the pathogenesis of these neurodevelopmental findings, but believe that they are unlikely to reflect primarily psychosocial effects. The later walking may reflect some abnormal process of neural development, perhaps involving myelination of motor tracts. Normal myelination of hippocampal pathways extends into adolescence and this, or some perturbation, has been suggested as a mechanism for the delayed appearance of positive schizophrenic phenomena (Benes, 1989) in adulthood. It is possible that delayed motor milestones were a manifestation of similar mechanisms, and tempting to speculate further that the pathogenesis of the early motor delays, the twitching and grimacing seen in adolescence, the poor performance in physical activities and even the motor abnormalities reported in unmedicated schizophrenia are all related.

The data on bladder and bowel control were crude and retrospective. They were examined as tangential markers of the autonomic abnormalities found in high risk research (Mednick & Schulsinger, 1968) and it was not surprising that no effect was found as reported abnormalities in high risk studies were subtle, including measures of electrodermal reactivity.

Educational Test Results

The finding of poor educational performance predicting later schizophrenia reinforces evidence from several types of epidemiological studies in favour of there being a premorbid deficit in intelligence (Aylward et al., 1984; Jones et al 1994a). There has, however, been little consensus as to the presence of a pattern of deficits specific to schizophrenia, although a differential deficit in performance (non-verbal) versus verbal skills has been a popular theme (Aylward et al., 1984). The present results lend a little support to this; verbal skills were less "significantly" predictive than were the non-verbal scores. Inspection of the pattern of the odds ratios revealed no specific deficits associated with schizophrenia, although these sub-scales do not provide fine grained assessment of cognitive function. Vocabulary and reading scores were least predictive, another theme recurring in the literature.

The first principal component of the educational test scores was analogous to the "g factor" of general intelligence consistently identified by previous workers (Crawford et al., 1992). Treated as a repeated measure, it differentiated cases from controls. The effect appeared to be stronger at age 15 than at age 13, although formal statistical analysis of such an increase with age was inconclusive. Given the longitudinal nature of the data, with the same subjects involved at each age, and the population base of the study, these findings are compelling evidence in favour of pre-psychotic intelligence deficits in schizophrenia occurring at least between 8 and 15 years, irrespective of sex or social class. Moreover, the linear trend in the association between IQ and schizophrenia, with no evidence of a sub-group of cases with very low scores, is evidence that features of cognitive function may represent a continuous risk factor for the disorder.

Socio-behavioural Data

As early as age four years with the preference for solitary play, there was evidence that behavioural characteristics predicted later schizophrenia. This effect persisted at age six when, as in the controls, it had become less common. Similarly, the findings from the teachers' reports at 13 and 15, and the self-report questionnaire at age 13 all indicated a consistency in this tendency for children destined to become cases to be anxious in social situations and to be rather retiring and aloof, akin to the schizoid, asocial personality. There was some evidence, although we would be cautious in its interpretation (v.s.), that this timidity and asociality was more marked for girls, echoing other findings (Watt, 1978; Done et al 1994). However, there is no doubt that aspects of this, such as the early preference for solitary play and, later, appearing gloomy in class, were present in boys and girls.

There was no evidence of an excess of antisocial behaviour by the cases. Such behaviour preceeding schizophrenia, mainly in boys, has been reported from child guidance attenders (Robins, 1966) a sample where, being at high risk for behavioural abnormalities, findings may be difficult to generalize. Other studies have relied on spontaneous comments by teachers, where antisocial conduct may be particularly likely to be noted (Watt, 1978) compared with shyness, or have included open-ended comments where the same information bias may operate. Our own results may have been affected by sampling bias, although even the most extreme effects suggested by the confidence limits were not very large and, in general, these results for antisocial behaviours were resoundingly negative.

Behavioural ratings used by all general population studies have been relatively crude such that that the same behaviour may be classified differently in different investigations. However, the consistency, over more than ten years of development, of the problems with socialization found more commonly in the cases, and that it was rated by mothers, different teachers and the children themselves, indicates that this finding is likely to be valid. However, it is of interest that neither mothers nor teachers identified these attributes as problems in their own right, suggesting that the effects were subtle. The findings at age 15 of excess habit behaviours predicting cases was in accord with the literature. Robins (1966) found that habits, such as nail biting, differentiated male child guidance clinic attenders who were to develop schizophrenia from those who were healthy as adults.

The Longitudinal Assessment of Performance - The Deviance Score

This score was considered a tentative representation of the striking trend for cases to be predicted by poor performance throughout childhood and was an attempt to exploit the potential of the study for examining intra-individual change. Several caveats must be born in mind. Variables were chosen for study on the basis that they might predict schizophrenia. There are few things which people with schizophrenia do better than normals, although many workers have searched for some factor which may explain the persistence of the genetic predisposition in the gene pool. Some psychological factors have been identified, such as latent inhibition, but their meaning is unclear (Hemsley, 1991). Thus, it was predictable that cases would accumulate poor scores on the chosen variables. Several variables at different ages would have been correlated and, except for I.Q. and sociability at age 15, no attempt was made to examine statistical independence. The system used to weight the categorical scores so that the mean deviation was zero was of doubtful statistical validity and the resulting weighted scores might not represent biologically relevant weights; playing alone might not have the same relevance as social status. For these reasons few statistical tests were performed on the score as the results would be difficult to interpret.

The main point of the score was to allow visual representation of the group trends prominent in the tables of results using a score based on *individual* change, although the number of individuals with complete data for inclusion was small by age 15. However, the figure demonstrates that, despite beginning with an (arithmetic) advantage, the cases quickly accumulated disadvantage and continued to do so, despite the possibility of gaining ground at each age that the score was computed. This deviance from the mean performance of the risk-set occurred several years before psychosis, and was considerable. Random measurement error and regression to the mean would predict that individuals would not continue to diverge from the group mean and this behaviour must somehow be associated with "caseness".

Developmental Risk for Schizophrenia

Many of the associations demonstrated between adult schizophrenia and childhood factors in neurodevelopmental, social and cognitive areas replicate findings previously reported. Past analysis of categorical ratings of abnormality versus normality has tended to focus attention on the notion of a subgroup of cases who showed pre-psychotic deviance, with the assumption that other cases are normal. This approach ignores the wide range of scores found in the general population and the fact that categorical ratings are often artificial, applying arbitrary or poorly defined cut-off points. In the present study, we were fortunate in that the availability of continuous measures of behaviour, personality and educational achievement enabled a more detailed assessment of the distribution of developmental risk.

The epidemiological basis to this investigation allows conclusions to be drawn concerning the population at risk of schizophrenia, on the basis of defining which parts of that total population were responsible for the largest proportion of schizophrenia. Linear trends in the associations between cases and both educational test scores and behavioural ratings indicated that the notion of a distinct, developmentally deviant sub-group who later suffer from schizophrenia *may* not portray the extent of the true situation, certainly in terms of aspects of the risk in the population. Thus, in terms of asociality and I.Q., the risk of schizophrenia appeared to be distributed more evenly through the population, such that, for any member of the risk set, the lower the score in the educational tests, or the more anxious they were in social situations, the more likely they were to develop schizophrenia as adults. The risk of schizophrenia within the general population was not confined to a particular group in terms of these characteristics. As schizophrenia is so rare, larger numbers (i.e. a larger population at risk), or a population-based case control study, would be required to examine the exact nature and distribution of this risk, for example whether it was truly linear. However, evidence of trends was consistent; in the majority of cases where they were examined, the odds ratio associated with the middle tertile of a distribution was intermediate between the baseline odds and the third tertile.

The consideration of developmental risk for schizophrenia may, therefore, be analagous to, for instance, blood pressure and risk of stroke. If blood pressure were measured only with an instrument registering either high or normal (whatever the definition), stroke may be found to be associated with a sub-group of individuals with hypertension. This strategy ignores the fact that many cases will have, so called, normal values and, more importantly, that the risk of stroke associated with blood pressure is linear over a wide range of values; the higher the blood pressure, the greater the risk of having a stroke.

This in no way indicates that the linear associations demonstrated in the present study are causal, nor excludes aetiological heterogeneity. However, they do allow consideration of how genetic and enviromental aetiological factors may operate in terms of a liability-threshold model. One possibility is that there is no specific causal factor for schizophrenia, but that the normal genetic and environmental determinants of behaviour, cognition and neurodevelopment also determine the risk of schizophrenia. Familiality of schizophrenia could be the result of the complex mix of effects involved in these processes also tending to cluster in families. However, as this risk would operate throughout the population, the incidence of schizophrenia would be expected to be rather higher than is observed unless further, necessary events occur.

It is more likely that specific causal factors are involved. Their effect(s), which we have demonstrated must occur early in life, probably effecting neural develoment, are betrayed in the associations we have demonstrated. Thus, a subject who would have had a high IQ score had their developmental progress been unimpeded, scores a little lower due to the effect of a particular gene or environmental factor and, perhaps having rather poorer information processing than they might have done, is a little less competent in social situations. Nevertheless, this subject may still function well within the normal range and would escape detection by a test designed to detect abnormality defined in terms of the group average. Another subject who, without the specific causal factor, would have been at the lower end of the normal range of functioning would be pushed into the realms of pathological functioning by the occurrence of this same event. This subject would be detected by the test described above. All cases would be prone to this process and, as a group, their functioning would slip towards the lower end of normal. Under such a model, a higher proportion of subjects with schizophrenia than previously thought may have suffered attenuated development, although the majority of these will remain undetected by tests designed to detect gross abnormality.

This model would also offer an explanation of the overlap between cases and controls which is demonstrated in virtually all studies of schizophrenia, be they of neuropathology or of pre-psychotic social functioning. It explains why, in studies of monozygotic twins, the affected cotwins as a group may show little abnormality but when compared with their own twin in a paired analysis, predicted differences become apparent (Suddath et al., 1990). A similar explanation has recently been suggested for the overlapping distributions of sizes of cerebral structures in schizophrenia and controls (Jones et al., 1994b; see Chapter 13). Here again, it is suggested that a much larger proportion of schizophrenia than previously imagined may be associated with disease-related changes in cerebral structure.

What happens to the deviance during development? Results from the deviance scale indicate that, whatever the size of the developmental abnormality, it tends to increase with age. It is possible that the fundemental difference between children destined for schizophrenia and other children, analogous to "the lesion" in developmental neuroanatomical models of schizophrenia, is not static, regardless of whether its manifestation changes with the maturity of the rest of the brain, as suggested by Weinberger (1987). Cortical structure and function are dependent upon one another. It is feasible that abnormal experience and abnormal fine structure develop hand-in-hand in a cascade fashion, particularly as abnormal function in terms of social behaviour will influence environmental experience. Either intrinsic or extrinsic events may initiate such a cascade of aberrant development, although current evidence is in favour of initial structural pathology (Akbarian et al., 1993 a&b) which may, whatever its cause, represent predisposition to psychosis (Jones & Murray, 1991). Whether or not this sequence of events proceeds far enough to produce positive psychotic phenomena would depend on an interaction between the environment, constitution, the current state of neurodevelopment and, possibly, chance events. The characteristic distribution of age at onset of these phenomena would be one consequence of this model where deviance increases over time.

Specificity of the Findings

It is interesting to speculate on the adult outcomes of subjects in the control group with high scores on the deviance score. Returning to the results themselves, some indication that the findings on the individual variables are relatively specific to schizophrenia amongst other psychological problems comes from Rodgers' work concerning the childhood characteristics of survey members who scored as "cases" on the short version of the PSE administered when they were 36 (Rodgers & Mann, 1986; Rodgers 1990 a&b). Women were more than twice as likely to be ascribed CATEGO ID levels of 5 or more (8.6% vs 3.8%) in sharp contrast to the sex ratio for schizophrenia, and PSE cases appeared to come from poorer homes. Of other variables investigated here, enuresis, habits and antisocial behaviour at 15 predicted caseness but the effect was stronger for women. Poor educational attainment did not predict PSE score in men. It would appear that items identified in the present study were not just markers for psychiatric problems in general.

In conclusion, this preliminary analysis of child development prior to adult onset schizophrenia has replicated a body of literature by demonstrating that children destined to develop schizophrenia in adult life can be differentiated from their peers across a variety of characteristics beginning with early milestones of motor and speech development. Initial events in schizophrenia must occur early. The epidemiological base of the study indicated that incidence of schizophrenia was not confined to a sub-group of the population in terms of childhood educational performance and sociability, but appeared to arise with increasing frequency as ability declined in these domains. Such tentative conclusions require replication but, if true, provide a further, longitudinal dimension to the schizophrenia phenotype yet to be explained in terms of basic neurobiology. Continuing investigations in this and other longitudinal investigations, particularly if results can be pooled, will facilitate such replication and will allow further exploration of the developmental antecedents of schizophrenia.

ACKNOWLEDGEMENTS

We are grateful to Prof MEJ Wadsworth for facilitating this investigation within the MRC National Survey of Health and Development, and to the technical and scientific staff of The Survey for their help. The past work of Dr Sheila Mann, who collected a great deal of clinical information, is gratefully acknowledged. PJ was supported by a U.K. Medical Research Council Training Fellowship.

APPENDIX

Details of the Variables Analyzed as Exposures

1. Socio-economic status. Several indices of socio-economic status were available through childhood.

Birth. Occupational group of father.
Municipal characteristics of place of birth, i.e. city/urban/rural.
Population size (from 1961 census) of administrative area of birth.
Age 4. A composite measure of material home circumstances was available (Rodgers, 1978). This was based on health visitors' reports, and was derived from eight variables concerning the state of housing and crowding therein, the cleanliness of the child and the child's clothes and the mother's "mothering skills", i.e. her management and understanding of her child in terms of the helath visitors' experience. The resulting total score was re-coded from one (the poorest circumstances) to four (the best), representing an ordered categorical variable.
Age 15. Occupational group of father was available coded according to the Registrar General's Classification.
2. Educational Achievement: Cognitive Test Scores. Results of cognitive tests were available for ages 8, 11 and 15 years. Both the tests and their development are described in detail by Pidgeon for the 8 and 11 year sets (Pidgeon, 1964) and those taken at 15 years (Pidgeon, 1968) Briefly, at age 8 four tests were given: a 60 item non-verbal picture test, a 35 item reading comprehension test (sentence completion), a 50 item word reading test, a 50 item vocabulary test (same words as above). At age 11 four tests yielded verbal, non-verbal, arithmetic, reading and vocabulary scores: an 80 item verbal and non-verbal test, a 50 item arithmetic test (problems and mechanical sums), a 50 item word reading test, a 50 item vocabulary test (same two tests as at age 8). At age 15 years three tests gave similar scores to those at 11: the group ability test - a 65 item verbal and non-verbal test, the Watts-Vernon reading test (Also given at age 26), a 47 item mathematics test.
Thus, there were non-verbal and verbal scores available at all three ages, mathematics/arithmetic at 11 and 15, vocabulary at 8 and 11 and reading at 8, 11, 15 and 26 years.
3. Early milestones and later physical development. During the health visitor interview at age 24 to 26 months, mothers were asked to recall the age to the nearest whole month that the survey member had:
sat alone
stood alone
walked alone
talked - saying more than names of familiars
cut the first tooth.

Health visitors noted if they found evidence that the survey member had not reached any of these milestones. Mothers were also asked to recall the birth weight of their child.

General physical development was assessed objectively during the medical examinations and height and weight were available at ages 7 and 11 years. Signs of puberty were noted during the medical exam and girls were questioned regarding menstruation. A composite measure of time of puberty for boys (infantile, early, advanced, mature) and girls (menarche at 142 to 153 months or prior to 142 months, 154 to 165 months, or 166 months or later) was created at age 15 years and was used in this analysis.

Assessment of day-time and night time bladder control was made at ages 4, 6 and 11 years and coded as dry, occasionally wet, usually wet and always wet. Bowel control was coded as controlled by - 12 months, 18 months, 6 years, after 6 years.

4. Social and behavioural characteristics. The earliest data on social behaviour came from maternal reports of play preferences at age 4 and 6 years. Mothers were asked whether the child usually played alone, with siblings, with other children, or in other (unspecified) circumstances.

At age 13 the children themselves completed the Pintner Aspects of Personality Inventory (Pintner et al., 1937; Pintner & Forlano, 1938). Four continuous measures were available for analysis. These were based on a previous principal components analysis of the three scales derived from this test (Rodgers, 1990 a&b) and comprised:-

1. Emotional stability (range 0-13, mean 3.9) - based on items such as "I often feel sad for no reason at all' and "I worry about the little mistakes I make".
2. Sociability (range 0-8, mean 4.8) - e.g. "I make friends easily", "I feel at home at parties".
3. Negative attitudes to others (range 0-11, mean 3.7) - e.g. "I find that very few people can be trusted" "I often get blamed for things I didn't do".
4. Aggressive behaviour (range 0-7, mean 3.7) - e.g. "I feel I have a right to fight for what I want," "I sometimes feel like hitting people".

At ages 13 and 15, questionnaires were completed by survey members' teachers who were asked to make global assessments in areas such as sensitive/highly strung, aggressive, shy. More specific ratings of certain behaviours, habits and attitudes (e.g. to school work) were also made. Children were assessed on a three point scale, (less than class mates, same as classmates, more than classmates). This information was available in both a raw and in a processed form. The latter was based upon principal components analysis, which gave three scales comprising continuous data with approximately normal distributions for the first two, the third being positively skewed:

Anxious behaviour (range 13-32, mean 20.5) - e.g. "timid child," "frightened of rough games," "always 'washed out'."

Antisocial bevhaviour (range 13-35, mean 18.9) - e.g. "poor or lazy worker," "frequently disobedient", "frequently evades the truth."

Habit behaviours (range 0-6, median and mode zero) - e.g. "nail-biter," "frequently twitches or grimaces."

REFERENCES

Akbarian S, Viñuela A, Kim JJ et al (1993) Disrupted distribution of nicotinamide-adenine dinucleotide phosphate-diaphorase neurons in temporal lobe of schizophrenics implies abnormal cortical development. Archives of General Psychiatry, 50, 178-189.

Akbarian S, Bunney WE, Potkin SG et al (1993) Altered distribution of nicotinamide-adenine dinucleotide phosphate-diaphorase cells in frontal lobe of schizophrenics implies distruption of cortical development. Archives of General Psychiatry, 50, 169-177.

Ambelas A. (1992) Preschizophrenics: adding to the evidence, sharpening the focus. British Journal of Psychiatry, 160, 401-404.

American Psychiatric Association: Diagnostic and statistical manual of mental disorders, Third Edition - Revised. Washington, DC: American Psychiatric Association, 1987.

Atkins E, Cherry N, Douglas JWB, Kiernan KE & Wadsworth MEJ (1981). The 1946 birth cohort: An account of the origins, progress. and results of the National Survey of Health and Development. In S.A. Mednick& A.E. Baert (eds.) "Prospective Longitudinal Research: An Empirical Basis for the Primary Prevention of Psychosocial Disorders. London: OUP.

Aylward, E., Walker, E. & Bettes, B. (1984) Intelligence in schizophrenia: meta-analysis of the research. Schizophrenia Bulletin, 10, 430-459.

Barker DJP & Osmond C (1986) Childhood respiratory infection and chronic bronchitis in England and Wales. British Medical Journal, 293, 1271-1275.

Barker DJP, Bull AR, Osmond C & Simmonds SJ (1990) Fetal and placental size and risk of hypertension in adult life. British Medical Journal 301, 259-262.

Barker DJP, Winter PD, Osmond C, Margetts B & Simmonds SJ (1989) Weight in infancy and death from ischaemic heart disease. Lancet, ii, 577-580.

Benes FM (1989) Myelination of cortico-hippocampal relays during late adolescence. Schizophrenia Bulletin, 10, 430-459.

Breslow NE & Day NE (1980) Statistical Methods in Cancer Research Vol 2. Section on analysis of continuous data in case control studies. pp. 227-228. Lyon: WHO.

Buka, S.L.,Tsuang, M.T. & Lipsitt, L.P. (1993) Pregnancy/delivery complications and psychiatric diagnosis. A prospective study. Archives of General Psychiatry, 50, 151-156.

Cannon-Spoor HE, Potkin SG & Wyatt RJ (1982) Measurement of premorbid adjustment in chronic schizophrenia. Schizophrenia Bulletin, 8 (3) 470-484.

Clare A. (1980) Psychiatry in Dissent. Controversial issues in thought and practice. 2nd ed. pp. 184-196. London: Tavistock.

Colley JRT, Douglas JWB & Reid DD (1973) Respiratory disease in young adults: influence of early childhood lower respiratory tract illness, social class, air pollution and smoking. British Medical Journal, 3, 195-198.

Crawford et al. (1992) Assessment of Premorbid Intelligence in Schizophrenia. British Journal of Psychiatry, 161, 69-74.

Crow TJ (1992) Maternal viral infection hypothesis. British Journal of Psychiatry, 161, 570-571.

Crow TJ & Done DJ (1992) Prenatal exposure to influenza does not cause schizophrenia. British Journal of Psychiatry, 161, 390-393.

Done J., Johnstone E.C., Frith C.D., Golding J., Shepard P.M. & Crow T.J. (1991) Complications of pregnancy and delivery in relation to psychosis in adult life: data from the British Perinatal Mortality Survey. British Medical Journal, 302, 1576-1580.

Done DJ, Crow TJ, Johnson EC & Sacker A (1994) Childhood antecedents of schizophrenia and affective illness: social adjustment at ages 7 and 11. Unpublished manuscript.

Douglas JWB & Cherry N. (1977) Does sex make any difference? Times Educational Supplement, 9th December, 3261,16-17.

Douglas JWB, Ross JM & Simpson HR. (1968) "All our futures" London: Peter Davies.

Douglas JWB (1964) "The Home and the School" London: MacGibbon & Kee.

Dunn J. & Plomin R. (1986) Determinants of maternal behaviour towards 3-year-old siblings. British Journal of Developmental Psychology, 4, 127-137.

Erlenmeyer-Kimling L, Cornblatt B, Friedman D et al (1982) Neurological, electrophysiological and attentional deviations in children at risk of schizophrenia. In FA Henn and H Nasrallah (Eds.) Schizophrenia as a Brain Disease. pp. 61-98. New York: OUP.

Fine, PEM., Adelstein, AM., Snowman, J., Clarkson, JA., Evans, SM. (1985) Long term effects of exposure to viral infections in utero. British Medical Journal, 290, 509-511.

Fish B. (1977) Neurobiological antecedents of schizophrenia in children. Archives of General Psychiatry, 34, 1297-1313.

Fish B, Marcus J, Hans SL, Auerbach JG & Perdue S. (1992) Infants at risk for schizophrenia: sequelae of a genetic neurointergrative defect. Archives of General Psychiatry, 49, 221-235.

Foerster A, Lewis SW, Owen MJ & Murray RM (1991) Pre-morbid adjustment and personality in psychosis. Effects of sex and Diagnosis. British Journal of Psychiatry, 158, 171-176.

Gittleman-Klein R & Klein DF (1969) Premorbid social adjustment and prognosis in schizophrenia. Journal of Psychiatric Research, 7, 35-53.

Godfrey KM, Barker DJP, Peace J, Cloke J & Osmond C (1993) Relation of fingerprints and shape of the palm to fetal growth and adult blood pressure. British Medical Journal 307, 405-409.

Hemsley DR (1991) What have cognitive deficits to do with schizophrenia? In G. Huber (Ed.) "Idiopathische Psychosen". pp11-125. Stuttgart: Scattauer.

Hirsch S & Leff JP. (1975) Abnormalities in the parents of schizophrenics. Maudsley Monograph 22. Oxford: OUP.

Jones P.B. & Murray R.M. (1991) The genetics of schizophrenia is the genetics of neurodevelopment. British Journal of Psychiatry, 158, 615 - 623.

Jones P.B., Bebbington P, Foerster A, Lewis SW, Murray RM, Russell A, Sham PC, Toone BK, Wilkins S. (1993) Premorbid social underachievement in schizophrenia. Results from the Camberwell Collaborative Psychosis Study. British Journal of Psychiatry, 162, 65 - 71

Jones PB, Guth CW, Lewis SW & Murray (1994a) Low intelligence and poor educational achievement precede early onset schizophrenic psychosis. In: AS David & J Cutting (Eds.) "The Neuropsychology of Schizophrenia". Hove: Lawrence Erlbaum.

Jones P.B., Harvey I, Lewis SW, Toone BK, van Os J, Williams M & Murray RM (1994b) Cerebral ventricle dimensions as risk factors for schizophrenia and affective psychosis. An epidemiological approach to analysis. Psychological Medicine. In the press.

Jones PB, Rodgers B, Murray RM & Marmot M (1994c) Child developmental risk factors for adult schizophrenia in the British 1946 birth cohort. Manuscript.

Kendell RE (1972) Schizophrenia: the remedy for diagnostic confusion. British Journal of Hospital Medicine, 8, 383-390.

Kraepelin E (1896). "Dementia Praecox" pp 426-441 of the 5th edition of Psychiatrie Barth: Leipzig. Translated (1987) by J Cutting and M Shepherd. In "The Clinical Roots of the Schizophrenia Concept". Cambridge: CUP.

Kraepelin, E. (1919) "Dementia Praecox and Paraphrenia". Edinburgh: Livingstone. Translated 1971, New York, Robert E. Krieger Publishing Corporation.

Lewis S.W., Owen M.J. & Murray R.M. (1989) Obstetric complications and schizophrenia: Methodology and mechanisms. In: "Schizophrenia - A Scientific Focus". (eds. Schulz S.C. & Tamminga C.A.), p. 56-68. Oxford University Press: New York.

Lewis G, David A, Andréasson S & Allebeck P (1992) Schizophrenia and city life. Lancet, 340, 137-140.

Lucas A. (1991) Programming by early nutrition in man. In "The Childhood Environment and Adult Disease". Ciba Foundation Symposium 156. Chichester: John Wiley and Sons.

Manly BFJ (1986) Multivariate Statistical Methods: A Primer. pp 59-71 & 72-84. London: Chapman Hall.

Martyn CN, Barker DJP & Osmond C (1988) Motorneurone disease and past poliomyelitis in England and Wales. Lancet 1: 1319-1322.

Mednick SA & Schulsinger F. (1968) Some premorbid characteristics related to breakdown in children with schizophrenic mothers. In D Rosenthal & SS Kety (Eds.) "Transmission of Schizophrenia" pp 267-291. New York: Pergamon Press.

Mednick SA, Machon RA, Huttenen MO & Bonnett D (1988) Adult schizophrenia following prenatal exposure to an influenza epidemic. Archives of General Psychiatry, 45, 188-192.

Miettinen OS (1969) Individual matching with multiple controls in the case of all or none responses. Biometrics, 22, 339-355.

O'Callaghan E., Larkin C. & Waddington J.L. (1990) Obstetric complications in schizophrenia and the validity of maternal recall. Psychological Medicine, 20, 89-94.

Pearson K. (1901) On lines and planes of closest fit to a system of points in space. Philosophical Magazine, 2, 557-572.

Pidgeon DA (1964) Tests used in the 1954 and 1957 surveys. In JWB Douglas "The home and the school" pp129 - 132. London: MacGibbon & Kee.

Pidgeon DA (1968) Appendix: Details of the fifteen year tests. In: JWB Douglas, JM Ross & HR Simpson "All our futures" pp 194 - 197. London: Peter Davies.

Pintner R, Loftus JJ, Forlano G & Alster B. (1937) Aspects of personality inventory: Test and manual. Yonkers: World Book Co.

Pintner R & Forlano G. (1938) Four retests of a personality inventory. Journal of Educational Psychology, 29, 93-100.

Plomin R, Reiss D, Hetherington EM and Howe GW (1994) Nature and nurture: genetic contributions to measures of the family environment. Developmental Psychology 30 (1) 32-43.

Poskitt EME & Cole TJ (1977) Do fat babies stay fat? British Medical Journal, 1, 7-9.

Pullen CR & Hey EN (1982) Wheezing, asthma and pulmonary dysfunction 10 years after infection with respiratory syncytial virus in infancy. British Medical Journal, 284, 1665-1669

Roberts GW (1990) Schizophrenia: a neuropathological perspective. British Journal of Psychiatry, 157, 1-10.

Robins LN (1966) *"Deviant Children Grown Up. A Sociological and Psychiatric Study of Sociopathic Personality"*. Baltimore: Williams and Wilkins.

Rodgers B (1978) Feeding in infancy and later ability and attainment: a longitudinal study. Developmental Medicine and Child Neurology, 20, 421-426.

Rodgers B (1990a) Adult affective disorder and early environment. British Jurnal of Psychiatry, 157, 539-550.

Rodgers B (1990b) Behaviour and personality in childhood as predictors of adult psychiatric disorder. Journal of child psychology and psychiatry, 31 (3), 393-414.

Rodgers B & Mann SA (1986) The reliability and validity of PSE assessments by lay interviewers: a national population survey. Psychological Medicine, 16, 689-700.

Royal College of Obstetricians and Gynaecologists and the Population Investigation Committee (1948) Maternity in Great Britain. London: OUP.

Rutter ML & Giller H. (1983) *Juvenile Delinquency: Trends and Perspectives.* Penguin: Harmondsworth.

Rutter M. (1984) Psychopathology and development: 1. childhood antecedents of adult psychiatric disorder. Australian and New Zealand Journal of Psychiatry, 18, 225-234.

Rutter, M.L. & Hersov, L. (1985) Child and adolescent psychiatry: Modern approaches. Second Edition. London: Blackwell.

Selten J-PCJ & Slaets JPJ (1994) Second trimester exposure to 1957 A_2 influenza epidemic is not a risk factor for schizophrenia. Schizophrenia Research, 11 (2), 95.

Sham P, Jones PB, Russell A, Gilvarry K, Bebbington P, Lewis S, Toone B & Murray R (1994) Age at onset, sex, familial psychiatric morbidity in schizophrenia. Report form the Camberwell Collaborative Psychosis Study. British Journal of Psychiatry. In the Press.

Sham, PC., O'Callaghan, E., Takei, N., Murray GK., Hare, EH. & Murray, RM. (1992). Increased risk of schizophrenia following prenatal exposure to influenza. British Journal of Psychiatry, 160, 461-466.

Suddath R.L., Christison G.W., Torrey E.F., Casanova M.F. & Weinberger D.R. (1990) Anatomical abnormalities in the brains of monozygotic twins discordant for schizophrenia. New England Journal of Medicine, 322, 789-794.)

Susser E & Lin SP (1992) Schizophrenia after exposure to the Dutch Hunger Winter of 1944-1945. Archives of General Psychiatry, 49, 983-988.

Tienari P, Sorri A, Lahti I, Naarala M, Wahlberg K, Moring J, Pohjola J & Wynne LC (1987) Genetic and psychosocial factors in schizophrenia: The Finnish Adoptive Family Study. Schizophrenia Bulletin, 13 (3), 477-484.

Wadsworth MEJ (1987) Follow-up of the first national birth cohort: findings forn the Medical Research Council National Survey of Health and Development. Paediatric and Perinatal Epidemiology, 1, 95-117.

Wadsworth MEJ (1991) The Imprint of Time. Childhood history and adult life. Oxford: Clarendon Press.

Walker E & Lewine RJ (1990) Prediction of adult-onset schizophrenia from childhood home movies of the patients. American Journal of Psychiatry, 147, 1052-1056.

Walker EF, Grimes KE, Davis DM & Smith AJ (1993) Childhood precursors of schizophrenia: facial expressions of emotion. American Journal of Psychiatry 150, 1654-1660.

Watt NF. (1978) Patterns of childhood social development in adult schizophrenics. Archives of General Psychiatry, 35, 160-165.

Watt, N. & Lubensky, A. (1976) Childhood roots of schizophrenia. Journal of Consulting and Clinical Psychology, 44, 363-375.

Weinberger, D.R. (1987) Implications of normal brain development for the pathogenesis of schizophrenia. Archives of General Psychiatry, 44, 660-669.

Wing JK, Cooper JE & Sartorius N. (1974) The measurement and classification of psychiatric symptoms. London: CUP.

SUBTYPES OF SCHIZOPHRENIA: DIAGNOSTIC AND CONCEPTUAL ISSUES

Pekka Tienari[1] and Lyman C. Wynne[2]

[1] Department of Psychiatry, Oulu University, Oulu, Finland
[2] Department of Psychiatry, University of Rochester School of Medicine and Dentistry, Rochester, New York

Of all the major psychiatric syndromes, schizophrenia is the most difficult to define and describe. Ever since Eugen Bleuler coined the term "schizophrenia" in 1911, controversy has raged over the question of whether the diverse clinical manifestations of schizophrenia are all derived from a single underlying etiopathological process or, alternatively, clinical subtypes of schizophrenia can be satisfactorily differentiated and linked to two or more distinctive disease entities or to distinctive disease processes. In recent years the research focus has shifted from "classical" subtyping to types of functions or domains of psychopathology that are hypothesized to be related to some but not all of the patients who are diagnosed as schizophrenic.

Actually, in the nineteenth century, forms of psychopathology had been identified that later became clumped together as subtypes of the broader concepts of dementia praecox and schizophrenia. The controversy of whether these clinical phenomena should be clumped together or split apart as distinctive entities has a long history (McGuffin, Farmer, and Gottesman, 1987). One early view was that all of the psychoses were expressions of a single disease entity, which Griesinger (1867) called Einheitspsychose (unitary psychosis).

The alternative was to separate out and classify several mental "diseases" on the basis of symptoms, onset, and outcome. Bleuler (1911) reviewed the early history of the precursors of his concept of schizophrenia (pages 5-6): In 1860 Morel coined the term démence précoce (dementia praecox) for a disorder of adolescent and young adult persons who were affected by a deteriorating psychotic course. A more narrowly delimited disease entity was labeled catatonia by Kahlbaum in 1863. In 1871 Hecker delineated a symptom picture that he called hebephrenia, and in 1894 Sommer included deteriorating paranoid syndromes in the concept of "primary dementia."

Then in 1896 Emil Kraepelin proposed that these "deteriorating psychoses" be brought together as subtypes of "a distinct disease" that he called dementia praecox (taking over Morel's term). Dementia praecox, because of its more chronic deteriorating course, was differentiated from manic depressive psychosis, with a remitting or episodic course.

Neural Development and Schizophrenia, Edited by S.A. Mednick and J.M. Hollister, Plenum Press, New York, 1995

In 1919 Kraepelin narrowed the concept of dementia praecox to exclude paraphrenia, which he viewed as not showing the "dullness and indifference which so frequently form the first symptoms of dementia praecox" (page 283) and as starting in middle life rather than adolescence. With respect to the criterion of a chronic, deteriorating course for schizophrenia, Eugen Bleuler (1911) observed, and Kraepelin (1919) later agreed, that some, perhaps many cases, "could be cured permanently or arrested for a very long period" (Bleuler, 1911, p. 7).

Both Bleuler and Kraepelin were undecided about the question of subdividing schizophrenia. Although Kraepelin hypothesized that the differing clinical manifestations all arose from unspecified underlying metabolic processes, in 1919 he stated: "I consider it an open question whether the same morbid process is not after all the cause of the divergent forms, though differing in the point of attack and taking a varying course" (page 1). Bleuler spoke of the "group of schizophrenias" as "tentatively" divided into four subtypes: paranoia, catatonia, hebephrenia, and simple schizophrenia. On the other hand, he believed that there were certain "specific permanent or fundamental symptoms" characteristic of schizophrenia that were "present in every case and at every period of the illness" (p. 13), suggesting that subtyping was not really of primary importance. The "fundamental" symptoms included disturbances of associations, changes in emotional reactions, a tendency to prefer fantasy to reality, and autism (withdrawal from reality into an inner world of fantasy). In Bleuler's view, some of the most frequent and striking symptoms were "accessory" (secondary): for example, hallucinations, delusions, catatonia, and abnormal behaviors.

Kraepelin's and Bleuler's ambivalence about clumping versus splitting of the schizophrenic syndrome into one versus more than one disease entity has remained unresolved over the subsequent decades. Two models for conceptualizing this problem have prevailed. In the first model a single etiopathological process is believed to underlie all of the primary manifestations of a single disease entity called schizophrenia; clinical and test differences among patients are thought to reflect factors such as neurodevelopmental variations in the regions of the brain that are affected, variations in the life circumstances of patients, and variations in the modifying and protective effects of genetic and experiential strengths. The diverse clinical manifestations of neurosyphilis have been cited as an example of this model. Researchers who have compared schizophrenics as a total group versus nonschizophrenic controls have explicitly, or sometimes only implicitly, adopted this model. The model is still applicable when investigators have defined "true" schizophrenia as having narrowed clinical boundaries within which all patients are hypothesized as being affected by the same pathologic process. For example, Weinberger (1987) has rejected the notion of subtypes on the grounds that the distributions of anatomical studies tend to be normal, not bimodal or polymodal; he has hypothesized that a primary neurodevelopmental process gives rise to a single disease or pathologic continuum.

As formulated by Carpenter et al. (1993), the second model for schizophrenia views the illness as a clinical syndrome consisting of two or more disease entities, each with its own etiology and pathophysiology but with shared clinical manifestations. Mental retardation, in which a number of discrete disease entities have been found within the syndrome, is an example of this model. As Carpenter et al. (1993) have pointed out, if model 1 (homogeneity) is correct, then schizophrenia-control comparisons will be robust, but if model 2 is correct, these comparisons will be weakened because only a portion of the experimental cohort will have the underlying disease vulnerability in question.

Over the past century, many divergent concepts about the core features and the most meaningful subdivisions of schizophrenia have been advocated in different countries and by different psychiatrists. Radical differences of opinion persist to the present day. Many researchers have used the broad clinical concept as their starting point but then have often gone on to examine subgroups of schizophrenics without ever agreeing upon which subdivision was optimal. Here we shall review some of the main subtyping efforts and comment on their relative merits.

"TRUE" SCHIZOPHRENIA VERSUS SCHIZOPHRENIA-LIKE DISORDERS

Repeated efforts have been made to identify clinical features that characterize what is believed to be "true" schizophrenia. Sometimes these approaches have basically followed model 1, as described above; the patients excluded from the "true" schizophrenia grouping are not studied in the same detail and are not linked to a second hypothesized process. More often, the "false" or "schizophrenia-like" patients have been linked to hypothetical psychological phenomena, not to a biological pathophysiology.

For example, Jaspers (1913) made a distinction between chronic, "process" schizophrenia, with a unifying clinical characteristic of "ununderstandability," contrasted with more understandable "psychogenic reactions." However, he did not specify a hypothesis about the nature of the "process" in "true" schizophrenia.

Later, Scandinavian psychiatrists and American research psychologists have proposed that a similar categorization should be used to differentiate "good-prognosis" and "poor-prognosis" cases. In the late 1930s, Langfeldt (1939), using followup data on patients in Oslo, made a distinction between "true" schizophrenia, which had a poor prognosis and a presumptive biological basis, and "schizophreniform" (schizophrenia-like) states, which had a good prognosis and were often precipitated by psychological stressors. Although the distinction between good and poor prognosis cases has influenced a considerable body of research, other investigators have found that the differentiating criteria did not predict outcome so accurately as had been hoped.

Kurt Schneider (1959) working from the 1930s to the 1950s, tried to make the diagnosis more reliable by identifying a group of symptoms that he believed were characteristic of schizophrenia, but were rarely found in other disorders. Unlike Bleuler's fundamental symptoms, Schneider's symptoms were not assumed to be the expression of any underlying, central psychopathological process. "Among many abnormal modes of experience that occur in schizophrenia, there are some that we put in first rank of importance, not because we think of them as basic disturbances, but because they have special value in helping us to determine the diagnosis of schizophrenia. When any one of these modes of experience is undeniably present and no basic somatic illness can be found, we make the diagnosis of schizophrenia. Symptoms of first-rank importance do not always have to be present for a diagnosis to be made" (1959). This last point is important. Some of these first-rank symptoms are included in the diagnostic criteria for schizophrenia in DSM-III-R (American Psychiatric Association, 1987) and ICD-10 (World Health Organization, 1992).

THE ACUTE/CHRONIC SUBDIVISION

A primary comparison has been made repeatedly between two basic concepts-- acute schizophrenia and chronic schizophrenia. This distinction paves the way for the description of the many clinical pictures encountered in practice, and has been the starting point for discussion of some of the main theories and arguments about schizophrenia.

Essentially, the acute/chronic distinction rests upon differences in the constellation of presenting symptoms, and in the type of premorbid adjustment, type of onset, and the subsequent course of illness. In acute schizophrenia, the predominant clinical features are delusions, hallucinations, and interference with thinking. Features of this kind are often called florid or "positive" symptoms. Some patients recover from acute illness, while others progress to the chronic syndrome. By contrast, the main symptomatic features of chronic schizophrenia tend to be the so-called "negative" symptoms of apathy, lack of drive, poverty of amount and content of speech, and social withdrawal.

As a general, but by no means entirely consistent pattern, the chronic syndrome is especially prominent in those patients whose onset of psychotic symptoms has emerged insidiously, with a so-called poor-premorbid adjustment, and with a more persistently impaired long-term course of illness; often it has been assumed that these patients are a more genetically or biologically determined subgroup of patients. In contrast, those who have a sudden, precipitous onset of psychotic symptoms with a good-premorbid adjustment more often, but not always, have a remitting or episodic course of illness. It has been generally assumed that what has been called "acute schizophrenia" is more "reactive," more susceptible to stressful life events, and more likely to be psychogenically induced than is true for the so-called poor-prognosis, "process," or chronic schizophrenic patients. Once the chronic syndrome is established, many patients eventually recover partially, but relatively few patients recover completely.

Brief Psychotic Disorders

Marginal to patients who have been called acute schizophrenics, there are still other cases that sometimes have been screened for preliminary inclusion with schizophrenia for purposes of certain studies. One such group includes patients with acute "organic" and drug-induced psychotic disorders. Another is what is called in DSM-III-R "brief reactive psychosis," a syndrome without prodromal or residual symptoms, with the active disturbance lasting not more than a month, apparently precipitated by stress, and presenting with prominent emotional turmoil. "Schizophreniform disorder" is a syndrome defined as having a duration between that for brief reactive psychosis and for schizophrenia; the phase of "characteristic," psychotic, "positive" symptoms is the same as in schizophrenia there may be prodromal and/or residual "negative" symptoms if the total duration of the episode is less than 6 months and more than one month.

The classificatory importance of the prodromal/residual symptoms is evident when one recognizes that "true" schizophrenia may be diagnosed with DSM-III-R criteria when the active psychotic symptoms are present for as briefly as one week--extended to one month in both DSM-IV (American Psychiatric Association, 1994) and ICD-10 (World Health Organization, 1992). During the rest of the 6-month period that is required for the diagnosis of DSM-III-R schizophrenia only nonpsychotic prodromal or residual symptoms need be present. However, these symptoms are nonspecific and are found commonly, but unreliably, before or after most psychotic episodes. The result has been that diagnoses of brief reactive psychosis and schizophreniform disorder are rarely made with DSM-III-R criteria, in contrast to the frequency with which the subgroup of "acute schizophrenia" was diagnosed in years past.

"CLASSICAL" SUBTYPING

The "classical,"Kraepelinian subtypes of schizophrenia (hebephrenic, catatonic, and paranoid) are relatively easy to identify in their prototypical forms. Patients with hebephrenic schizophrenia often appear silly and childish in their behavior. Affective flattening and thought disorder are prominent. Delusions are common, but poorly organized. Hallucinations are common, but not elaborated.

Catatonic schizophrenia is characterized by motor symptoms and by changes in activity varying between excitement and stupor. Hallucinations, delusions, and affective symptoms occur but are usually less obvious. Although the catatonic subtype is still listed in diagnostic manuals, it has been seen rarely in industrialized, urban settings during the last three decades. Catatonia now appears to be more appropriately viewed as a temporary phase of psychotic illness, not specifically a subtype of schizophrenia.

In paranoid schizophrenia, the clinical picture is dominated by well-organized paranoid delusions. Thought processes and mood are relatively unaffected, and the patients may appear normal until abnormal beliefs are uncovered.

The simple subtype, which has not been consistently accepted, is an insidious but progressive development of the characteristic "negative" features of schizophrenia (for example, blunting of affect, loss of volition) without being preceded by overt psychotic symptoms.

Unfortunately, these primary subgroups cannot be clearly or reliably distinguished in clinical practice from mixed-type, or "undifferentiated," schizophrenics. No support for the classical subtyping was found cross-culturally in the International Pilot Study of Schizophrenia (World Health Organization, 1973). Nevertheless, even in the upcoming DSM-IV (American Psychiatric Association, 1994), the "traditional" clinical subtyping survives in terms of the main schizophrenia subtypes: paranoid, disorganized (formerly hebephrenic), catatonic, and undifferentiated. The ICD-10 (World Health Organization, 1992) adds the simple type. In DSM-II (American Psychiatric Association, 1968), five subtypes were listed but then were dropped in DSM-III (American Psychiatric Association, 1980): simple type, acute schizophrenic episode, latent type, schizoaffective type, and childhood type.

"STANDARDIZED" DIAGNOSES

The research consensus over the last 25 years has been that the splitting into such a great diversity of subtypes has not been useful. Therefore, many researchers have preferred to identify a core group of patients using operational or "standardized" criteria. An important example of a standardized diagnosis is obtained through CATEGO (Wing, Cooper, and Sartorius, 1974), a computer program designed to process data from the Present State Examination (PSE). The narrowest syndrome (S+) is diagnosed mainly on the symptoms of thought intrusion, broadcast or withdrawal; delusions of control; and voices discussing the patients in the third person or commenting on his or her actions. Unfortunately, CATEGO has been found to be excessively overinclusive of patients who have too little else in common.

The Feighner Criteria (Feighner et al. 1972), another example of a standardized diagnostic system, were developed in St. Louis to identify patients with a poor prognosis. The criteria are reliable but restrictive, leaving many cases without a diagnosis.

The Research Diagnostic Criteria (RDC; Spitzer et al., 1978) were developed from those of the Feighner Criteria. The main difference is in the length of history required before the diagnosis of schizophrenia can be made: two weeks, instead of the 6 months in Feighner's criteria. In turn, the DSM-III (1980) was derived in considerable part from the RDC. DSM-III, and its 1987 and 1994 revisions, is a diagnostic system intended for broad clinical use but incorporating some of the operational features of the earlier research approaches. The ICD-10 (1992) now shares some of the characteristics of the DSM systems, but certain minor differences remain.

Thus, with respect to schizophrenia, researchers still are searching for more satisfactory ways to subtype the broad range of phenomena that have been regarded by various investigators as relevant. In addition to the acute/chronic and good prognosis/poor prognosis dichotomies that have already been discussed, other major subdivisions include: (a) psychotic/nonpsychotic; (b) paranoid/nonparanoid; (c) affective/nonaffective; (d) familial/sporadic; and (e) positive/negative.

THE PSYCHOTIC/NONPSYCHOTIC SUBDIVISION

Beginning with Eugen Bleuler, there has been a persistent, important question as to whether certain nonpsychotic patients share the same biological and/or pathophysiological dysfunctions as patients with the more "characteristic" psychotic symptoms. Patients who resemble those with "typical" schizophrenia, but who fail to meet strict criteria for diagnosis of the psychotic form of the illness, fall into three groups.

The first group consists of people who from an early age have behaved oddly and have shown features resembling those seen in schizophrenia (for example, ideas of reference, persecutory beliefs, and unusual styles of thinking) but without the definite and more characteristic, floridly psychotic symptoms of schizophrenia. When long-standing, these disorders can be classified in the "odd" cluster of DSM-III-R personality disorders (schizotypal, paranoid, and schizoid personality disorders). In ICD-10, schizotypal disorder is grouped with schizophrenic and delusional disorder, not as a form of personality disorder.

The second group is composed of people who develop nonpsychotic, predominantly schizotypal symptoms after a period of relatively normal development. Bleuler (1911) spoke of these patients as having "simple schizophrenia." Although this subtype term has been retained in ICD-10, that manual states that this is "a difficult diagnosis to make with any confidence" (page 95). In DSM-III-R these patients are not explicitly classified and probably are usually designated as schizoid personality disorder or as schizotypal personality disorder.

The third group of nonpsychotic patients on the margins of schizophrenia are those persons who have shown the full clinical picture of schizophrenia in the past but have progressed to a stage with long-term, nonpsychotic, "negative" symptoms. In both DSM-III-R and ICD-10 these cases are classified as "residual schizophrenia," which is better thought of as a late stage of the illness, not as a subtype in the usual sense.

Still another term for nonpsychotic schizophrenic illness has been "latent" schizophrenia. Because of data from the Danish Adoption Study (Kety et al. 1968), Spitzer and colleagues (1979) introduced the concept of "schizotypal personality disorder," using more explicit criteria than had been applied to "latent schizophrenia." Although "latent schizophrenia" was abandoned in DSM-III (1980), it has recently been revived by Kety and Ingraham (1992). They have found in their recent analysis of the Danish Adoption Study data that, genetically, patients with latent schizophrenia--as they have diagnosed it--share genetic similarities with more typical schizophrenics.

By now, a number of other studies have established that there is genetic overlap between so-called typical schizophrenia and schizotypal personality disorder. However, Torgersen et al. (1993) and Kendler et al. (1993b) both have concluded that, in addition to the overlap, there is also a difference between the familial aggregation of schizotypal and schizophrenic persons. Thus, the question remains as to whether schizotypal disorder should be best included as a subtype of schizophrenia or as a distinctive clinical entity, apart from schizophrenia.

Borderline States

In the United States there was formerly much interest in states or syndromes intermediate between schizophrenia and the neuroses and personality disorders. Prior to DSM-III (1980), the term "borderline states" was used in three main ways. First, a "core borderline syndrome" was characterized as an enduring entity with vacillating involvement with others, overt or acted-out expressions of anger, depression, and absence of indications of consistent self-identity (Grinker, Werble, and Drye, 1968).

Second, a borderline state was regarded as mild form of schizophrenia. This usage resembled Bleuler's concept of latent schizophrenia; it also covers the nonpsychotic portion of the "schizophrenia spectrum" referred to in some genetic studies, as well as the concept of ambulatory, "pseudoneurotic" schizophrenia (Hoch and Polatin, 1949).

Third, the usage that is retained today is defined operationally in DSM-III-R as borderline personality disorder, a pervasive pattern of instability of mood, interpersonal relationships, and self-image. Researchers now agree that this disorder is not genetically related to schizophrenia and appears to more closely linked to the spectrum of mood disorders.

THE PARANOID/NONPARANOID DISTINCTION

There has not been a consistent agreement about what the criteria should be for the paranoid subtype of schizophrenia. Especially, there has been a question as to whether persons with paranoid symptoms should be included in this subtype if their delusional or hallucinatory experiences are fragmentary and nonsystematized. Most diagnosticians believe that paranoid schizophrenics, as well as patients with paranoid psychosis, tend to have well-organized and "systematized" delusions and hallucinations. However, past studies have not consistently used this distinction. Also, there has been an inconsistent tendency to exclude patients from the paranoid subtype if they have disorganized speech or behavior. This exclusionary criterion was not included in DSM-III (1980) but was introduced in DSM-III-R (1987).

A few research clinicians, especially Tsuang and Winokur (1974), have started with poor-prognosis schizophrenics, identified using the narrow Feighner criteria, and then have differentiated paranoid versus hebephrenic subtypes of patients. Followup findings showed that the paranoid patients did better than the hebephrenic patients on a number of clinical measures, for example, with more motor symptoms and more tangential thinking in the hebephrenic patients. Kendler et al. (1984) confirmed that, using the Tsuang-Winokur criteria, as well as DSM-III RDC, and ICD-9, short- and long-term outcomes were better for paranoid than nonparanoid schizophrenia. On the other hand, Kendler et al. (1988) found no difference in the risk for psychiatric disorders in the relatives of probands with different subtypes of schizophrenia. They concluded that the subtypes of schizophrenia appear "valid" from a prognostic but not from a familial standpoint.

THE AFFECTIVE/NONAFFECTIVE DISTINCTION

In 1933, Kasanin explicitly introduced the subtype of schizoaffective schizophrenia. Although this category became popular, especially in the U.S., many researchers felt that this subtype broadened the concept of schizophrenia excessively and provided too much overlap with manic-depressive or bipolar disorder. Therefore, efforts have been made to subdivide the schizoaffective patients into those who are more like typical schizophrenics versus those who are more like manic-depressives.

The problem was further complicated by the failure in DSM-III (1980) to provide any criteria whatsoever for schizoaffective disorder, which was split off into a DSM-III group of categories called "Psychotic Disorders Not Elsewhere Classified." In DSM-III-R, schizoaffective disorder has been defined as a disturbance during which, at some time, there is either a major depressive or manic syndrome concurrent with the psychotic symptoms that are characteristic of schizophrenia, but there has also been at least 2 weeks when these delusions or hallucinations occur in the absence of prominent mood disturbance, and all of the episodes of a mood syndrome have been brief relative to the total duration of the active and residual phases of the disturbance.

Recent research, for example, by Kendler et al. (1993a) shows that schizoaffective disorder, as defined in DSM-III-R, appears to segregate with schizophrenia in family studies, even though both ICD-10 and DSM-IV still list schizoaffective disorder separately from schizophrenia, as if these are discrete disease entities. Currently, most researchers prefer to group schizoaffective disorder, narrowly defined as in DSM-III-R, together with schizophrenia.

Another important aspect of the affectivity dimension is that with the DSM-III narrowing of the diagnostic criteria for schizophrenia, there was a broadening of the diagnosis of bipolar and manic-depressive disorder, so that some of the same psychotic symptoms found in schizophrenia were now recognized as also present in bipolar psychoses. It seems certain that a considerable number of patients previously diagnosed as schizophrenics, particularly in the United States, have in more recent years been diagnosed as bipolar psychotics.

Previously, many of these bipolar patients would have been diagnosed as having so-called good-prognosis schizophrenia, or as an acute schizophrenic episode followed by remission. Although there has been a strong tendency to regard schizophrenia as primarily a chronic illness since the advent of DSM-III, with the minimum of 6 months duration, there continues to be a question as to whether patients with a nonremitting or deteriorating course are biologically different from those with partial or complete remissions.

THE FAMILIAL/SPORADIC DISTINCTION

The variable of familial history has been used to classify patients in terms of their relatives' histories, rather than their personal clinical characteristics. In one such approach patients have been classified as "familial" (those with a schizophrenic first-degree relative), versus "sporadic" (those with a negative family history for schizophrenia). Several investigators have differences between patients with familial versus sporadic schizophrenia (Kendler and Hays, 1982; Reveley et al., 1984; Shur, 1982; and Walker et al., 1982). Although it is tempting to equate familial with genetic schizophrenia and sporadic with exogenous forms of the illness, the indirect family history method has low sensitivity and misclassifies a considerable proportion of familial cases as sporadic. Kendler (1988) found that the familial versus sporadic distinction has low statistical power to detect etiological heterogeneity, requiring larger sample sizes than are ordinarily available.

Other investigators, using the "high-risk" methodology, have attempted to examine relatives personally and to classify subjects in terms of degree of presumed genetic risk based upon schizophrenia spectrum illness of the parents. For example,

Cannon et al. (1993) have shown that genetic risk for schizophrenia interacts with obstetric complications in predicting selectively to morphological abnormalities of the brain.

Methodologically rigorous studies clearly demonstrate that schizophrenia substantially aggregates in families (Kendler and Diehl, 1993). Also, familial factors that predispose to schizophrenia also increase the risk for schizophrenia-related personality disorders and probably for some forms of nonschizophrenic nonaffective psychosis. Results from a new twin study (Onstad et al., 1991) and updates from two adoption studies (Kety and Ingraham, 1992; Tienari et al., 1991) continue to support the hypothesis that genetic factors play a major role in the etiology of schizophrenia.

Nevertheless, this aggregation does not seem sufficient for a useful classificatory criterion of genetic versus sporadic cases. Despite the statistical evidence of family aggregation, there are many "sporadic" cases of schizophrenia without a discernible family history of the illness. Genetically-related criteria are hazardous to apply because, as Kendler and Diehl (1993) have stated: "gene carriers need not manifest the illness (incomplete penetrance), affected individuals need not have the gene (environmental forms or phenocopies), diagnostic uncertainties cannot be avoided, and different families may carry different susceptibility genes (genetic heterogeneity)" (page 261).

POSITIVE/NEGATIVE SYMPTOMS

Especially during the last decade, there has been a great deal of research and controversy associated with an effort to dichotomize schizophrenic symptoms as positive versus negative (Andreasen, 1982). As noted above, this distinction overlaps to a considerable extent with the acute/chronic subtyping, but is based upon symptoms seen cross-sectionally in time, rather than upon the course of illness. Positive-symptom patients with active delusions, hallucinations, incoherence of thinking, and disorganized behavior, have been contrasted with negative-symptom schizophrenics who have flat affect, poverty of speech, social withdrawal, and loss of initiative and interests.

In practice, although some patients can be recognized as having "positive" schizophrenia versus "negative" schizophrenia," most patients show a mixture of positive and negative symptoms. This is an example of the difficulty, recently pointed out by Andreasen and Carpenter (1993), that arises if one tries to test the hypothesis that there are two or more disease entities within the present concept of schizophrenia. They observe that this construct (described above as model 2) is excellent for exploratory studies, but the multiple clinical criteria for each entity complicate the interpretation of group differences.

DOMAINS OF PSYCHOPATHOLOGY, NOT DISEASE ENTITIES

A number of current researchers have abandoned trying to classify schizophrenic patients in terms of disease entities with multiple criteria applied to schizophrenia as a whole (model 1) or to the subtypes that have been discussed above (model 2). Instead, in a model 3 as proposed by Carpenter et al., (1989, 1993), more specific, delimited domains of psychopathology are selected that are hypothetically linked to a delimited neurophysiologic or neuroanatomic process. Several such models for reducing the heterogeneity of schizophrenia have been proposed (for example, Pogue-Geile and Keshavan, 1991; Tsuang et al., 1990).

In an effort to identify a specific domain of psychopathology of this kind that appears to have a neuroanatomic basis, Carpenter et al. (1988) have introduced the term "deficit syndrome." This concept refers to negative symptoms that are sustained over time and are not attributable to other causes such as medication, primary depression, or institutionalization. Other investigators seeking to identify distinctive domains of schizophrenic psychopathology have concluded that a three-compartment model appears to be the most satisfactory (Kay and Sevy, 1991; Lenzenweger et al., 1991; Arndt et al., 1991; Barnes and Liddle, 1990). In addition to the deficit syndrome, they have identified the domains of hallucinations/delusions and of cognitive/attentional impairments as having distinctive characteristics.

The strategy of hypothesizing links between specific symptom complexes and specific pathophysiological processes is illustrated in the distinction between Type I and Type II schizophrenia that has been proposed by Crow (1980, 1985). He modified the positive/negative distinction in formulating a hypothesis about the underlying role of dopamine. Type I is said to have an acute onset, mainly positive symptoms, and good social functioning during remissions. It has a good response to neuroleptics, with biochemical evidence of dopamine overactivity. In contrast, Type II is said to have an insidious onset, mainly negative symptoms, and poor outcome. It has a poor response to neuroleptics without evidence of dopamine overactivity. Also, some investigators believe that in Type II there is evidence of more structural change in the brain (especially ventricular enlargement).

Crow's proposition can be viewed, as Carpenter et al. (1993) have pointed out, not as a distinction between putative disease entities each defined by multiple criteria, but with a starting point defined in terms of a single, central criterion--the presence or absence of irreversible negative symptoms, the deficit syndrome. A falsifiable hypothesis is then proposed in which this domain of psychopathology is linked to a discrete etiologic mechanism. This exemplifies the third model for reducing heterogeneity, an approach that appears to generate testable hypotheses more readily than do models 1 and 2.

As an alternative to identifying psychopathological domains clinically, another approach that appears highly promising for reducing heterogeneity is to define subgroups homogeneous for physiological markers that correlate with, or may underlie a schizophrenic process of interest. An example is the use of smooth-pursuit eye-tracking dysfunction (Holzman, 1985). Such markers can be observed not only in many schizophrenic probands but also in the symptomatically well biological relatives of schizophrenic probands.

SUMMARY

The question has remained unresolved, even in the classifications of DSM-IV and ICD-1O, as to the most appropriate boundaries for schizophrenia, together with the problem of heterogeneity and subtyping within this syndrome. We have provided an overview of those subdivisions that have generated the most research, and that currently continue to be relevant even though the specific details of classificatory criteria have shifted back and forth over time.

The subtyping of schizophrenics and the redefining of the boundaries of schizophrenia is obviously of great relevance to researchers who wish to have a preliminary way of generating samples of patients who then can be evaluated for linkage studies, for studies of biological markers, and for studies of gene/environment interaction. The problem is complicated by the fact that there is still disagreement as to the extent that genetic heterogeneity may exist. If more than one major gene is involved, then perhaps certain subtypes or dichotomies (as described above) may turn out to be relevant to distinctions that are made by biological markers and/or by genetic linkage studies.

A fundamental recommendation for any study of schizophrenia is that researchers should specify the explicit criteria that they are using for making their diagnostic distinctions, both for the overall category of schizophrenia and for subtypes. Over the years, the same terms have been used with frequent changes in definitions or with no definitions explicitly offered. This inconsistency has substantially impeded clarification of problems concerning how both genetic and environmental factors contribute to vulnerability and strengths, to the onset of clinical psychotic illness, and to the course of the illness.

An important new research emphasis is to hypothesize links between specific domains of psychopathology, such as the deficit syndrome, identified as present in all subjects in a study and then to assess for neuroanatomic and other correlates of this domain. It is not possible to conclude that this conceptual and research model will be productive, but it does have the distinct advantage of generating falsifiable hypotheses (Carpenter et al., 1993). Alternatively, physiologic markers, such as eye-tracking dysfunction, can be used to reduce syndromal heterogeneity.

REFERENCES

American Psychiatric Association, 1968, "DSM-II: Diagnostic and Statistical Manual of Mental Disorders" (2nd ed.), American Psychiatric Association, Washington DC.

American Psychiatric Association, 1980, "DSM-III: Diagnostic and Statistical Manual of Mental Disorders" (3rd ed.), American Psychiatric Association, Washington DC.

American Psychiatric Association, 1987, "DSM-III-R: Diagnostic and Statistical Manual of Mental Disorders" (rev. ed.), American Psychiatric Association, Washington DC.

American Psychiatric Association, 1994, "DSM-IV: Diagnostic and Statistical Manual of Mental Disorders" (4th. ed.), American Psychiatric Association, Washington DC.

Andreasen, N.C., 1982, Negative versus positive schizophrenia: definition and validation, Arch. Gen. Psychiat. 36:1325.

Andreasen, N.C. and Carpenter, W.T.,Jr., 1993, Diagnosis and classification of schizophrenia, Schiz. Bull. 19:199.

Arndt, S., Alliger, R.J., and Andreasen, N.C., 1991, The distinction of positive and negative symptoms: the failure of the two- dimensional model, Brit. J. Psychiat. 158:317.

Barnes, T.R.E. and Liddle, P.F., 1990, Evidence for the validity of negative symptoms, Mod. Probl. Pharmacopsychiat. 24:43.

Bleuler, E., 1911 (English ed., 1950), "Dementia Praecox or the Group of Schizophrenias," International Universities Press, New York.

Cannon, S.A.,Parnas, J., Schulsinger, F., Praestholm, J., and Vestergaard, A., 1993, Developmental brain abnormalities in the offspring of schizophrenic mothers: I. contributions of genetic and perinatal factors, Arch. Gen. Psychiat. 50:551.

Carpenter, W.T.,Jr. and Buchanan, R.W., 1989, Domains of psychopathology relevant to the study of etiology and treatment of schizophrenia, in: "Schizophrenia: Scientific Progress," S.C. Schultz and C.A. Tamminga, eds., Oxford University Press, New York.

Carpenter, W.T.,Jr., Buchanan, R.W., Kirkpatrick, B., Tamminga, C., and Wood, F., 1993, Strong inference, theory testing, and the neuroanatomy of schizophrenia, Arch. Gen. Psychiat. 50:825.

Carpenter, W.T.,Jr., Heinrichs, D.W., and Wagman, A.M.I.,1988, Deficit and nondeficit forms of schizophrenia: the concept, Am. J. Psychiat. 145:578.

Crow, T.J., 1980, Molecular pathology of schizophrenia: more than one disease process? Brit. Med. J. 280:66.

Crow, T.J., 1985, The two-syndrome concept: origins and current status, Schiz. Bull. 11:471.

Feighner, J.P., Robins, E., Guze, S.G., Woodruff, R.A., Winokur, G., and Munoz, R., 1972, Diagnostic criteria for use in psychiatric research, Arch. Gen. Psychiat. 26:57.

Griesinger, W., 1867, "Mental Pathology and Therapeutics," New Sydenham Society, London.

Grinker, R.R., Werble, B., and Drye, R.C., 1968, "The Borderline Syndrome: A Behavior Study of Ego-functions," Basic Books, New York.

Hoch, P.H. and Polatin, P., 1949, Pseudoneurotic forms of schizophrenia, *Psychiat. Quart.* 23:249.

Holzman, P.S., 1985, Eye movement dysfunctions and psychoses, *Internatl. Rev. Neurobiol.* 27:179.

Jaspers, K, 1913, "Allgemeine Psychopathologie," Springer, Berlin.

Kasanin, J., 1933, The acute schizoaffective psychosis, *Am. J. Psychiat.* 13:97.

Kay, S.R. and Sevy, S., 1991, Pyramidical model of schizophrenia, *Schiz. Bull.* 16:537.

Kendler, K.S., 1988, The sporadic v. familial classification given aetiological heterogeneity: II. power analyses, *Psychol. Med.* 18:991.

Kendler, K.S., and Diehl, S.R., 1993, The genetics of schizophrenia: a current genetic-epidemiologic perspective, *Schiz. Bull.* 19:261.

Kendler, K.S., Gruenberg, A.M., and Tsuang, M.T., 1984, Outcome of schizophrenic subtypes defined by four diagnostic systems, *Arch. Gen. Psychiat.* 41:149.

Kendler, K.S., Gruenberg, A.M., and Tsuang, M.T., 1988, A family study of the subtypes of schizophrenia, *Am. J. Psychiat.* 145:57

Kendler, K.S., and Hays, 1982, Familial and sporadic schizophrenia: a symptomatic, prognostic, and EEG comparison, *Am. J. Psychiat.* 139:1557.

Kendler, K.S., McGuire, M., Gruenberg, A.M., O'Hare, A., Spellman, M., and Walsh, D., 1993a, The Roscommon family study: I. methods, diagnosis of probands, and risk of schizophrenia in relatives, *Arch. Gen. Psychiat.* 50:527.

Kendler, K.S., McGuire, M., Gruenberg, A.M., O'Hare, A., Spellman, M., and Walsh, D., 1993b, The Roscommon family study: III. schizophrenia-related personality disorders in relatives, *Arch. Gen. Psychiat.* 50:781.

Kety, S.S. and Ingraham, L.J., 1992, Genetic transmission and improved diagnosis of schizophrenia from pedigrees of adoptees, *J. Psychiat. Res.* 26:247.

Kety, S.S., Rosenthal, D., Wender, P.H., and Schulsinger, F., 1968, The types and prevalence of mental illness in the biological and adoptive families of adopted schizophrenics, *J. Psychiat. Res.* 6:345.

Kraepelin, E., 1896, "Psychiatrie," Barth, Leipzig.

Kraepelin, E., 1919, "Dementia Praecox and Paraphrenia," Livingstone, Edinburgh.

Langfeldt, G., 1939, "The Schizophreniform States," Munksgaard, Copenhagen.

Lenzenweger, M.F., Dworkin, R.H., and Wethington, E., 1991, Examining the underlying structure of schizophrenic phenomenology: evidence for a three-process model, *Schiz. Bull.* 17:515.

McGuffin, P., Farmer, A.E., and Gottesman, I.I., 1987, Is there really a split in schizophrenia? The genetic evidence, *Brit. J. Psychiat.* 150:581.

Onstad, S., Skre, I., Torgersen, S., and Kringlen, E., 1991, Twin concordance for DSM-III-R schizophrenia, *Acta Psychiatr. Scand.* 83:395.

Pogue-Geile, M.F. and Keshavan, M., 1991, Negative symptomatology in schizophrenia: syndrome and subtype status, *in:* "Negative Schizophrenic Symptoms: Pathophysiology and Clinical Implications," J.F. Greden and R. Tandon, eds., American Psychiatric Press, Washington DC.

Reveley, A.M., Reveley M.A., and Murray, R.M., 1984, Cerebral ventricular enlargement in "non-genetic" schizophrenia: a controlled twin study, *Brit. J. Psychiat.* 144:89.

Schneider, K., 1959, "Clinical Psychopathology," Grune and Stratton, New York.

Shur, E., 1982, Family history and schizophrenia: characteristics of groups with and without positive family histories, *Psychol. Med.* 12:591.

Spitzer, R.L., Endicott, J., and Gibbon, M., 1979, Crossing the border into borderline personality and borderline schizophrenia, *Arch. Gen. Psychiat.* 36:17.

Spitzer, R.L., Endicott, J., and Robinson, E., 1978, Research diagnostic criteria: rationale and reliability, *Arch. Gen. Psychiat.* 35:773.

Tienari, P., 1991, Interaction between genetic vulnerability and family environment: the Finnish adoptive family study of schizophrenia, *Acta Psychiatr. Scand.* 84:460.

Torgerson, S., Onstad, S., Skre, I., Edvardsen, J., and Kringlen, 1993, "True" schizotypal personality disorder: a study of co- twins and relatives of schizophrenic probands, *Am. J. Psychiat.* 150:1661.

Tsuang, M.R., Lyons, M.J., and Faraone, S.V., 1990, Heterogeneity of schizophrenia: conceptual models and analytic strategies, *Brit. J. Psychiat.* 156:17.

Tsuang, M.R. and Winokur, G., 1974, Criteria for subtyping schizophrenia: clinical differentiation of hebephrenic and paranoid schizophrenia, *Arch. Gen. Psychiat.* 31:43.

Walker, E. and Shaye, J., 1982, Familial schizophrenia: a predictor of neuromotor and attentional abnormalities in schizophrenia, *Arch. Gen. Psychiat.* 39:1153.

Weinberger, D.R., 1987, Implications of normal brain development for the pathogenesis of schizophrenia, *Arch. Gen. Psychiat.* 44:660.

Wing, J.K., Cooper, J.E., and Sartorius, N., 1974, "Measurement and Classification of Psychiatric Symptoms," Cambridge University Press, Cambridge.

World Health Organization, 1973, "Report of the International Pilot Study of Schizophrenia, Vol. 1," World Health Organization, Geneva.

World Health Organization, 1992, "The ICD-10 Classification of Mental and Behavioral Disorders: Clinical Descriptions and Diagnostic Guidelines," World Health Organization, Geneva.

FETAL VIRAL INFECTION AND ADULT SCHIZOPHRENIA: EMPIRICAL FINDINGS AND INTERPRETATION

Ricardo A. Machón,[1,2] Sarnoff A. Mednick,[2] and Matti O. Huttunen[3]

[1] Loyola Marymount University, Los Angeles
[2] University of Southern California, Los Angeles
[3] University of Helsinki, Finland

INTRODUCTION

We have put forth the hypothesis that an important part of the genetic predisposition to schizophrenia is expressed as a disruption of fetal brain development probably occurring in the second trimester of gestation. The hypothesized disruption of brain development may involve errors in the migration, positioning, orientation and connection of young neurons. These errors of development may also be triggered by teratogens (such as a maternal viral infection) which impact the fetus during a critical period of gestation (Mednick, Machón, Huttunen & Bonett, 1988; Mednick, Cannon, Barr and Lyon, 1991).

These hypotheses stem from a series of studies we have conducted in Scandinavia. The oldest of these projects involved the study of a cohort of 207 offspring of schizophrenic women who we have been following for the past 32 years (Mednick & Schulsinger, 1968). Offspring with schizophrenic mothers are at "high risk" for schizophrenia. These offspring are now 46 years old (on the average) with 31 of them now being diagnosed as schizophrenic (Parnas et al., 1993). One of the factors which best predicts their later schizophrenia are midwife reports (from the 1940's) of their severe difficulties in pregnancy and delivery. Reviews of the literature have consistently noted that schizophrenics tend to have a history of a significant excess of perinatal complications (McNeil, 1988; Mednick, Cannon & Barr, 1991). For those at genetic risk, these perinatal difficulties are also significantly related to structural brain anomalies assessed by imaging techniques (Cannon, Mednick & Parnas, 1989). We have additionally studied the pregnancies and deliveries of a large consecutive birth sample of infants in Helsinki at high risk for schizophrenia and noted an elevation in maternal flu-like symptoms occurring in the latter half of the pregnancy. These symptoms were further associated with an increase in delivery difficulties and poor postnatal status (Wrede et al., 1980).

These Helsinki findings encouraged us to examine the impact of viral infections

Neural Development and Schizophrenia, Edited by S.A. Mednick and J.M. Hollister, Plenum Press, New York, 1995

during gestation on the risk of adult schizophrenia. We decided to conduct this research in the context of a major influenza epidemic for a number of reasons:

1. Most importantly, an influenza epidemic frequently has a short duration with relatively definite beginning and ending dates. We can therefore observe which part of gestation overlaps the height of an epidemic. This allows us to determine whether a narrow critical period of gestation exists and what its temporal boundaries are.

2. Influenza epidemics are frequent events, making it possible to retrospectively find severe epidemics in which exposed fetuses will now be at an age for developing schizophrenia.

3. Influenza epidemics tend to be world-wide, making it possible to attempt to replicate the findings for a given epidemic in other national settings.

THE HELSINKI INFLUENZA EPIDEMIC STUDY

In 1957 the citizens of Helsinki experienced a severe Type A2/Singapore influenza epidemic. This epidemic was well-studied by epidemiologists; they defined the beginning and ending dates of the epidemic by the number of working days missed because of illness. By this criterion they determined that the epidemic began 8 October and ended 14 November 1957.

We recorded all of the inpatient psychiatric hospital diagnoses of a population, born in the County of Uusimaa (encompassing greater Helsinki) between 15 November, 1957 and 14 August, 1958 who had been "exposed prenatally" to the influenza during various months of their fetal life. Control subjects comprised those individuals born during the same months as the index cases, but in the preceding six years (1951-1957).

The index year cohort and controls were paired by month of birth. For example, index year subjects born 15 November, 1957 to 14 December, 1957 were in their ninth month of fetal life during the epidemic exposure; their controls were born 15 November to 14 December in the years 1951 through 1956. The index and control pairings were created in a similar fashion for the other eight months.

In order to control for an equal period of risk for psychopathology (since the controls were between one and six years older than the index cases), we only accepted psychiatric admissions through the age of 26 years and 56 days, the age of the youngest in the index cohort.

Figure 1 presents the percent of psychiatric admissions with schizophrenic diagnoses for the index (influenza exposed) and controls as a function of fetal trimester of exposure. The differences between the index and control groups were not significantly different for the first or third trimesters. Subjects exposed to the influenza in the second trimester had a significantly higher proportion of schizophrenia diagnoses (34.6%) than their controls (20.8%) (Chi square [1] = 7.69, $p < .01$). Within the index group, the second trimester exposed subjects evidenced a significantly higher proportion of schizophrenia diagnoses than the pooled first (20.0%) and third (24.6%) trimester exposed subjects (Chi square [1] = 3.93, $p < .05$). These results appear to be reliable, being replicated in several psychiatric hospitals within Uusimaa and among males and females.

We also examined these data as a function of population-based schizophrenia rates. We identified the index schizophrenics born in the city of Helsinki proper in order to calculate these population-based rates of schizophrenia. Figure 2 presents these population statistics for the index subjects through the age of 26 and age of 30, respectively. By the age of 26 years, the rate of schizophrenia for the second-trimester exposed subjects (11.6/1,000) was significantly higher than the combined first- (5.8/1,000) and third (6.2/1,000) trimester rates (Chi square [1] = 4.82, $p < .05$)

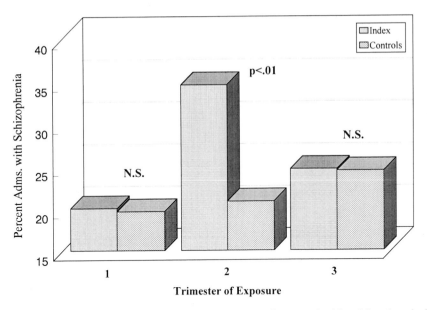

Figure 1. Percent of psychiatric admissions who were diagnosed with schizophrenia for Index and Control groups as a function of fetal trimester of exposure.

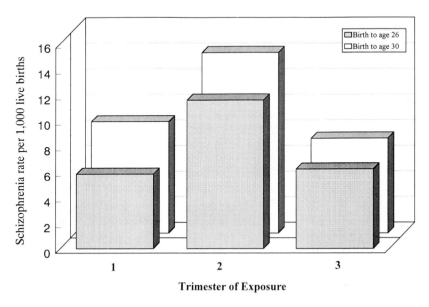

Figure 2. Population based rates of schizophrenia for Index group from birth to age 26 and age 30, respectively, as a function of fetal trimester of exposure.

193

(Mednick, Machón, Huttunen & Bonett, 1988). By the age of 30 years, the rate of schizophrenia for the second-trimester exposed subjects (14.1/1,000) was significantly higher than the combined first- (8.7/1,000) and third (7.4/1,000) trimester rates (Chi square [1] = 8.06, p < .005) (Mednick, Machón & Huttunen, 1990).

The above mentioned results were intriguing but had certain limitations:

1. The data were drawn from only one city.

2. The study was restricted to a single epidemic. Thus, a variety of co-varying factors could not be controlled.

3. There was not a large number of schizophrenics found in the index year (total n=72).

THE DANISH FORTY YEAR STUDY

In the light of the above mentioned limitations, our research group then undertook a replication and extension of the Helsinki findings in Denmark (Barr, Mednick & Munk-Jorgensen, 1990). We extended the period of the Helsinki influenza study to 40 years of births of schizophrenics and 40 years of influenza (1911-1950). We included a complete national population of ever-hospitalized schizophrenics (more than 7500) using perhaps the most complete and accurate national psychiatric register in the world. We also examined all influenza epidemics occurring during these 40 years.

The data included: 1. the number of hospital schizophrenics born each month per 1,000 live-born in Denmark; and 2. the number of cases of influenza per month (1910-1950) per 1,000 population reported to the Danish Ministry of Health.

Each of the 40 Januarys was assigned to one of three groups: one-third with the highest levels of influenza, one-third with average levels of influenza and one-third with the lowest levels of influenza. The same type of grouping was completed for the other 11 months and the highest, the medium and the lowest influenza months were pooled yielding three groups of months with the highest, medium and lowest prevalence of influenza controlled for calendar month and season of exposure.

Each month was also assigned a score. This score indicated how much the birth rate of schizophrenia deviated from the average level for that month across the 40 years. We then computed the rates of schizophrenia for each of the 9 months of gestation following high, medium and low influenza months. We will describe one analysis of these data.

Question? Were unusually high influenza months followed by births of unusually large rates of schizophrenia?

Fetuses exposed during unusually high influenza months during their **6th month** of gestation, had a significantly elevated risk of succumbing to schizophrenia in adulthood. No such relationship was observed for those exposed in the sixth month during low- or medium-influenza months.

The relationship between schizophrenia and other infectious diseases have also been examined. Barr et al. (1991), in Denmark, repeated his analyses examining 28 infectious illnesses other than influenza. No other illness during gestation evidenced a significant association with an increased rate of births of schizophrenia. O'Callaghan et al. (1993), in the United Kingdom, completed a similar analysis for 16 other infectious diseases. No other significant association with schizophrenia was observed.

REPLICATION ATTEMPTS

The Helsinki Influenza study and the Danish Forty Year study have inspired several attempts at replication. Table 1 presents a summary of the literature examining the 1957 influenza epidemic. These studies have largely replicated the second trimester effect first reported in our 1988 publication, in several different nations, continents and hemispheres, and encompassing several research designs. The two studies (Bowler & Torrey, 1990; Crow & Done, 1992) failing to replicate the effect have been criticized on the grounds of severe methodological restrictions which render their results difficult to interpret (Mednick, Huttunen & Machón, 1994). Several studies with sizable sample sizes have shown a **sixth month effect** as well. Table 2 summarizes the studies which have examined multi-influenza epidemics other than the 1957. These have also largely shown a second trimester and sixth month effect.

Table 1. Summary of 1957 Influenza Epidemic Studies: Replication Attempts

Author	Year	City or Nation	Finding
Mednick et al.	1988	Helsinki	Second trimester
Kendell & Kemp	1989	Scotland	1/2 Replication
		Edinburgh	Replication- 6th month
Bowler & Torrey	1990	U.S.A.	Non-replication
O'Callaghan et al.	1991a	U.K.	Replication- 6th month
Kunugi et al.	1992	Tokyo	Replication- 6th month
Waddington	1992	Ireland	Replication
Crow & Done	1992	U.K.	Non-replication
Machón & Mednick	1993	Finland	Replication- 6th month
Fahy et al.	1993	U.K.	Replication
Welham et al.	1993	Queensland, Austr.	Replication
Adams, Kendell et al.	1993	England,	Replication
		Denmark,	Replication
		Scotland	Replication
Beckmann et al.	1993	Germany	Replication

Table 2. Summary of Multi-Influenza Epidemic Studies: Replication Attempts

Author	Year	City or Nation	Finding
Barr et al.	1990	Denmark	Replication- 6th month (40 years)
Sham et al.	1992	U.K.	Replication (22 years)
Morris et al.	1993	Ireland	Replication 3rd trimester (50 years)
Takei et al.	1993	U.K.	Replication (27 years)
Welham et al.	1993	Brisbane, Austr.	Replication (2 of 3 epidemics)

INFLUENZA *EXPOSURE* VERSUS INFLUENZA *INFECTION*

Note that there are two instances in Table 1 of a failure to replicate the second trimester findings. The Crow & Done (1992) study is especially interesting since it was completed in the context of a major British birth cohort study, born in a week in March 1958. *At the time of delivery,* all women in this study were asked to **recall** whether they had suffered an influenza infection during the pregnancy and if so in which month.

Crow & Done found that maternal reports, at the time of delivery, of influenza infection during pregnancy were **not** related to an elevated level of schizophrenia in the offspring. This study has been criticized for surprisingly low ascertainment of both schizophrenia and influenza (O'Callaghan et al., 1991b; Mednick, Huttunen and Machón, 1994).

In order to better understand the Crow & Done results, we conducted a study in Copenhagen in the context of an ongoing perinatal project. We routinely asked women in their 25th week of pregnancy whether they had suffered a persistent cough or high fever during the pregnancy. To assess accuracy of recall, we asked these same women the same questions at the time of delivery (as in the Crow & Done study). 50% (12 of 24) of those who had reported a high fever in the 25th week failed to report the fever at the time of delivery. 85% (33 of 39) of those who had reported a persistent cough at the 25th week failed to report the cough at the time of delivery. At the time of delivery, a large proportion of women failed to recall symptoms of influenza reported earlier in their pregnancy (Voldsgaard et al., in press). The apparent unreliability of retrospective assessment seems to be part of the basis of Crow & Done's failure to find a relationship.

The studies cited in Tables 1 and 2 have two serious problems:

Problem One

In the studies cited, the stage of gestation of the fetus at the time of the epidemic was estimated from their date of birth. For pre- and post-term babies this estimate is incorrect. Since, in some studies, a tendency towards prematurity has been observed among the births of subjects who developed schizophrenia, this is likely to result in some inappropriate assignment of subjects to trimester of gestation of exposure to the epidemic.

Problem Two

In all of these studies (except the Crow and Done, 1992), the increased risk for schizophrenia was associated with second-trimester **exposure** to the epidemic. The timing of the second trimester of gestation is calculated from the date of birth. The period of exposure to the epidemic is defined as the temporal **overlap** of the second trimester with the height of the epidemic. None of these studies, however, determined whether any of the mothers had actually suffered any infection.

We have now carried out a series of analyses in order to address the above mentioned problems: To estimate the stage of gestation more precisely (Problem One), we examined the excellent Helsinki antenatal clinic records for our subjects. These records permitted us to estimate the stage of gestation from the date of last menstruation.

To determine whether any of the Helsinki mothers actually experienced an influenza **infection** (Problem Two), we examined Helsinki antenatal clinic files for each of the Helsinki-born schizophrenics who were exposed to the 1957 epidemic during their first, second or third trimester of gestation. The prenatal clinic printed-forms include a consistently answered question about infections and symptoms since the last clinic visit. These are completed by an obstetrical nurse. Visits of the pregnant women to the clinics were frequent.

Of the schizophrenics exposed to the 1957 epidemic in their first or third trimesters of gestation, twenty percent of their mothers were noted in the antenatal clinic files to have suffered from an influenza infection. This is approximately the background population rate of influenza infection. Of the schizophrenics who were exposed to the epidemic **in the second trimester**, however, 86.7% had a notation made by the obstetrical nurse indicating that their mothers had suffered an influenza infection during the second trimester of gestation.

We interpreted these findings as follows:

1. There were schizophrenics born in Helsinki before the 1957 epidemic.
2. There would have been some schizophrenics born in Helsinki in 1957 and 1958 without the epidemic.
3. Children with maternal infection had an increased risk of developing schizophrenia.
4. We hypothesized that because of maternal influenza in the second trimester, the epidemic was associated with a <u>surplus</u> of schizophrenics born between 1957 and 1958.
5. It follows that the surplus second trimester schizophrenics should have all suffered a maternal influenza infection, as was observed.

POSSIBLE MEDIATING FACTORS

Why is maternal second trimester influenza infection associated with a reliable increase in the risk of adult schizophrenia in the offspring? We have considered several hypotheses:

Pregnancy and Birth Complications (PBCs)

We were nudged in the direction of this area of research by our repeated finding of an excess of PBCs among schizophrenics (Mednick, Cannon & Barr, 1991). As early as 1970, we published a paper suggesting that perinatal difficulties increased risk for schizophrenia by damaging vulnerable areas of the hippocampus.

Thus, we hypothesized that one possible etiological pathway might involve maternal influenza producing an abnormality in the fetus which then would increase the risk of serious delivery complications. To test this, we examined the excellent Helsinki Hospital records of the deliveries of the Helsinki schizophrenics. The specific index of delivery complications was based on overall judgement of the obstetrician, but reflected many specific items. In contrast to our expectation, rather than being worse, the second trimester schizophrenics evidenced significantly **less** complicated deliveries than controls.

Our hypothesis that maternal influenza during gestation may increase the risk of delivery complications was not supported. These data support an etiological model of **replacement** rather than **interaction**. That is, some individuals may develop schizophrenia as a result of PBCs, while others may develop schizophrenia as a result of influenza infection in their mothers during the second trimester of gestations (see Laing et al., Chapter 9).

Not all whose mothers had a second trimester influenza infection became schizophrenic. One possibility is that the infection must hit during a **very** narrow window of neural development. This would explain the relatively small number becoming schizophrenic.

Genetic Predisposition

Another possibility we have mentioned is some kind of second hit. It does not seem to be delivery complications. We explored the possibility that it might be genetic vulnerability. Those who have both genetic liability to schizophrenia and influenza may be at very high risk.

We predicted therefore, that a greater proportion of second trimester schizophrenics would have first degree relatives with schizophrenia than would first or third trimester schizophrenics.

We identified the first degree relatives of the Helsinki schizophrenics and checked for any psychiatric diagnoses in three registers:

1. Psychiatric hospitals
2. National pension register
3. Psychoactive drugs register

Preliminary results showed that the first degree relatives of second trimester schizophrenics did not differ significantly from first or third trimester schizophrenics or controls in rates of either schizophrenia; affective psychoses; or severe mental disorder. The hypothesis that influenza must combine with increased genetic vulnerability was also not supported.

DIFFERENTIATING CLINICAL SYMPTOM PATTERN

It has been hypothesized that the basic disorder of the schizophrenic spectrum is schizotypal personality disorder and that schizophrenia results from the addition of further risk factors. We considered the hypothesis that second trimester influenza produces a personality organization or symptom pattern such as schizotypal personality disorder, that might place the individual at increased risk for schizophrenia. Therefore, we thought that examining the symptoms may be a useful strategy.

The diagnosis of schizophrenia probably includes a number of clinically differentiated subgroups. A subgroup of schizophrenics who share a specific narrow etiology is likely to exhibit a distinctive restricted clinical pattern. We reasoned that a second trimester influenza infection must be regarded as a relatively specific etiological factor. We examined the second trimester Helsinki schizophrenics to see if there was a pattern of symptoms which were distinctive for them. We interviewed index and control subjects and factor analyzed their interview and hospital record symptom reports. The following third order factors resulted:

1. Flat affect
2. Delusions of jealousy
3. Verbally hostile
4. Anhedonia
5. Metonyms
6. Hallucinations
7. Delusions of reference
8. Suspicious.

Analyses of variance results revealed that the second trimester schizophrenics had significantly higher levels of symptom factors 2 (Delusions of jealousy), 7 (Delusions of reference), and 8 (Suspicious) than did schizophrenics exposed in the first or third trimester or controls born in the same months.

We also examined other clinical characteristics based on hospital chart ratings. Figure 3 presents population based rates of schizophrenia comparing index schizophrenics rated as "Suspicious" or "Not Suspicious" as a function of trimester of exposure. The reader will note that those first or third trimester exposed rated as "Suspicious" have comparable rates of schizophrenia as those rated as "Not Suspicious". Among the second trimester exposed, however, those subjects rated as "Suspicious" evidenced significantly elevated rates of schizophrenia as compared to those rated as "Not Suspicious".

STUDIES CURRENTLY IN PROGRESS

1. In collaboration with Ted Jones at University of California, Irvine, we are presently studying the brains of second trimester abortuses of schizophrenic women.

2. We are also preparing to examine the neurointegrative functioning of infants whose mothers suffered a serologically verified influenza and mycoplasma pneumonia infection in the second trimester.

3. We are additionally attempting to identify the part of the second trimester fetal brain recognized by antibodies from schizophrenic and normal women who have a serologically verified influenza infection.

4. We are soon preparing to conduct MRI studies of the brains of the Helsinki influenza infected schizophrenics.

5. For all of Finland, we are currently investigating specific symptom patterns associated with second trimester exposure to influenza.

REFERENCES

Adams, W., Kendell, R.E., Hare, E.H. and Munk-Jorgensen, P., 1993, Epidemiologic evidence that maternal influenza infection contributes to the etiology of schizophrenia, *British Journal of Psychiatry*, 163:522-534.

Barr, C.E., Mednick, S.A. and Munk-Jorgensen, P., 1990, Exposure to influenza epidemics during gestation and adult schizophrenia: A 40-year study, *Archives of General Psychiatry*, 47:869-874.

Barr, C.E., Mednick, S.A. and Munk-Jorgensen, P., 1991, Prenatal infection and schizophrenia in the offspring: A survey of 28 diseases. Paper presented at the third International Congress on Schizophrenia Research, Tucson, Arizona.

Beckmann, J., 1993, Neuropathology findings in schizophrenics, paper presented at NATO-sponsored meeting on Neurodevelopment in Schizophrenia: Theory and Research, held in Lucca, Tuscany, Italy.

Bowler, A.E. and Torrey, E.F., 1990, Influenza and schizophrenia: Helsinki vs. Edinburgh, *Archives of General Psychiatry*, 47:876-877.

Cannon, T.D., Mednick, S.A. and Parnas, J., 1989, Genetic and perinatal determinants of structural brain deficits in schizophrenia, *Archives of General Psychiatry*, 46:883-889.

Conrad, A.J. and Scheibel, A.B., 1987, Schizophrenia and the hippocampus: The embryological hypothesis extended, *Schizophrenia Bulletin*, 13:577-587.

Crow, T.J. and Done, D.J., 1992, Prenatal exposure to influenza does not cause schizophrenia, *British Journal of Psychiatry*, 161:390-393.

Fahy, T.A., Jones, P.B., Sham, P.C., Takei, N., and Murray, R.M., 1993, Schizophrenia in Afro-Caribbeans in the UK following prenatal exposure to the 1957 A2 influenza pandemic, *Schizophrenia Research*, 9:132.

Huttunen, M.O., Machón, R.A. and Mednick, S.A., 1994, Prenatal factors in the pathogenesis of schizophrenia, *British Journal of Psychiatry*, 164 (suppl. 23):15-19.

Kendell, R.E. and Kemp, I.W., 1989, Maternal influenza in the etiology of schizophrenia, *Archives of General Psychiatry*, 46:878-882.

Kunugi, H., Nankos, S. and Takei, N., 1992, Influenza and schizophrenia in Japan, *British Journal of Psychiatry*, 160:274-275.

Machón, R.A. and Mednick, S.A., in press, Adult schizophrenia and early neurodevelopmental disturbances, *Confrontations Psychiatriques*.

McNeil, T.F., 1988, Obstetric factors and perinatal injuries, *in*: "Handbook of Schizophrenia," M.T. Tsuang and J.C. Simpson, eds., Elsevier, Amsterdam.

Mednick, S.A., Cannon, T.D. and Barr, C.E., 1991, Obstetrical events and adult schizophrenia, *in*: "Fetal Neural Development and Adult Schizophrenia," S.A. Mednick, T.D. Cannon, C.E. Barr and M. Lyon, eds., Cambridge University Press, Cambridge, U.K.

Mednick, S.A., Cannon, T.D., Barr, C.E and Lyon, M., 1991, "Fetal Neural Development and Adult Schizophrenia," Cambridge University Press, Cambridge, U.K.

Mednick, S.A., Huttunen, M.O. and Machón, R.A., 1994, Prenatal influenza *infections* and adult schizophrenia, *Schizophrenia Bulletin*.

Mednick, S.A., Machón, R.A. and Huttunen, M.O., 1990, An update on the Helsinki influenza project, *Archives of General Psychiatry*, 47:292.

Mednick, S.A., Machón, R.A., Huttunen, M.O. and Bonett, D., 1988, Adult Schizophrenia following prenatal exposure to an influenza epidemic, *Archives of General Psychiatry*, 45:189-192.

Mednick, S.A and Schulsinger, F., 1968, Some premorbid characteristics related to breakdown in children with schizophrenic mothers, *Journal of Psychiatric Research*, 6:267-91.

Morris, M., Cotter, D., Takei, N., Walsh, D., Larkin, C., Waddington, J.L. and O'Callaghan, E., 1993, An association between schizophrenic births and influenza deaths in Ireland in the years 1921-1971, *Schizophrenia Research*, 9:137.

Nasrallah, H.A., 1991, Neurodevelopmental aspects of bipolar affective disorder, *Biological Psychiatry*, 29:1-2.

O'Callaghan, E., Sham, P., Takei, N., Glover, G. and Murray R.M., 1991a, Schizophrenia following prenatal exposure to 1957 A2 influenza epidemic, *The Lancet*, 337:1248-1250.

O'Callaghan, E., Sham, P., Takei, N., Glover, G. and Murray, R.M., 1991b, Schizophrenia and influenza. *Lancet*, 338:118-119.

O'Callaghan, E., Sham, P., Takei, N., Murray, G., Glover, G., Hare, E. and Murray, R.M., 1993, Schizophrenic births in England and Wales and their relationship to infectious diseases, *Schizophrenia Research*, 9:138.

Parnas, J., Cannon, T.D., Jacobsen, .B., Schulsinger, H., Schulsinger, F., and Mednick, S.A., 1993, Lifetime DSM-III-R diagnostic outcomes in the offspring of schizophrenia mothers. Results from the Copenhagen High Risk Study, *Archives of General Psychiatry*, 50:707-714.

Sham, P.C., O'Callaghan, E., Takei, N., Murray, G.K., Hare, E.H., and Murray, R.M., 1992, Schizophrenia following pre-natal exposure to influenza epidemics between 1939 and 1960, *British Journal of Psychiatry*, 160:461-466.

Stagaard, M., Moos, T. and Mollgard, K., 1991, Is the genetic vulnerability to schizophrenia linked to abnormal development of the ventricular system and the brain barrier systems in the human fetal brain?, *in*: "Fetal Neural Development and Adult Schizophrenia," S.A. Mednick, T.D. Cannon, C.E. Barr and M. Lyon, eds., Cambridge University Press, Cambridge, U.K.

Takei, N., O'Callaghan, E., Sham, P., Glover, G. and Murray, R.M., 1993, Does prenatal influenza divert susceptible females from later depressive psychosis to schizophrenia?, *Schizophrenia Research*, 9:141.

Voldsgaard, P., Mednick, S.A., Christensen, H., Bredkjaer, S., and Schulsinger, F., in press, The Crow et al. influenza-schizophrenia study: Accuracy of maternal reports obtained at the time of delivery.

Waddington, J.L., 1992, The declining incidence of schizophrenia controversy: A new approach in a rural Irish population. Paper presented at the annual meeting of the Royal College of Psychiatrists, Dublin, Ireland.

Welham, J.L., McGrath, J.J., and Pemberton, M.R., 1993, Schizophrenia: Birthrates and three Australian epidemics, *Schizophrenia Research*, 9:142.

Wrede, G., Mednick, S.A., Huttunen, M.O. and Nilsson, C.G., 1980, Pregnancy and delivery complications in the births of an unselected series of Finnish children with schizophrenic mothers, *Acta Psychiatrica Scandinavica*, 62:369-381.

HOW CAN WE JUDGE WHETHER OR NOT PRENATAL EXPOSURE TO INFLUENZA CAUSES SCHIZOPHRENIA?

John McGrath[1], David Castle[2], and Robin Murray[2]

[1] Clinical Studies Unit
Wolston Park Hospital
Wacol, Australia

[2] Institute of Psychiatry
De Crespigny Park
London, United Kingdom

In 1787, William Perfect referred to the then contemporary view that "instances of insanity are at this day more numerous in the kingdom than they were at any former period" and, in discussing a particular case, wondered whether the cause was "the epidemic catarrh, more generally known by the name of influenza, which raged with such violence in the year of 1782" (Perfect, 1787. p118). Since William Perfect first suggested a relationship between influenza and insanity, similar theories have been intermittently proposed, often following major epidemics of influenza. For example, Menninger (1928) claimed that many of the cases of psychosis which followed the severe 1918/19 influenza pandemic were indistinguishable from dementia praecox. Since then influenza itself has been partly tamed by means of vaccination and antibiotic treatment of secondary infection. However, the controversy over whether influenza can cause schizophrenia is raging with renewed violence.

The reason for this resurgence of interest was, of course, the report by Mednick et al., (1988) which claimed that those individuals exposed to the 1957 influenza pandemic in Helsinki in their second trimester of gestation, had an increased risk of later receiving a diagnosis of schizophrenia. Several research groups set out to try and replicate the finding. The first report, from Kendell and Kemp (1989) characterised much of the debate to follow, with a positive replication emerging from one data set (Edinburgh) and a negative finding for a larger data set covering the whole of Scotland. Kendell, the senior author, concluded that prenatal influenza and schizophrenia were unrelated, only to change his mind when he and his colleagues analysed more comprehensive data for Scotland four years later (Adams et al., 1993).

What criteria exist that allow us to review the intervening literature and to conclude whether or not influenza really is a contributory "cause" of schizophrenia? How can we judge if there actually is an association between two variables of interest, and how can we infer that one variable is the cause of the other? Hill (1965) and Susser (1991) have described criteria that can help guide these decisions. The criteria include: strength, consistency, specificity, biological gradient, time order, coherence and plausability. None of the criteria "prove"an association, nor causation. Support for each criterion strengthens the cases for an association; the absence of such support weakens the cases, but does not exclude a true association. Thus, the criteria provide a framework in which we can examine the evidence in a systematic fashion.

It is, however, important to temper the application of these criteria to schizophrenia with two caveats. Firstly, it is likely that schizophrenia is aetiologically heterogeneous; no single risk modifier can be expected to explain all of the variance. Secondly, the nosological boundaries of the group of illnesses commonly subsumed under the label "schizophrenia" are far from clear. Thus, the main outcome variable (schizophrenia present or absent) lacks the clarity of many diseases for which the epidemiological criteria of causality were initially described (e.g. lung cancer, infectious diseases, etc.).

CONSISTENCY

Consistency, one of the most important criteria for causality, has been subdivided by Susser (1991) into replicability and survivability. Replicability refers to the number of times an association is confirmed, preferably by different groups at different times, while survivability takes into account aspects of the research design that add credence to a particular study (e.g. larger sample size). The assessment of relicability rests on the assumption that negative findings reach publication as frequently as positive replications, which may not always be the case.

The published studies can be divided into those ecological studies carried out at the population level and, to date, two studies examining birth cohorts. An association between prenatal exposure to the 1957 A2 influenza pandemic and schizophrenia (either male, female or both) has been supported by data from Denmark (Mednick, Machón, Huttunen, & Bonett, 1988; Mednick, Machón, & Huttunen, 1990; Adams, Kendell, Hare, & Munk-Jorgensen, 1993), England and Wales (O'Callaghan, Sham, Takei, Glover, & Murray, 1991; Adams, Kendell, Hare, & Munk-Jorgensen, 1993; Fahy, Jones, & Sham, 1992), Scotland (Adams, Kendell, Hare, & Munk-Jorgensen, 1993), Japan (Kunugi, Nanko, & Takei, 1992) and Australia (McGrath, Welham, Pemberton & Murray, 1994). Two studies did not find an association (Torrey, Bowler, & Rawlings, 1992; Selten and Slaets, 1994) and one was equivocal (Kendell and Kemp, 1989). These studies are summarised in Table 1.

Several groups have examined influenza epidemics in general. Most of these multi-epidemic studies (see Table 2) have reported positive associations for England and Wales (Sham, O'Callaghan, Takei, Murray, Hare, & Murray, 1992; Takei, Sham, O'Callaghan, Glover, & Murray, 1993), England alone (Adams, Kendell, Hare, & Munk-Jorgensen, 1993), and Denmark (Barr, Mednick, & Munk-Jorgensen, 1990; Takei et al., 1994b) with the exception of Scotland (Adams et al., 1993). Two studies which have examined schizophrenia and a range of infectious diseases have contributed modest support for an association between schizophrenia and influenza (Torrey et al., 1988; Watson et al., 1984). McGrath et al., (1994), in Australia, found an association for the 1954 A1 epidemic, but not the 1959 A2 epidemic. Adams et al., (1993) did not replicate the Danish findings of Barr et al., (1990), despite the fact that the data sets employed by the two groups overlapped considerably. It is important to note that the English data used by Adams and colleagues and by Sham and colleagues overlaps considerably, thus lessening the weight afforded to these replications.

Table 1. Schizophrenia and the 1957 Influenza epidemic

Reference	Location	Base sample size *	Comments regarding association between exposure and increased risk of schizophrenia
Mednick et al., (1988, 1990)	Helsinki Finland	1,781 (subset)	Second trimester exposure associated to increased risk of being admitted to a psychiatric hospital with schizophrenia.
Kendell and Kemp (1990)	Edinburgh Scotland	2,371 13,540	Edinburgh data showed an association with 6th month exposure for the 1957 data which was not found for Scotland.
Torrey et al., (1992)	10 U.S. States	43,814	No associations found
O'Callaghan et al., (1991)	England & Wales	1,670 (subset)	Associations between exposure during the 5th month, especially for females
Crow et al., (1991)	United Kingdom	Birth cohort ofspring of 16268 mothers†	No associations found using record linkage with a large birth cohort.
Kunugi et al., (1992)	Japan	836 (subset)	Association with exposure during second trimester
Fahy et al., (1993)	Afro-Caribbeans in England	1,722	Association between exposure during second trimester found in Afro-Caribbean patients.
McGrath et al., (1994)	Queensland Australia	7,858	Associations between exposure during second trimester after the 1957 (mainly females) epidemics.
Adam et al., (1993)	Denmark Scotland England	18,723 16,960 22,021	1957 data demonstrate 2nd trimester association for all English patients, males and female Scottish patients, but only female Danish patients.
Cannon et al., (1994)	Ireland	Birth cohort of 980 †	No excess of cases of schizophrenia in the 'exposed' group versus the 'non-exposed' group.
Selten and Slaets (1994)	Holland	4634 (subset)	No associations found.

* The total number of cases of schizophrenia on which the assessment was based
† Birth cohorts examined for cases of schizophrenia in those 'exposed and non-exposed' to influenza prenatally.

Table 2. Influenza and schizophrenia; evidence from multi-epidemic studies

Reference	Location	Epidemic/s	Base sample size*	Comments regarding association between exposure and increased risk of schizophrenia
Watson et al., (1984)	Minnesota, USA	1916-1958	3,246	Associations found with diphtheria, pneumonia and influenza.
Torrey et al., (1988)	10 states of the USA	1920-1955	2,519	Associations found with measles, polio, varicella-zoster, but only trend level association with influenza.
Barr et al., (1992)	Denmark	1911-1950	7,239	Association found for exposure during sixth month of gestation.
Sham et al., (1992)	England & Wales	1939-1960	14,830	Association between exposure during 3rd and 7th months.
McGrath et al., (1994)	Queensland Australia	1954 1957 1959	7,858	Associations between exposure during second trimester after the 1954 (mainly males) and the 1957 (mainly females) epidemics. No associations found after the 1959 epidemic.
Adam et al., (1993)	Denmark Scotland England	1911-1965 1932-1960 1921-1960	18,723 16,960 22,021	General association between epidemics and Schizophrenia only found in the English data (lag of -2 and -3 months)
Takei et al., (1994a)	England & Wales	1938-1965	3,827	Association between second trimester exposure

* The total number of cases of schizophrenia on which the assessment was based

An intriguing relative consistency is that in five of the 6 studies in which the sexes were examined separately, the positive association found was mainly, or exclusively in females (Mednick et al., 1990; O'Callaghan, Sham, Takei, Glover, & Murray, 1991; McGrath et al., 1994; Adams, Kendell, Hare, & Munk-Jorgensen, 1993; Takei et al., 1994a, 1994b).

Takei et al., (1994a) who reviewed these studies were unsure whether there is a relatively sex-specific effect of influenza on female foetuses, or whether a similar effect occurs in males but is obscured by other aetiological factors (eg perinatal complications) operating in males.

Thus, most, but not all of the population based studies that examined associations between prenatal exposure to influenza and subsequent schizophrenia, have been positive. However, all of these studies suffer from the same design weakness - we cannot be sure that the mothers whose children later developed schizophrenia actually had influenza during the crucial stage of pregnancy. All they show is that the mothers were pregnant during a documented influenza epidemic. Aggregating data at the population level can introduce biases, which may lead to an "ecological fallacy." Associations that appear sound when assessed for populations (at the ecological level), can disappear at the level of the individual. Aggregating data can distort associations and putative causative pathways. In order to increase the "survivability" of the association, it is necessary to examine the offspring of women who were known to have had influenza at the supposedly critical period.

Several investigators have pointed out that a variable may impact simultaneously with influenza epidemics (e.g. cold weather) that is more closely related to the modification of risk, leaving the epidemics as mere risk indicators (not causally related). Barr, Mednick, & Munk-Jorgensen, (1990) and Adams, Kendell, Hare, & Munk-Jorgensen, (1993) have examined climatic factors as potential confounding variables, but neither group could demonstrate any consistent pattern that would implicate such variables. It remains possible that the risk-increasing factor is not influenza per se, but some maternal behaviour consequent upon being infected(e.g. the consumption of analgesics or other medications).

Mednick and colleagues (1993) examined the antenatal records of patients with schizophrenia who were in utero during the 1957 epidemic. Women attending the antenatal clinics in Helsinki in the 1950's were routinely asked if they had had any infections since their last clinic visit. Approximately 20% of the mothers of those schizophrenic patients who were in the first and third trimesters during the 1957 epidemic, reported having influenza, compared to 87% of mothers of schizophrenic patients who were in their second trimesters during the epidemic. This study does provide some support for the association between the variables of interest at the level of the individual, and, more specifically, for the second trimester "window of vulnerability" proposed by Mednick (Mednick et al., 1988). However, the sample is small, and the lack of a well control group makes it impossible to assess the key question - does prenatal influenza increase the odds ratio of the exposed offspring developing schizophrenia? In order to address this question, a more representative population sample is required. As far as we know, only two studies have addressed this design issue.

Crow and Done (1992) had access to a unique dataset, the National Child Development Survey. This representative cohort included all children born in the United Kingdom during one week in March 1958; by sheer chance, such offspring would have been in the second trimester during the 1957 epidemic. After the birth, midwives had given the mothers a long questionnaire including one item on whether they had had influenza during the pregnancy. Using the the National Mental Health Enquiry, Crow and Done (1992) attempted to identify all members of the cohort who were admitted to a psychiatric hospital in England and Wales up to 1986. Among the offspring of the 945 women who reported having had influenza during the second trimester, only three cases of schizophrenia (broadly defined) were identified, not above expectation. Curiously, Crow and Done found a trend towards an increased risk of affective psychosis among those exposed to the epidemic during their second trimester. However, this cohort study is not without its own limitations. O'Callaghan et al. (1991) have commented on the unreliability of diagnoses derived from case notes, and also on the unexpectedly low rates of women who actually reported influenza during their second trimester. The first comment can equally be applied to many of the other studies reported above. As to the second, Mednick et al., (personal communication) have demonstrated that women giving birth cannot recall accurately whether or not they had suffered influenza several months previously. In addition, some of the mothers of the cohort members may have had subclinical influenza infection. Ideally, future studies should document serological evidence of an antibody response to influenza exposure. Finally, because the Mental Health Enquiry ceased in 1986, only that subset of cases who required admission for schizophrenia before the age of 27 years could have been identified.

A follow-up study of 980 individuals born in Dublin during the 1957 influenza epidemic has been carried out by Cannon et al., (1994). Within the cohort, 476 individuals were born to mothers who complained of symptoms of influenza during pregnancy and 504 were born to mothers who did not suffer symptoms of influenza. This cohort was originally collected by Coffey et al. (1959) as an investigation into the relationship of maternal influenza and congenital deformities. Cannon and colleagues were able to trace and interview 238 from the "influenza-exposed" group and 287 from the "non-exposed group". The names and dates of birth of the cohort members were also matched against Dublin psychiatric hospital records. Four cases of schizophrenia were identified by these methods - two from the "exposed' group and two from the "non-exposed". The authors conclude that an "influenza" effect on schizophrenia, if present, is not of sufficient magnitude to be detected in a sample of this size.

In summary, the association between influenza and schizophrenia has some, but not overwhelming, consistency. The relative replicability of findings at a population level has not been confirmed in the two cohort studies which have been carried out. These negative findings require careful consideration when considering explanatory hypotheses, and, indeed, may point the way towards fruitful avenues for research.

STRENGTH OF ASSOCIATION

The stronger the association between a supposed cause and the effect, the greater the likelihood that a causal relationship exists between them. There are several ways to assess the effect size of the association between the proposed influenza risk factor and schizophrenia. For example, using data from the Queensland study, McGrath and colleagues (McGrath et al., 1994) identified an association for exposure to the 1954 A1 epidemic and an increased rate of preschizophrenic births four months after the onset of epidemic. During the index period (the month of November) 24 cases of schizophrenia were identified against an estimated background of 2,563 "non-schizophrenics". The non-epidemic comparison months (all Novembers from the 10 surrounding non-epidemic years) identified 109 cases of schizophrenia against a background of 25,208 "non-schizophrenics". Those born in the index month had an odds ratio of about 2.2 (95% CI 1.4 to 3.4) of developing schizophrenia compared to those born in the comparison months.

Several groups have tried to estimate how many extra cases of schizophrenia can be attributed to influenza. Barr et al., (1990) suggested that the relationship between schizophrenia and influenza accounted for, at most, 4% of all cases of schizophrenia. Takei et al., (1993), using data from those born in England and Wales between 1938 and 1965, concluded that prenatal exposure to influenza caused a 14% increase in the number of females who subsequently developed schizophrenia. Sham et al., (1992) estimated there was a 1.4% increase in cases of schizophrenics for every 1000 deaths attributed to influenza in the two to three months before birth. However, one must recognise that influenza deaths are only a tangential indicator of the number of pregnant women contracting influenza. The true effect may therefore have been underestimated.

In addition, one must remember that major influenza epidemics occur only once every few years, and usually last only a matter of weeks. The proposed risk modifying exposure is restricted to those born in a brief window of dates several months after the peak of the epidemic. It could be argued that the epidemic effect may be only "the tip of the iceberg" and that there may be a risk modifying effect of respiratory viruses in general extending over the year. There are no data to support or reject such a proposal, but if correct, the effect size of such a risk factor may be larger than that suggested by the studies of epidemics.

In summary, the strength of the association between the variables of interest is modest, and it appears that influenza is a minor risk modifier for schizophrenia. However, a small association does not equate with an inconsequential association.

SPECIFICITY

Specificity has been subdivided into specificity of cause and specificity of effect (Susser, 1991). Does the putative causal factor result in only one specific outcome, and is the outcome the result of only one cause? Where found, specificity of either cause or effect adds considerable credence to an association. (e.g. the close association between mesothelioma and earlier asbestos exposure). The most frequent clinical outcome that follows a pregnant woman contracting the influenza virus is influenza in the mother, with no obvious adverse effects on the foetus. Could prenatal exposure to influenza lead to other disorders, and in particular, neurological disorders? One study (Mattock, Marmot & Stern, 1988) proposed an association between prenatal exposure to the 1919-1920 influenza pandemic and an increase risk of Parkinson's disease in later life, but to our knowledge, this study has not been replicated. Takei et al., (1994c) have made a preliminary report of a weak association between non-specific mental handicap and prenatal exposure to influenza about the fourth month of pregnancy. They reason that exposure at this earlier period may produce more severe cortical damage than that associated with schizophrenia. However, once again the study requires replication.

Is the association specific to influenza? In terms of specificity of cause, Watson, Kucala, Tilleskjor, & Jacobs, (1984) and Torrey, Rawlings, & Waldman, (1988), O'Callaghan, Sham, Takei, Glover, Murray, Hare & Murray (1993) have examined a wide range of infectious diseases for an association between prenatal exposure and later schizophrenia, and found consistency only for influenza. Adams et al., (1993) assessed measles as well as influenza, but once again, the only consistent finding emerged for influenza. However, few diseases come in such huge brief epidemics, and thus studies of most other infectious diseases do not have the same statistical power as those examining influenza.

It could be argued that within the narrow context of the role of infection and schizophrenia, a moderate degree of specificity of cause has emerged for the association between influenza and schizophrenia. Overall the proposed association between influenza and schizophrenia lacks specificity, but specificity would be unexpected in a multifactorial disorder such as schizophrenia. Thus, the fact that many smokers do not suffer myocardial infarction does not invalidate the evidence that smoking is a significant risk factor for coronary artery disease. In other words, it could be argued that the lack of specificity carries less weight in this scenario.

TEMPORALITY

For one factor to cause a certain outcome, it must precede that outcome - in this case, the influenza has to precede the schizophrenia. The temporal order of the association between prenatal influenza and later schizophrenia seems beyond doubt. Although the age of onset of florid schizophrenia is most commonly in early adult life, a wealth of evidence indicates that subtle precursors of this disorder can be traced back to the earliest years of life (Murray, Lewis, Owen, & Foerster, 1988).

BIOLOGICAL GRADIENT

Biological gradient, or dose response, states that more exposure should lead to more outcomes, as in exposure to toxins and carcinogens. Most of the population studies have reported a positive association between indicators of the severity of influenza epidemics (e.g. deaths, days off sick, etc.) and the number of births of preschizophrenics. At the level of the individual, there is nothing to suggest that a more severe "dose" of prenatal influenza exposure increases the chance of schizophrenia in the offspring. Indeed, Knight (1991) has argued that the Crow and Done (1992) negative findings suggest the opposite - that offspring of women who were so sick as to remember their infection did not have an increased risk of developing schizophrenia. The Queensland study demonstrated that the 1959 epidemic was longer and resulted in higher mortality than the 1957 epidemic, but, unlike the 1957 epidemic, no association with increased rates of schizophrenia was found (McGrath, Welham, Pemberton & Murray, 1994).

COHERENCE AND PLAUSABILITY

If an association between variables appears plausible from the perspective of current science, then this adds some weight to causality. The absence of such plausibility certainly makes an association much more difficult to accept. However, the history of science is replete with examples of correct hypotheses that lack plausibility because of an incomplete contemporary knowledge base (e.g. the earth is spherical rather than flat). Also, creative scientists can nearly always generate a "plausible sounding" hypothesis, especially in a field with a relatively limited information base like schizophrenia.

The proposed association between prenatal influenza and schizophrenia can be readily incorporated within the neurodevelopmental hypothesis of schizophrenia. This theory draws considerable, but not incontrovertible support (see Castle and Gill, 1992), from a range of sources including studies of the antecedents of schizophrenia, neuropathology, structural neuro-imaging, and the presence of minor physical anomalies (Murray, O'Callaghan, Castle & Lewis, 1992). Because it is proposed that an early teratogenic effect of influenza results in a neurodevelopmental defect, which subsequently manifests itself as schizophrenia, the hypothesis is "coherent" and "plausible" within a body of current scientific thought. However, theories which are plausible within the framework of a fashionable paradigm have a habit of being wrong. For example, the miasma theory of disease (i.e. that emanations from stagnant and dirty water caused disease) ultimately proved incorrect even though it correctly predicted that proper sanitation and the drainage of swamps near villages would reduce disease.

The neurodevelopmental theory of schizophrenia may provide a time-frame during which the risk factor impacts: however, the intervening segments of the causal chain need "plausible" hypotheses. Direct foetal infection by the influenza virus is unlikely (Wright, Gill, & Murray, 1993). If non-specific epiphenomena of influenza infection (maternal fever, circulatory changes, stress responses, changes in nutrition, etc.) were pathogenic, they should also lead to an association between schizophrenia and other infectious diseases; however, as discussed above with respect to specificity, this does not appear to be the case. In order to explain the findings, some researchers have implicated auto-immune reactions as the 'direct' teratogen, and suggested that only certain mothers have the prerequisite immune response to produce the noxious antibody (Wright, Gill, & Murray, 1993). The problem with these theories is that each additional layer of complexity invites dissection with Ockam's razor.

One approach to the search for biological plausibility lies in the detailed analysis of those cases of schizophrenia born after influenza epidemics for other clinical and pathological variables (e.g. age of onset, minor physical anomalies, structural brain abnormalities, etc.) or potential confounding aetiological factors (e.g. family history of psychosis, pregnancy and birth complications). For example, Mednick (1993) has presented data suggesting that certain symptom clusters (e.g. suspiciousness) predominate in those cases of schizophrenia born several months after an influenza epidemic. A preliminary analysis of all first admissions to hospitals in England and Wales with schizophrenia, also suggests that those (particularly females) who were in their fifth month of gestation at the time of an influenza epidemic are particularly likely to receive a diagnosis of paranoid subtype (Takei et al., 1994d). In addition, Takei and colleagues, (1994d) have examined the CT scans of 83 UK born schizophrenics. The patients were divided into four groups on the basis of their date of birth: those who had been in their fifth month of gestation at a time when the prevalence of influenza had been 1) very low 2) low 3) high 4) very high. Intriguingly, increased risk of exposure to influenza at this period of gestation was associated with increased area of the Sylvian Fissures, particularly on the left.

Evidence from animal models can also add weight to the argument of causality. With respect to influenza and schizophrenia, the offspring of pregnant mice infected with influenza have been examined for hippocampal pyramidal cell disarray, a featured described in some patients with schizophrenia. To date, the results have been inconclusive (Cotter et al., 1994). If further studies are positive then appropriate animal models may be linked to influenza experiments in order to tease out potential mechanisms (e.g effect of maternal antibodies on the developing brain, etc.).

CONCLUSIONS

How well do the available data meet the epidemiological criteria for the assessment of causality? The finding of an association between the 1957 epidemic and schizophrenic births has, in the main, been replicated at the population level. The association between schizophrenic births and influenza epidemics in general, adds weight to the association as does the relative consistency of the finding of a greater female than male effect. The lack of support from the two cohort studies erodes the case for an association.

The exact mechanism of the proposed association is yet to be elucidated, but the \g hypotheses draw coherence from available theories of schizophrenia and of ...urodevelopment in general. The risk modifying exposure (influenza) precedes the outcome variable (schizophrenia). The strength of the association is small. Overall, the specificity is poor, but the lack of associations with infections other than influenza provides moderate specificity of cause. The strength and specificity of associations between putative aetiological variables and schizophrenia would be diluted by the multi-factorial nature of the outcome variable. Overall, the case that prenatal influenza causes schizophrenia is far from proven, but has sufficient credibility to merit further research.

Is the strength of the case sufficient to start planning some type of public health interventions (e.g. vaccination, education about the dangers of infections during pregnancy, etc.)? The answer is clearly no. Even if an association is present (i.e. influenza does cause schizophrenia) the mechanism by which this occurs is unknown. There is the potential that a premature intervention would have negative consequences or even lead to an increased incidence of schizophrenia; if the teratogenic element is the maternal antibody reaction rather than a direct effect of the virus, then vaccination may conceivably potentiate problems by precipitating a more aggressive antibody response.

In order to either strengthen or reject the case, it will be necessary for epidemiological researchers to improve the design of future studies. However, it seems unlikely that the issue of whether prenatal influenza does indeed cause schizophrenia will be resolved conclusively by epidemiological means. Indeed, a recent commentary in the Lancet (Skrabanek, 1993) has indicated the perils of relying wholly on epidemiological data. The focus of research is therefore likely to move to biological and experimental studies.

ACKNOWLEDGMENTS

The authors are indebted to Drs. P. Jones, P. Sham, N. Takei and M. Cannon for their helpful comments on this chapter. The tables and extracts from the text are reproduced with kind permission of the Australian and New Zealand Journal of Psychiatry.

REFERENCES

Adams, W., Kendell, R.E., Hare, E.H., & Munk-Jorgensen, P. (1993), Epidemiological evidence that maternal influenza contributes to the aetiology of schizophrenia: An analysis of Scottish, English and Danish data, *Brit J Psychiatry*, 163:522-534.

Barr, C.E., Mednick, S.A., & Munk-Jorgensen, P. (1990), Exposure to influenza epidemics during gestation and adult schizophrenia. A 40-year study, *Arch Gen Psychiatry*, 47:869-874.

Cannon, M., Cotter, D., Sham, P.C., Larkin, C., Murray, R.M., Coffey, V.P., O'Callaghan, E. (1994), Schizophrenia in an Irish sample following prenatal exposure to the 1957 influenza epidemic: A case-controlled, prospective follow-up study, *Schizophrenia Research*, 11:95

Castle, D. & Gill, M. (1992), Maternal viral infection and schizophrenia, *British Journal of Psychiatry*, 161:273-274.

Coffey, V.P. & Jessop, W.J.E. (1959), Maternal influenza and congenital deformities. A prospective study, *Lancet*, ii:935-938.

Cotter, D., Farrell, M., Takei, N., Sham, P., Larkin,C., Oxford, J. S., Murray, R.M. & O'Callaghan,E. Does prenatal exposure to influenza induce pyramidal cell disarray in mice? Submitted.

Crow, T.J., Done, D.J., (1992), Prenatal exposure to influenza does not cause schizophrenia, *British Journal of Psychiatry*, 161:390-393.

Fahy, T.A., Jones, P.B., & Sham, P.C. (1992), Schizophrenia in afro-Carribeans in the UK following prenatal exposure to the 1957 A2 influenza epidemic, *Schizophrenia Research*, 6:98-99.

Hill, A.B. (1965), Environment and disease: An association or causation?, *Proceedings of the Royal Society of Medicine*, 58:295-300.

Kendell, R.E. & Kemp, I.W. (1989), Maternal influenza in the etiology of schizophrenia, *Arch Gen Psychiatry*, 46:878-882.

Knight, J. (1991), Schizophrenia and influenza. *Lancet*, 338:390.

Kunugi, H., Nanko, S., & Takei, N. (1992), Influenza and schizophrenia in Japan, *British Journal of Psychiatry*, 161:274-275.

Mattock, C., Marmot, M., & Stern, G. (1988), Could Parkinson's disease follow intra-uterine influenza? A speculative hypothesis, *Journal of Neurology, Neurosurgery, and Psychiatry*, 51:753-756.

McGrath JJ, Pemberton M, Welham JL, Murray RM. (1994) Schizophrenia and the influenza epidemics of 1954, 1957 and 1959: A southern hemisphere study, *Schizophrenia Research*, in press.

Mednick, S.A., Machón, R.A., & Huttunen, M.O. (1990), An update on the Helsinki influenza project, *Archives of General Psychiatry*, 47:292.

Mednick, S.A., Machón, R.A., Huttunen, M.O., & Bonett, D. (1988), Adult schizophrenia following prenatal exposure to an influenza epidemic, *Arch Gen Psychiatry*, 45:189-192.

Mednick, S.A. (1993), Fetal viral infection and adult schizophrenia: Empirical findings and interpretation. Paper presented at NATO Advanced Study Institute - Neural Development and Schizophrenia: Theory and Research. Italy, 22nd September.

Menninger, K.A. (1928), The schizophrenic syndromes as a product of acute infectious disease, *Archives of Neurology and Psychiatry*, 20:464-481.

Murray, R.M., O'Callaghan, E., Castle, D., J., Lewis, S.W. (1992), A neurodevelopmental approach to the classification of schizophrenia, *Schizophrenia Bulletin*, 18:319-332.

Murray, R.M., Lewis, S.W., Owen, M.J., & Foerster, A. (1988), The neurodevelopmental origins of dementia praecox, *in:* P. Bebbington & P. McGuffin, eds., "Schizophrenia: The Major Issues (pp. 90-106). London: Heinemann.

O'Callaghan, E., Sham, P., Takei, N., Glover, G., & Murray, R. (1991), Schizophrenia and influenza. *Lancet*, 338:118-119.

O'Callaghan, E., Sham, P., Takei, N., Glover, G., & Murray, R.M. (1991), Schizophrenia after prenatal exposure to 1957 A2 influenza epidemic, *Lancet*, 337:1248-1250.

O'Callaghan, E., Sham, P., Takei, N., Glover, G., Murray, G., Hare, E. & Murray, R.M. (1993), Schizophrenic births in England and Wales and their relationship to infectious diseases, in press.

Perfect, W. (1787), "Select Cases in the Different Species of Insanity," Rochester: London, p118.

Selten, J-P.C.J., Slaets, J.P.J. (1994), Second-trimester exposure to 1957 A2 influenza is not a risk factor for schizophrenia. The Dutch national register, *British Journal of Psychiatry*, in press.

Sham, P.C., O'Callaghan, E., Takei, N., Murray, G.K., Hare, E., & Murray, R.M. (1992), Schizophrenia following pre-natal exposure to influenza epidemics between 1939 and 1960, *British Journal of Psychiatry*, 160:461-466.

Skrabanek, P. (1993), The epidemiology of errors, *Lancet*, 342:1502.

Susser, M. (1991), What is a cause and how do we know one? A grammar for pragmatic epidemiology, *American Journal of Epidemiology*, 133:635-648.

Takei, N., Sham, P., O'Callaghan, E., Glover, G., & Murray, R.M. (1994a), Prenatal influenza and schizophrenia: Is the effect confined to females?, *American Journal of Psychiatry*, 151:117-119.

Takei, N., Mortensen, P.B., Klæning, U., Murray, R. M., Sham, P.C., O'Callaghan, E. & Munk-Jørgensen, P. (1994b), Relationship between in utero exposure to influenza epidemics and risk of schizophrenia in Denmark, in press.

Takei, N., Murray, G. O'Callaghan, E., Sham, P.C., Glover, G. & Murray, R.M. (1994c), Prenatal exposure to influenza epidemics and risk of mental retardation. Submitted.

Takei, N. (1994d), personal communication.

Torrey, E.F., Bowler, A.E., & Rawlings, R. (1992), Schizophrenia and the 1957 influenza epidemic. *Schizophrenia Research*, 6:100.

Torrey, E.F., Rawlings, R., & Waldman, I.N. (1988), Schizophrenic births and viral diseases in two states, *Schizophrenia Research*, 1:73-77.

Watson, C.G., Kucala, T., Tilleskjor, C., & Jacobs, L. (1984), Schizophrenic birth seasonality in relation to the incidence of infectious diseases and temperature extremes, *Archives of General Psychiatry*, 41:85-90.

Wright, P., Gill, M., & Murray, R.M. (1993), Schizophrenia: Genetics and the maternal immune response to viral infection, *American Journal of Medical Genetics (Neuropsychiatric Genetics)*, 48:40-46.

DISRUPTION OF FETAL BRAIN DEVELOPMENT BY MATERNAL ANTIBODIES AS AN ETIOLOGICAL FACTOR IN SCHIZOPHRENIA

Peter Laing,[1][*] John G. Knight,[2] Pádraig Wright[3] and William L. Irving[4]

[1] Department of Immunology, University Hospital, Queens Medical Centre, Nottingham, United Kingdom
[2] Department of Psychological Medicine, University of Otago, Dunedin, New Zealand
[3] Genetics Section, Institute of Psychiatry and Kings College Hospital, London, United Kingdom
[4] Department of Microbiology, University Hospital, Queens Medical Centre, Nottingham, United Kingdom
[*] Correspondence

ABSTRACT

Various immunological abnormalities have been described in schizophrenics and in their family members. Usually these have been confined only to a subgroup of schizophrenics, and have been interpreted as evidence that some schizophrenia is caused by autoimmune processes occurring in postnatal life. However, recent discoveries indicate that the neuropathology of schizophrenia has a developmental basis, which is consistent with reports that maternal exposure to influenza in mid gestation increases the risk of subsequent schizophrenia in the offspring. The capability of influenza viruses to elicit autoimmune reactions to brain tissue in man and animals, and the proven causative role of maternal autoantibodies in various disease-states of the fetus and neonate, suggest a new interpretation of the immunological data: i.e. that the association of autoimmune phenomena with schizophrenia represents a familial manifestation of a maternal tendency to produce anti-brain autoantibodies which disrupt the development of the fetal brain. This view is supported by animal studies which demonstrate the teratogenic and behavioural effects of maternally administered anti-brain antibodies on the developing fetus.

INTRODUCTION

The genetic predisposition to schizophrenia, and the recent discoveries of brain abnormalities at the macroscopic, cellular and molecular levels in schizophrenics (Kendler, 1988; Roberts and Bruton, 1990; Bloom, 1993; Arnold et al., 1991) exclude the notion that this disorder is merely a 'functional' psychosis, and confirm that whatever causes schizophrenia is strongly influenced by biological factors. In the light of the increasing evidence of biological mechanisms, psychogenic theories of schizophrenia which posit that schizophrenia is caused primarily by psychological effects of adverse life experiences are becoming increasingly untenable (Knight et al., 1992), and have given way to the more plausible view that schizophrenia is a disease of the brain. In recent years many diseases which were once believed to have endocrine, infectious or psychogenic etiologies have been shown to have an autoimmune or immunopathological basis (e.g. Graves' disease, insulin dependent diabetes, rheumatoid arthritis, and multiple sclerosis) establishing autoimmunity alongside infection, neoplasia etc., as a major category of disease causation (Knight et al., 1987; Steinman, 1993). Since schizophrenia also shares certain epidemiological and pathological characteristics with diseases of proven autoimmune etiology, this has led several authors to postulate that schizophrenia itself may be an autoimmune disease (DeLisi et al., 1985; Abramsky and Litvin, 1978; Knight, 1982a; Knight et al., 1987; Pert et al., 1988). Thus, genetic predisposition, absence of clinical symptoms at birth, age-at-onset characteristics, discordance in monozygotic twins, chronicity and remission/relapse are all features of schizophrenia which are closely paralleled by autoimmune diseases such as Graves' disease, insulin-dependent diabetes, and multiple sclerosis (Knight, 1982a).

The most widely held immunological theory of schizophrenia is the autoimmune hypothesis, and in recent years a considerable body of literature has emerged on this subject. Here we will examine this literature, and will offer a radical and testable reinterpretation of the data. We will suggest that a subset of schizophrenia results from the production of autoantibodies against brain proteins during pregnancy which cross the placenta and disrupt the development of the fetal brain. This hypothesis is most applicable to schizophrenia following maternal influenza, since influenza is known to precipitate autoimmune phenomena. However, it is also applicable to schizophrenia in general since it is possible that some mothers produce the putative autoantibodies constitutively or sporadically in response to other infectious triggers, and not only following infection with influenza.

THE AUTOIMMUNE HYPOTHESIS OF SCHIZOPHRENIA

The Immunogenetics of Schizophrenia. The genetics of schizophrenia shares several features in common with the genetics of autoimmune diseases. Most studies of the inheritance of schizophrenia indicate the existence of a strong genetic predisposition (Kendler, 1988). The notion that a disease can be determined genetically poses certain problems if that disease can confer reproductive disadvantage, as is the case with schizophrenia - schizophrenics having fewer offspring than normal (Jonsson, 1991; Ritsner et al., 1992). For example, why therefore haven't the schizophrenia genes been eliminated from the human population by natural selection? The question was first posed by Slater who suggested that the schizophrenia genes might confer survival advantage against infectious disease (Huxley et al., 1964). This hypothesis was tested in a ten year study in the UK which measured the prevalence of infectious diseases in family members of schizophrenics in two general practices (Carter, and Watts, 1971). It was found that the first degree relatives of schizophrenics were less likely to suffer from several viral infections, including influenza, yet were no different in their susceptibility to bacterial infections - supporting the notion of heterozygote advantage for the schizophrenia genes. The concept of an advantageous effect of a potentially deleterious gene is clearly illustrated by the familiar example of the heterozygote advantage of the sickle cell hemoglobin gene (Vogel and Motulsky, 1986). Thus, in its homozygous state this gene causes sickle cell-hemoglobinuria, whereas heterozygotes are free of sickle-cell disease but benefit from this gene by being resistant to malaria as evident from the natural selection of this gene in malaria-endemic regions. However, perhaps the best example of genes which confer resistance against infectious disease, yet which may also have deleterious consequences, is provided by the genes of the major histocompatibility complex (MHC), which includes the genes encoding the human leukocyte antigens (HLA) (Tiwari and Terasaki, 1985; Nepom, 1988; Todd and Bottazzo, 1993).

In mammalian species, including man, there are qualitative and quantitative differences between individuals in the immune response to any given microbial or synthetic antigen. These differences are influenced by highly polymorphic 'immune response genes', many of which (though not all) lie in the MHC. The main evolutionary reason for the extreme polymorphism and heterozygosity of this group of genes appears to be resistance against infectious disease: i.e. such variation between individuals of a population will ensure that any given infectious disease will be survived by at least some members of that population (Riley and Olerup, 1992). Thus, certain human leukocyte antigen genes (HLA genes), which reside in the MHC, confer a degree of resistance against infectious diseases such as malaria - HLA B59 (Hill et al., 1993), and influenza - HLA A2 (McMichael et al., 1977; Silver et al., 1992). Natural selection of certain MHC genes by infectious disease is also evident in the descendants of survivors of fatal epidemics of typhoid and yellow fever among Dutch emigrants to South America (de Vries et al., 1979). However, these advantageous connections of HLA and MHC antigens with infectious disease, though long suspected, have become evident only recently, and in general HLA antigens are more strongly implicated in the genetic determination of autoimmune diseases (Tiwari and Terasaki, 1985).

Since pathogenic microbes are under considerable pressure from natural selection to evade the immune response, the protective antigens of many such microbes have come to resemble host constituents to facilitate evasion of the immune system: e.g. the capsular polysaccharide of the group-B meningococci - which is structurally and immunologically identical to the polysialic acid moiety of NCAM - the neuronal cell-adhesion molecule (Husmann et al., 1990). This is also true of the influenza haemagglutinin whose peptidic elements are fundamentally similar to host proteins (Ohno, 1991) including certain brain antigens (Shaw et al., 1986). Thus, an effective immune response against a microbial antigen confers a certain risk of cross-reaction against host antigens (i.e. autoimmunity). A great many HLA-associated diseases have transpired in recent years to have an autoimmune or probable autoimmune pathogenesis (Roitt, 1988). Thus, the function of the MHC genes seems to be to establish an optimal compromise between defence against infection and the avoidance of autoimmune disease (Adams, 1987).

The strongest and best established association yet to be recorded between possession of specific HLA antigens and the occurrence of a disease is provided by narcolepsy-cataplexy which is a neuropsychiatric disorder consisting of daytime drowsiness and cataplexy or sleep paralysis, in which almost 100% of affected individuals possess the class-II HLA antigens DR2 and DQw1 (Lock et al., 1987). More-recently the HLA association has been defined more precisely as attributable to DRw15/DQw6/Dw2 and DQB1*0602 (Aldrich, 1993; Olerup et al., 1990). Like schizophrenia, narcolepsy has a strong genetic predisposition, 30% of index cases having an affected relative (Yoss, and Daly, 1960), yet genetic factors appear not to be solely responsible for the disease since discordance in monozygotic twins has been recorded, and because only about 1 in 500 individuals having HLA DR2 and DQ1 develop narcolepsy (Lock et al., 1987; Montplaisir and Poirier, 1987). Despite this strong genetic predisposition, many narcoleptics do not have an affected parent, indicating incomplete penetrance of the disease determining genes and/or the operation of multiple co-dominant genes, features which are characteristic of the inheritance of the autoimmune diseases (Knight, and Adams, 1982b), (and of schizophrenia, Knight et al., 1990). In view of these findings, and the associations between narcolepsy and autoimmune diseases (including SLE, pernicious anaemia, multiple sclerosis, insulin dependent diabetes and thyroid diseases) (Parkes, 1989), it is strongly suspected that narcolepsy is an autoimmune disease. The pathology of narcolepsy is incompletely characterized, but, not unlike schizophrenia, involves disturbances of monoaminergic (and cholinergic) transmission - albeit in different brain regions to those implicated in the pharmacology and neuropathology of schizophrenia (Aldrich, 1993). Nevertheless, since schizophrenia may also be considered a disease of the brain, and since schizophrenia also has a strong genetic predisposition, it is prudent therefore to consider whether the genetic determination of schizophrenia may be influenced by HLA genes, as is that of narcolepsy. Studies of HLA-disease association in schizophrenia have so-far concentrated on Class-I HLA antigens and have in the main yielded conflicting results. Although an association of paranoid schizophrenia with HLA A9 was replicated by McGuffin and colleagues in two separate studies (1986, 1989), the separate analysis of the subspecificities of A23 and A24 which comprise A9 has led to conflicting reports, one group finding an association with A24 (e.g. Asaka et al., 1981), and others not finding such an association (Alexander et al., 1990).

A fundamental problem in the interpretation of HLA-disease associations is the occurrence of linkage disequilibrium whereby crossing-over occurs less frequently between certain HLA genes than would be predicted by chance (Tiwari and Terasaki, 1985). Thus, an apparent association of one HLA gene with the disease in question can, in fact, be due to a stronger association with a linked HLA gene in the same haplotype which is more closely associated with the disease - often resulting in very weak apparent associations in the early stages of an investigation. Also, the antigens chosen for study may fail to include the disease-gene(s) or genes in linkage-disequilibrium with it. For example, the earliest HLA-associations recognised for insulin-dependent diabetes implicated the antigen HLA B8, but further studies demonstrated stronger associations with DR3/DR4 and now with certain HLA DQ alleles (Nepom, 1988; Todd, 1990; Braun, 1992). So far, there have been relatively few studies of the class-II/D-locus antigens in schizophrenia, despite their important role in the determination of immune responsiveness and their strong associations with certain autoimmune diseases and with narcolepsy.

The tendency to mutual exclusivity of schizophrenia and rheumatoid arthritis is another factor which would suggest a possible involvement of class-II HLA antigens in the genetic predisposition to schizophrenia. Thus rheumatoid arthritis is associated with HLA DR4 and HLA DR1 (Gregersen, 1993). Given the exclusivity of rheumatoid arthritis and schizophrenia which has been replicated in several studies (Eaton et al., 1992), and the fact that both of these diseases have a strong genetic predisposition, it is possible that genes which predispose to rheumatoid arthritis (such as DR4 and DR1) protect against schizophrenia. The opposite scenario is equally possible - i.e. that genes that predispose to schizophrenia (as yet unidentified) protect against rheumatoid arthritis. Since rheumatoid arthritis is an immunopathologically mediated disease, and since the existence of protective effects of some HLA antigens against certain autoimmune diseases is a well established finding (Todd, 1990), either of the above scenarios (i.e. rheumatoid arthritis genes protecting against schizophrenia or vice-versa) could indicate an involvement of HLA-D locus antigens in the genetic determination of schizophrenia. The few studies which have been performed of D-locus antigens in schizophrenia to date provide some support for the view that D-locus antigens are involved. Thus, in a large study of Japanese subjects involving many HLA class-I and class-II (including D-locus) antigens, Miyanaga et al. found that only HLA DR8 conferred a significantly increased risk of schizophrenia (relative risk four-fold) (Miyanaga et al., 1984). Also, Ganguli et al. (1987) found an association of schizophrenia with DRw6 in African Americans.

If HLA DR4 were to exert a protective effect against schizophrenia, which could be postulated on the basis of the exclusivity of rheumatoid arthritis and schizophrenia, then *association* of schizophrenia with other D-locus antigens would be expected to give rise to relatively weak associations such as those observed by Miyanaga et al., and Rabin et al., -- perhaps any of several other D-locus antigens being permissive of schizophrenia. Our suggestion that it is maternal immune responsiveness (e.g. to influenza) which determines schizophrenia is entirely consistent with the HLA data. The disease-associated HLA genes would be possessed by the mother but not necessarily by the schizophrenic offspring. (Although, according to this hypothesis, schizophrenics and their siblings would express the relevant genes at a higher frequency than randomly selected individuals). In accord with this prediction, our own preliminary investigations indicate that HLA B44 is over-represented in the mothers of schizophrenics when there is evidence of maternal disease transmission, (Wright et al., 1993). Although B44 is a class-I HLA antigen, it could - by virtue of the linkage disequilibrium of HLA genes - be a surrogate marker of a D-locus mediated disease mechanism, as appears to be the case with HLA B8 in insulin-dependent diabetes (Todd, 1990; Braun, 1992).

More-recently it has become possible to perform HLA typing at the genomic level using the polymerase chain reaction (PCR) (Mullis and Faloona, 1987). Unlike serological HLA typing, which has been used in virtually all studies of HLA in schizophrenia to date, typing by PCR allows explicit identification of individual allelic forms of the genes which encode the polypeptide chains of the heterodimeric D-locus antigens. Using this technique, Nimgaonkar et al. found a decreased representation of an allele of the HLA DQB1 gene in African Americans with schizophrenia, i.e. DQB1*0602 (Nimgaonkar et al., 1993). This further supports the involvement of D-locus antigens in the genetic determination of schizophrenia. However, further studies of class-II HLA antigens in schizophrenics and (more importantly) in their mothers are clearly needed.

Class-III genes of the major histocompatibility complex have also been suggested as markers of the genetic predisposition to schizophrenia - a sevenfold increased risk being reported in association with the C4BQ0 'null' allele (i.e. a non-expressed form of the gene) (Rudduck et al., 1985). This allele, is also associated with various autoimmune disorders - notably with the rheumatic/connective-tissue disease systemic lupus erythematosus (SLE). However, recent studies from our laboratories (Knight, Dawkins et al., unpublished) and a recent study by Fananas et al. (1992) have failed to substantiate this finding.

An increased incidence of C4BQ0 has recently also been reported in autism (Warren et al., 1991). The neuropathology of autism, like that of schizophrenia, exhibits evidence of perturbed brain development (Kemper and Bauman, 1993). Warren et al. found an increased incidence of the C4BQ0 allele in autistic individuals and in their mothers, but not in their fathers (Warren et al., 1991). This mode of transmission would suggest to us that autism could involve maternal autoimmunity as an etiological factor. Although autism differs from schizophrenia in many important respects, it shares with schizophrenia evidence of a developmental origin, and an involvement of maternal viral infection as a risk factor. For example, congenital rubella, resulting from maternal infection, was a major cause of autism (e.g. following the 1964 epidemic in the USA) (Chess et al., 1971) until the introduction of the rubella vaccination. Although it is well-established that rubella virus crosses the placenta, and it is not therefore necessary to postulate a role for autoantibodies in the neurodevelopmental pathogenesis of rubella-autism, there remains non-rubella autism which is of obscure etiology. Perhaps maternal anti-brain autoantibodies play a role in the non-rubella cases of autism, although the differences between autism and schizophrenia in their C4BQ0 associations would suggest that if antibodies are involved in the pathogenesis of these disorders - then they originate via distinct pathogenetic mechanisms, and react with distinct antigens.

Autoimmune diseases are not invariably associated with HLA antigens. For example, endogenous posterior uveitis (a common cause of blindness) does not exhibit detectable HLA associations, although it appears to be a T-cell mediated autoimmune disease (Forrester, 1987). Also, genetic studies of autoimune diseases in animals show that the MHC accounts for only about one third of the genetic predisposition to the murine equivalent of SLE - a prototypic model autoimmune disease (Knight, and Adams, 1978; Knight, and Adams, 1982). Presumably therefore, as yet unidentified non-MHC genes also play an important role in the genetic predisposition to autoimmune diseases. In man, polymorphic forms of genes encoding the T-cell receptor have been implicated in the genetic predisposition to multiple sclerosis, which exhibits relatively weak HLA associations (Oskenberg et al., 1993). It will be of interest, therefore, to examine the role of T-cell receptor genes and other non-MHC immune response genes in the genetic predisposition to schizophrenia.

Familial association of schizophrenia with autoimmune diseases? Another feature of autoimmune diseases which has been examined in relation to schizophrenia is their tendency to associate in families. Thus, the first-degree relatives of probands with a given autoimmune disease tend to show evidence of the same disease, or (less frequently) of other specific autoimmune diseases. For example, the organ-specific autoimmune diseases affecting the thyroid (Graves' disease and myxedema), adrenal cortex (Addisons disease), and stomach (atrophic gastritis and pernicious anaemia) tend to associate in families, and in individuals, coexistence of these diseases occurring more-frequently than would be predicted by chance (Doniach et al., 1982). The overlap between these diseases is more evident when tissue-specific antibodies are measured, such individuals frequently showing evidence of subclinical organ-specific autoimmunity to one or more of the tissues in this group (Doniach et al., 1982; Roitt, 1988), although the antibodies themselves do not exhibit cross-tissue reactivity (Knight et al., 1984). Therefore, if schizophrenia were an organ-specific autoimmune disease of the brain, it might be anticipated that family members of schizophrenics, and perhaps schizophrenics themselves, should exhibit an increased incidence of other recognized organ-specific autoimmune disorders or their characteristic autoantibodies. In fact, an increased incidence of certain diseases known or suspected to have an autoimmune basis has been reported in the family members of schizophrenics - e.g. non-insulin dependent diabetes (Mukherjee and Schnur, 1989), and autoimmune thyroid disease (De Lisi et al., 1991). An increased incidence of various autoantibodies has also been documented in several studies by Rabin and colleagues (Ganguli et al., 1993b). Recently also, autoantibodies to DNA and Sm autoantigen (which are non-organ specific autoantibodies) have been reported with increased frequency in families with multiple cases of schizophrenia (Sirota et al., 1993a; Sirota et al., 1993b).

The influence of anti-psychotic medication is a problematic confounding variable in studies of the occurrence of autoantibodies in schizophrenics themselves. For example, the occurrence of anti-nuclear antibodies appears to be a medication artifact (Villemain et al., 1988; Chengappa et al., 1992; Ganguli et al., 1992). Also, the problem of agranulocytosis with clozapine appears to have a drug-induced immune mechanism (Lieberman et al., 1990; Pfister et al., 1992). High incidences of anti-phospholipid antibodies have also been reported in unmedicated as well as in medicated schizophrenics (Rabin and Ganguli, 1991; Amital Tephizla et al., 1992). Since these antibodies commonly occur following infection (McNeil et al., 1991), this could indicate the existence of an ongoing infectious process in schizophrenia. For example, autoantibodies against a 60 kDa heat-shock protein have recently been reported, which may indicate the existence of a bacterially-driven autoimmune reaction in schizophrenics (Kilidireas et al., 1992). However, unlike studies of the prevalence of autoantibodies in schizophrenics themselves, studies of their prevalence in the family members of schizophrenics are not subject to the confounding effects of neuroleptic medication, and are therefore potentially more-meaningful.

We suggest that the findings of autoimmune phenomena in the family members of schizophrenics and in schizophrenics themselves are manifestations of a heritable trait of immune responsiveness which, when expressed in a pregnant woman, can give rise to schizophrenia in the offspring. For example, a study by DeLisi and colleagues documented an association between delayed language development in first admission patients with schizophrenia, with a family history of (autoimmune) thyroid disease - notably in the mothers (De Lisi et al., 1991). Although thyroid autoimmunity is commoner in females (Denman, 1991), and this could perhaps provide a trivial explanation for this maternal association, it is equally possible that these observations are attributable to maternal antibodies. Thus, Chiovato et al. have recently observed that the transplacental passage of thyroid autoantibodies is associated with impaired neuropsychological development in the offspring (Chiovato et al., 1992), perhaps via the effects of these antibodies on fetal levels of thyroid hormones. It may also be significant that human autoantibodies against thyroglobulin cross-react with acetylcholinesterase - a surface protein of cholinergic synapses (Ludgate et al., 1989), since the intraperitoneal administration of antibodies against acetylcholinesterase in neonatal rats results in selective damage to the developing brain, temporarily ablating central cholinergic synapses (Rakonczay et al., 1993).

Evidence of Anti-Brain Autoimmunity in Schizophrenia. If schizophrenia has an autoimmune pathogenesis, then it should be possible to demonstrate antibody or cell-mediated autoimmunity to specific brain antigens in schizophrenics, or other characteristic immunological abnormalities. The evidence of autoimmune mechanisms in schizophrenia has been reviewed in detail by ourselves and others previously (DeLisi et al., 1985; Pert et al., 1988; Kirch, 1993; Ganguli et al., 1993b). Most of the investigations which have been performed to date have used methods which are capable of demonstrating immunological reactions of antibodies with discrete components of brain tissue or crude brain extracts. Thus, Heath et al. used immunoelectrophoresis (Heath et al., 1990) and several authors have used enzyme-linked immunosorbent assay (Sugiura et al., 1989). Although many such studies have reported potentially interesting positive findings, because of the diversity of methodological approaches, these reports remain unconfirmed by independent laboratories. The use of impure antigens in methods such as immunoelectrophoresis and ELISA would be appropriate if the antigen in question were an abundant component of brain tissue (e.g. as thyroglobulin is an abundant proteinaceous component of the thyroid gland). However, it is possible that pertinent antigens (e.g. neurotransmitter receptors) are present in crude tissue extracts at concentrations far below the thresholds of detection of these methods. It is therefore unlikely that they would be capable of detecting pathologically significant autoantibodies comparable to those which cause Graves' disease or myasthenia gravis for example, which are present in minute quantities in serum (Adams, 1980; Lindstrom et al., 1988). Moreover, some studies of immunological phenomena in schizophrenia, e.g. reports of elevated CD5[+] B-cell numbers (McAllister et al., 1989), and precipitin reactions on immunoelectrophoresis (Heath et al., 1990) have unfortunately not been replicated in similar studies by independent laboratories (Knight et al., 1990; Ganguli et al., 1993a). In this respect, the majority of the reports of autoimmune phenomena in schizophrenia remain unconfirmed. Despite these conflicting findings, recent reports by independent groups using the relatively simple technique of indirect immunofluorescence suggest a high prevalence of antibodies against neurones of the cerebral cortex in the serum of schizophrenic patients (Sugiura et al., 1989; Shima et al., 1991; Henneberg et al., 1993).

Another approach to the problem of detecting autoimmune reactions in schizophrenia is to select a candidate antigen on the basis of an etiological hypothesis, and then determine whether schizophrenics exhibit evidence of immunity against the antigen. However, perhaps because of the lack of compelling evidence or hypothesis which would favour any particular antigen over the tens of thousands of potential brain antigens, relatively few studies have adopted this design. Using this approach, Bergquist et al. found antibodies against dopamine in the CSF of schizophrenics using a solid phase ELISA with covalently immobilised dopamine conjugates (Bergquist et al., 1993). A small molecule such as dopamine is perhaps an unlikely target for an autoimmune reaction, since in general such small molecules cannot provide both T-cell and antibody antigenic determinants which are necessary for antibody production. It is possible that these findings indicate the existence of an ongoing immune response to dopamine-derived neuromelanin or neuromelanin-protein conjugates in schizophrenia which could be indicative of pathological immune responses in schizophrenia. Also, a report of failure to find anti-dopamine-receptor (D2) autoantibodies in schizophrenics (Kirchlach et al., 1987), has recently been contradicted by positive findings (Chengappa et al., 1993). Of course, the need for independent replication of all such studies is emphasized, before such phenomena can be considered established markers of schizophrenia.

Permeability of the Blood-Brain Barrier to Antibodies. One of the reasons that the autoimmune hypothesis of schizophrenia has not gained widespread acceptance derives from a belief that the blood brain barrier in adults is impervious to antibodies, and that the anti-brain antibodies found in some schizophrenics would not have access to their target antigens and could not therefore be involved in any pathologically significant disease process. This view is challenged by recent observations from the paraneoplastic autoimmune syndromes which are rare complications of ceratin cancers. These syndromes, which are distinct from metastatic and endocrine manifestations, arise as a consequence of the inappropriate expression of nervous system antigens by certain tumours (e.g. small cell lung carcinoma, ovarian and breast carcinomata) at sites remote from the brain, and manifest in various ways as encephalomyelitis with sensory neuropathy, cerebellar degeneration, etc. - depending on the nature of the offending antigen expressed by the tumour and upon its distribution in the nervous system (Posner, 1992). Lambert-Eaton myasthenic syndrome is an example of a paraneoplastic disorder associated with small cell lung cancer where the antibodies (directed against a presynaptic voltage-gated calcium channnel) have proven to be the disease causing agents (Vincent et al., 1989). Paraneoplastic autoimmunity can be very damaging, not only to the brain, but also to the tumour - cases of tumour regression having been ascribed to it (Darnell et al., 1991). However, although immunologically caused neurological or psychiatric disease is itself rarely evident in patients with these cancers, studies of patients with small cell lung carcinoma (SCLC) demonstrate that 30% of these individuals produce antibodies against brain tissue which reach their intracellular (nuclear) target antigens in brain neurones *in vivo* (Drlicek et al., 1992). Although these findings suggest that perhaps not all anti-nervous system antibodies elicited by SCLC are pathogenic, they do demonstrate that anti-brain antibodies produced remotely can reach the brain despite the existence of an apparently intact blood-brain barrier. This demonstrates that, at least in the case where antibodies are directed against brain antigens, that such antibodies can traverse not only the blood brain barrier - but also the plasma membrane of neurones to reach their target antigens *in vivo*.

The notion that the blood-brain barrier is *not* an absolute barrier to anti-brain antibodies is also supported by observations in rats where the intravenous administration of monoclonal antibodies against acetylcholinesterase resulted in their accummulation in brain tissue (Brimijoin et al., 1990). Perhaps anti-brain antibodies become trapped there in an analogous way to the trapping of glucose by phosphorylation once it enters a cell (i.e. the escape of anti-brain antibodies from the brain may be prohibited by their attachment to brain antigens, whereas non-specific antibodies are free to leave - unhindered by such attachments - achieving only a low steady state concentration). Also, the long-lived nature of neurones may make these cells especially vulnerable to the adverse effects of specific antibodies which react with their cellular constituents (i.e. a low steady state concentration of antibody having a chronic or cumulative effect).

The case that antibodies can cause psychosis is supported by recent observations from SLE, where 30-50% of patients exhibit neuropsychiatric manifestations (fits, depression, psychosis etc.) at some stage in their disease which are associated with production of anti-ribosomal-P autoantibodies (Bonfa et al., 1987; Schneebaum et al., 1991; Nojima et al., 1992). Although the nominal antigen of these antibodies has an intracellular distribution (i.e. ribosomal), the antibodies also cross-react with a cell surface antigen which is present on neurones (Koren et al., 1992) supporting the view that these antibodies are causally related to the neuropsychiatric pathology of SLE. Longitudinal studies by Elkon and colleagues demonstrate a close relationship of levels of anti-P with periods of psychosis in SLE patients (Bonfa et al., 1987), although anti-P is not a specific marker of psychosis since it can also be detected in patients with exclusively neurological symptoms (Schneebaum et al., 1991). Presumably however, if an autoantibody were directed against a regionally-specific brain antigen such as a dopamine receptor or transporter (as has been postulated for schizophrenia) then its effects might be correspondingly specific and related selectively to the activities of that neurotransmitter.

In addition to the ingress of peripherally-synthesized anti-brain antibodies in schizophrenia, it is also possible that antibodies are synthesized intrathecally as is the case in certain other neurological disorders such as multiple sclerosis. Thus, elevated levels of IgG (expressed as IgG/albumin ratio) have been reported in the CSF of schizophrenic patients in two separate studies (Kirch et al., 1985; Kirch et al., 1992), which may indicate the occurrence of intrathecal immunoglobulin synthesis in a subgroup of schizophrenics, although evidence of oligoclonal banding comparable to that seen in multiple sclerosis has not been found (Stevens et al., 1990). Preliminary findings of raised levels of CSF interleukin-2 have recently been reported in unmedicated schizophrenics (Licinio et al., 1993), supporting the view of an an ongoing immune response in the schizophrenic brain. This latter observation is of interest since IL2 used therapeutically to treat certain neoplastic diseases has severe neuropsychiatric side-effects, including psychotic symptoms (Hussain et al., 1993). These findings in the CSF of schizophrenics are potentially important and worthy of further study. However, perhaps because it is not routine practise to take CSF from schizophrenic patients, replication of these studies has not, to our knowledge, been undertaken in other centres.

Schizophrenia as a Para-Infectious Disorder? Viral encephalitis can give rise to symptoms which are clinically indistinguishable from those of schizophrenia, but so too can various other organic disease processes which are apparently unrelated to schizophrenia except in their psychiatric manifestations. A capacity to cause schizophrenia-like symptoms does not therefore necessarily implicate an infectious agent in the etiology of schizophrenia, although it may constitute grounds for the investigation of viruses as potential etiological agents. The discovery of the 'slow virus' prion diseases (kuru, Creutzfeld-Jakob disease etc.) (Gibbs and Gajdusek, 1972), and the recognition that certain viruses can persist in their hosts (including man) following an acute infection (e.g. herpesviruses, retroviruses) or if acquired in utero (e.g. rubella) have lent credence to the idea that schizophrenia could be the result of a slow or persistent virus infection (Torrey, 1973; Torrey, 1988). However, attempts to passage putative prions from schizophrenic brain in primates (Kaufmann et al., 1988), or to demonstrate or to isolate conventional viruses or retroviruses from schizophrenic brain or lymphocytes have been unsuccesful (King, and Cooper, 1989; Feenstra et al., 1989). However, since new viruses continue to be discovered (e.g. human herpes viruses 6 and 7, HIV, hepatitis C and E viruses have all been discovered in the past few years), and since it is likely therefore that that there are many human viruses still to be discovered, it is possible that a so-far undiscovered agent, or a known agent acting in an unconventional way, may be responsible for schizophrenia.

The Hit and Run Hypothesis. There may be other reasons for the failure to isolate specific viruses from schizophrenic brain. For example, the onset of schizophrenia could be triggered by a non-persistent virus infection, in which case it might be possible to isolate virus for a very limited period only (e.g. a few weeks), during or even before the onset of psychiatric morbidity. Schizophrenia could also be the result of an idiosyncratic reaction of susceptible individuals to various common virus infections as appears to be the case for acute disseminated encephalomyelitis and Guillain Barré syndrome (Spillane, and Wells, 1964; Cohen, and Lisak, 1987). It is also possible that schizophrenia could result from an insult to the brain caused by a virus acting at a site remote from the brain. For instance, several viruses are capable of infecting the brain in man causing encephalitis (e.g. herpes simplex), others can cause encephalitis without infecting the brain. Thus acute disseminated encephalomyelitis (ADEM) may be precipitated by infection or vaccination with various viruses (Cohen, and Lisak, 1987). Studies of the pathogenesis of ADEM following measles (as distinct from subacute sclerosing panencephalitis) by Johnson (1987) and Gendelman et al., (1984) indicate that ADEM is an autoimmune disorder directed at myelin antigens and not the result of infection of the brain by measles virus. This is probably also true for ADEM following influenza virus infection which can occasionally also be precipitated by influenza vaccine, which does not contain viable viruses, and which could not therefore result in infection of the brain (Spillane and Wells, 1964).

Further evidence of the capacity of influenza viruses to elicit autoimmunity to nervous system antigens is provided by the 1976 swine flu. The US Government sponsored vaccination programme of 1976-1977 against the 'swine' influenza (A/New Jersey/76 H1N1) resulted in a seven fold increased risk of occurrence of Guillain Barré syndrome (Safranek et al., 1991). Since infection by influenza virus from the inactivated vaccine can be excluded as a pathogenetic mechanism, and since most cases of non-vaccine associated Guillain Barré syndrome appear to be autoimmune in character mediated by antibodies reacting with glycolipid antigens of myelin (Gregson et al., 1993), it is very likely that the post-vaccinal Guillain Barré syndrome was also autoimmune. Interestingly, the viral strain implicated in the post-vaccine Guillain Barré syndrome was one of the strains which we found elicited anti-brain antibodies in rabbits (Laing et al., 1989). Naturally occurring Guillain Barré syndrome is often preceded by respiratory tract infections, but various other non-respiratory infections have also been implicated, notably *Campylobacter jejuni* - a common cause of gastroenteritis (Kaldor and Speed, 1984). The most common viral precipitants of Guillain Barré syndrome appear to be the Herpes viruses, cytomegalo- and Epstein-Barr; and *Mycoplasma pneumoniae* (Cook et al., 1987). These findings emphasize the point that the search for a single virus as the causative agent of schizophrenia may be futile if the pathogenesis of schizophrenia is comparable to that of ADEM or Guillain Barré syndrome, since it is possible that several, and perhaps many, infectious agents are responsible. These findings do not however imply that the search for a common (or major) pathogenic mechanism in schizophrenia is similarly futile, since it is possible that several viruses could precipitate the same autoimmune process against brain antigens leading to schizophrenia.

There is little evidence to suggest that schizophrenia is, formally speaking, a post-encephalitic disorder since the vast majority of schizophrenics have no history of encephalitis or other neurological disorders such as Guillain Barré syndrome. Also, the neuropathological correlates of schizophrenia are not indicative of an antecedent encephalitis. However, these factors may merely reflect the facts that ADEM is underdiagnosed (Cohen, and Lisak, 1987), or may reflect unrealistic expectations of the histological apearance of a transient encephalitis decades after the event: i.e. most studies of the neuropathology of encephalitis having been performed on fatal cases in the acute phase of the disease. Alternatively, schizophrenia might be attributable to the occurrence of subclinical post-infectious encephalomyelitis. Thus, animal studies indicate that 'encephalitis' at the subclinical (histological) level may be a relatively common phenomenon. In the rat model of multiple sclerosis known as experimental allergic encephalomyelitis (EAE), there is considerable variation among inbred strains (analogous to individuals in the human population) in their susceptibility to the disease which is induced by peripheral immunisation with myelin or its constituent antigens (Mason, 1991). Even strains which show no outward evidence of disease exhibit neuropathological evidence of encephalitis at the histological level following immunisation (i.e. perivascular extravasation of lymphocytes) resulting in permeabilisation of the blood-brain barrier to lymphocytes and antibodies (Linington et al., 1993). It is therefore possible that breaches of the blood-brain and blood-nerve barriers, comparable to the occurrence of subclinical EAE, could occur in man following infections. This would go some way to explaining the epidemiological similarities which have been noted between multiple sclerosis and schizophrenia (Stevens, 1988).

The non-respiratory symptoms of influenza can be reproduced by therapy with cytokines such as interleukin-2 or interferon alpha (Bocci, 1988) which suggests that these manifestations occuring in the context of influenza have an immunopathological rather than an infectious basis: i.e. being mediated by cytokines. A transient breach of the blood-brain barrier caused by the systemic activity of cytokines secreted during influenza would expose the ordinarily sequestered brain antigens to T-lymphocytes activated by sensitization to influenza virus antigens, creating a suitable scenario for the occurrence of anti-brain autoimmunity in predisposed individuals (i.e. in those having appropriate immune-response genes). For example, the auto-sensitization of the immune system to sequestered antigens is known to be the mechanism responsible for sympathetic opthalmia, where trauma to one eye results in a bilateral autoimmune attack on both eyes (Forrester, 1987; Roitt, 1988). Analogous sensitization of the immune system to *brain* antigens might explain the occurrence of schizophrenia years after closed head trauma (Wilcox and Nasrallah, 1987). The probability of immunological sensitization to brain antigens during influenza could be greatly increased by viral mimicry of host antigens. Thus, analogies in amino-acid sequence have been described between influenza virus antigens and brain proteins (Shaw et al., 1986) and PL (unpublished). Also, we have observed that inoculation of rabbits (Laing et al., 1989) and mice with certain influenza-A viruses gives rise to the production of autoantibodies against specific brain antigens. Damage to the target organ has also recently emerged to be a factor which can predispose to Graves' disease. Thus, therapeutic irradiation of the neck for lymphoma or laryngeal cancer is a risk factor for the subsequent occurrence of Graves' disease (Hancock et al., 1991).

Influenza, Schizophreniform Psychosis and Encephalitis Lethargica. In the era following the terrible 1918 pandemic of influenza-A, which was responsible for at least 20 million deaths, Menninger described many cases of schizophrenia which he judged were attributable to influenza (Menninger, 1928). However, according to present day criteria these individuals with 'schizophrenia' would have received a diagnosis of schizophreniform psychosis. Menninger's observations were not unique to the 1918 pandemic since each new pandemic of influenza is followed by a rash of reports of post-influenzal psychosis which appears to be a rare post-infectious complication of influenza (Sulkava et al., 1981). Indeed, at the time of writing, we are dealing with one such case, verified by serological diagnosis, in a pregnant woman in Nottingham. Although these observations fall short of implicating influenza in the etiology of schizophrenia, they do at least demonstrate that influenza can have severe adverse effects on the brain. Influenza also appears to be capable of exacerbating psychotic symptoms in schizophrenic and bipolar patients (Torrey, personal communication), a phenomenon which may depend on cytokine-mediated permeabilisation of the blood-brain barrier, or on the intercurrent boosting of pathogenic autoimmune processes. Also, post-influenzal depression is a common feature of the clinical syndrome of influenza (Murphy and Webster, 1990) which is taken for granted, yet which might also relate to influenza's capacity to cause pathological processes in the brain.

Influenza-A appears to have been the infectious agent responsible for encephalitis lethargica (von Economo's encephalitis) (Ravenholt and Foege, 1982; Boos and Esiri, 1986), which was a winter pandemic disease that was prevalent before and during the reign of the 1918 (H1N1) strain of influenza-A (1915-1926). Repeated attempts to demonstrate viral antigens in encephalitis lethargica brain tissue have been unsuccesful (Boos, and Esiri, 1986) which would favour the view that this disorder, like ADEM following measles and influenza, is autoimmune in character. The one virus antigens (influenza) in the post-mortem brain tissue of encephalitis lethargica patients (Gamboa et al., 1974) can be reinterpreted, in the light of our findings of influenza-virus induced anti-brain autoimmunity in rabbits (Laing et al., 1989), as being more-plausibly attributed to anti-brain antibodies in the influenza antiserum used by the authors to visualize influenza virus antigens. Encephalitis lethargica was frequently followed by bizarre neurological and psychiatric sequelae which often appeared only after an interval of several years. For example, Boyle has argued that the case-descriptions of Kraepelin and Bleuler from which our modern concepts of schizophrenia were developed included many individuals who may have been experiencing the sequelae of encephalitis lethargica according to von Economo's criteria (Boyle, 1990).

In the chronic phase of encephalitis lethargica, unlike schizophrenia, postmortem studies have demonstrated clear evidence of degenerative changes (gliosis, neuronal-loss and the occurrence of neurofibrillary tangles) (Boos and Esiri, 1986). These findings, among other considerations, would argue for distinct pathogenetic mechanisms for encephalitis lethargica and schizophrenia. However, it is still possible that these pathogenic mechanisms are related etiologically in a fundamental way. For example, infection with certain serotypes of group-A streptococci can give rise to autoimmune sequelae such as rheumatic fever, Sydenham's chorea or post-streptococcal glomerulonephritis, or indeed to combinations of these disorders, which - despite their clinical and pathological diversity - clearly have related autoimmune mechanisms (Bisno, 1985).

The autoimmune diseases are characterised by long and variable prodromal periods during which pathological processes are active although disease is not clinically evident: e.g. insulin dependent diabetes - where autoimmunity to beta-cell autoantigens such as glutamate decarboxylase (which is also also a brain antigen) can precede the onset of symptoms by several years (Baekkeskov et al., 1990). Also, in polyendocrine autoimmunity (the coexistence of two or more organ-specific autoimmune disorders in the same individual) the mean interval between the onset of each disease can be as much as seven years (Knight and Adams, 1982b). A long and variable prodromal period such as this would blur any expected temporal association between the offending infection and the onset of schizophrenia. Whether influenza would be expected to result in acute psychosis in the immediate post-infectious period, or in chronic schizophrenia years later might depend upon the quality and duration of any immune response to brain antigens. Thus, a predominantly cell-mediated (T-lymphocyte) response might result in encephalitis, whereas a predominantly antibody-mediated response against appropriate antigens might result in schizophrenia after a long interval without requiring the occurrence of clinically evident encephalitis. These statements are necessarily speculative, but serve to illustrate the degree of subtlety which may be required in evaluating and testing the autoimmune hypothesis of schizophrenia. It may be that the clinical syndrome of schizophrenia is the final common pathway of several disease processes, of which autoimmunity is but one. For example, fever can be elicited by many hundreds of different infectious agents, yet it is caused by the actions of a single immune molecule (interleukin-1) on thermoregulatory neurones in the brain. Despite the problems and reservations expressed here about the autoimmune hypothesis, we conclude with the view that the autoimmune hypothesis of schizophrenia as an explanation for the onset of schizophrenic symptoms in adult life is definitely tenable, and more plausible than viral or psychogenic theories of schizophrenia. However, although the autoimmune hypothesis can explain the precipitation of the clinical symptoms of schizophrenia, it lacks supportive evidence of postnatal pathological changes in the schizophrenic brain, and cannot explain recent findings of the developmental nature of the neuropathology of schizophrenia.

Evidence That Schizophrenia has a Developmental Basis. The brains of some schizophrenics exhibit subtle and occasionally gross anatomical and cytoarchitectonic abnormalities in neuroimaging and post mortem studies. For example, heterotopia of neuronal clusters in the pre-alpha layer of the entorhinal cortex, disarray of hippocampal pyramidal neurones, enlarged ventricles, misplaced neurones in the cortical subplate and asymmetric deviations in the sulcogyral pattern - all of which are evocative of perturbed brain development (refer to other chapters; Bloom, 1993). Recently, molecular evidence has also emerged which is consistent with this interpretation. Thus, decreased expression of the kainate site of the glutamate receptor (Kerwin et al., 1990), and abnormal expression of the microtubule associated proteins Map-2 and Map-5 have been reported (Arnold et al., 1991) in postmortem studies of schizophrenic brains. Some studies have also found significant gliosis in the schizophrenic brain - notably in the limbic system (Stevens, 1982) and corpus callosum (Nasrallah et al., 1983) albeit at lower levels than in neurodegenerative diseases like Alzheimer's disease, or the prion diseases, where the glia (predominantly astrocytes) proliferate and take the place of dead neurones. Although gliosis has not been a widely replicated finding, some postmortem studies which failed to find gliosis deliberately excluded schizophrenic brains from study if they exhibited evidence of organic brain disease, inflammation, atrophy or degenerative processes (e.g. the seminal paper of Jakob, and Beckmann, 1986). So it is uncertain whether the failure to find gliosis represents a genuine absence of gliosis in the schizophrenic brain, or whether it is a consequence of a conscious selection bias introduced to obtain a homogeneous sample of 'schizophrenic' brains uncomplicated by confounding variables such as coexisting brain pathology **presumed** to be unrelated to schizophrenia. Although such preselection is a valid strategy, the results of such studies can not be held to negate the possibility of inflammatory or degenerative changes such as gliosis being part of the neuropathology of schizophrenia. Since gliosis is a characteristic reaction to brain injury in postnatal life which is not evident following insults to the fetal brain (Roberts, 1990), and since gliosis is not definitively implicated in schizophrenia, the neuropathological concomitants of schizophrenia have been widely interpreted as evidence of a developmental pathogenesis: i.e. the insult(s) which gave rise to the brain abnormalities having occurred during fetal life - probably in mid gestation (Beckman and Jakob, 1991).

Given the recent data linking second trimester maternal influenza with subsequent schizophrenia in the offspring (see chapters 6 and 7) and the evidence that birth complications are a risk factor for subsequent schizophrenia (McNeil, 1991), the theme emerging from these diverse observations is of various kinds of interference with brain development giving rise to schizophrenia later in life. Although a causal relationship between these very early life events and the neuropathological concomitants of schizophrenia has not yet been established, it is natural to assume as a working hypothesis that schizophrenia represents the culmination of a pathological process which began several decades earlier in prenatal life. This interpretation is supported by evidence of various kinds of premorbid malfunctioning (such as retarded development) in a large fraction of schizophrenics (see Chapter 3). However, schizophrenia is an acquired disorder, and not all schizophrenics exhibit evidence of premorbid malfunctioning. Moreover, even those who do exhibit premorbid malfunctioning change ultimately to become frankly schizophrenic. In view of these factors it is likely that postnatal biological factors (e.g. virus infections, head trauma), as well as developmental factors, are important in the pathogenesis of schizophrenia, although corresponding evidence of postnatal pathology at the neuroanatomical level (e.g. gliosis) is equivocal.

The Mechanism of the Pro-Schizophrenic Effects of Maternal Influenza. Since the landmark study of Mednick and colleagues which first suggested that maternal exposure to influenza epidemics is a risk factor for the subseqent development of schizophrenia in the offspring (Mednick et al., 1988), this association has been established and confirmed by independent groups in several countries (see chapters 6 and 7). Although the findings have not been universally positive, a clear consensus has emerged that this phenomenon is genuine - even among authors who were initially skeptical (Adams et al., 1993). Although influenza is a systemic disease involving symptoms emanating from multiple tissues and organs (myalgia, headache etc.), and although complications such as encephalitis (mentioned above) and myocarditis may occur, these extrarespiratory features have an immunopathological rather than an infectious basis (Cohen, and Lisak, 1987). Unlike infections with measles and rubella viruses where viraemia provides the opportunity for hematogenous spread of virus to extrarespiratory tissues, there is no viraemic phase in influenza (Murphy, and Webster, 1990). Given this effective containment of influenza virus infection to the respiratory tract, and the fact that the placenta poses an effective barrier - even for many blood-borne viruses, can infection of the fetus by influenza virus be considered a likely mechanism for the pro-schizophrenic effects of gestational influenza? There are numerous case-reports in the literature which would suggest that this is possible. However, the majority of these case reports do not provide convincing evidence of transplacental passage or fetal infection (reviewed by Rushton et al., 1983). Several of them rely upon the immunohistochemical demonstration of influenza virus antigens in fetal tissues, e.g. in brain tissue (Conover and Roessmann, 1990), which we have shown is more likely to be attributable to the presence of autoantibodies elicited by influenza virus immunisation in the antisera used for immunohistochemical demonstration of viral antigens (Laing et al., 1989). There are nevertheless two studies which provide convincing evidence of transmission of influenza virus to the fetus, namely the reports of Yawn et al. (1971) (in which multi-organ failure secondary to influenza pneumonia may have been a factor facilitating viral spread) and that of McGregor et al. (1984). However, it should be noted that even in the context of fatal maternal pneumonia, transmission of influenza virus to the fetus is not inevitable (Ramphal et al., 1980). The case of McGregor et al. was confirmed both by virus isolation from amniotic fluid and by the demonstration of immunological sensitization of the fetus to influenza virus antigens - as evident from the presence of influenza-A specific IgM in the cord blood. However, in the reports of Yawn and McGregor, infection occurred close to term, i.e. too late to account for the mid-gestational (months 5-7) pro-schizophrenic effect implicated in epidemiological studies of influenza and also by neuropathological studies. Moreover, the clinical presentation as amniotic fluid infection syndrome (McGregor et al., 1984) would suggest a possible cervical route rather than placental transmission of infection. Also, although transplacental infection with influenza-A virus can be engineered to occur in ferrets, this requires intracardiac inoculation with unnaturally large quantities of virus (Rushton et al., 1983). It is therefore very unlikely that the pro-schizophrenic effects of maternal influenza can be accounted for by influenza virus infection of the fetus in man. We reason instead, by analogy to the extrarespiratory symptoms and complications of influenza, that the pro-schizophrenic effects of gestational influenza have an immunopathological basis.

THE TERATOGENIC ANTIBODY HYPOTHESIS OF SCHIZOPHRENIA

The teratogenic antibody hypothesis posits that the perturbed brain development of schizophrenia is caused by transplacentally transmitted maternal autoantibodies or alloantibodies against antigens which are present in fetal brain tissue. Since autoimmune diseases have a strong genetic predisposition, virtually all of the evidence which has been cited in support of the autoimmune hypothesis of schizophrenia (such as autoimmune phenomena in schizophrenics and their family members, linkage with immune response genes etc.) may be interpreted to support the teratogenic antibody hypothesis. However, the teratogenic antibody hypothesis can explain in addition the developmental nature of the neuropathological concomitants of schizophrenia. In its simplest form, the teratogenic antibody hypothesis implies that the autoimmune phenomena observed in schizophrenics themselves are epiphenomena reflecting an incidentally inherited genetic predisposition to produce anti-brain autoantibodies. Thus, it would suggest that studies of autoimmunity in schizophrenia should be redirected to investigate the *mothers* of schizophrenics rather than schizophrenics themselves. However, it should be noted that the autoimmune and teratogenic antibody hypotheses of schizophrenia may not be mutually exclusive.

Transplacentally Transmitted Antibodies as Agents of Disease

We have considered various mechanisms, other than infection of the fetus by influenza virus, whereby maternal influenza could have adverse effects on the fetus. For example maternal fever, if transmitted to the fetus as a rise in fetal body temperature, could conceivably have deleterious consequences for brain development. Similarly, maternal cytokines (such as the endogenous pyrogen interleukin-1) might have profound effects on the fetus, although there is no evidence that cytokines can cross the placenta. Also, if increased body temperature or interleukin-1 had adverse effects on the fetus, then virtually any pyrexial illness in mid pregnancy might be associated with the birth of a schizophrenic offspring, yet this does not appear to be the case. Also, re-activation of latent herpesviruses such as cytomegalovirus or varicella zoster by maternal influenza could result in fetal infection by these viruses which are capable of crossing the placenta, but the rarity of these infections during pregnancy would argue against this explanation.

Although it is usual that maternal infection with a given infectious agent results in protection of the fetus and neonate against that agent by virtue of the transplacental transmission of maternal IgG antibodies, in certain instances maternal infection can enhance the vulnerability of the offspring to infection via immunological mechanisms. For example, neonatal infections with dengue and hepatitis-B viruses involve (respectively) the transmission of maternal infection-enhancing antibodies, and the imposition of fetal immune tolerance to viral antigen (Kliks et al., 1989; Milich et al., 1993). If similar mechanisms were operative with influenza-A virus then the pro-schizophrenic effects of maternal influenza might be attributable to increased vulnerability of the offspring to subsequent postnatal influenza infection. However, there is no evidence to suggest that maternal influenza can increase fetal vulnerability to infection, nor is there evidence that maternal pyrexia *per se* has adverse effects on the human fetus. By contrast, there are several fetal/neonatal disease states which are known to be caused by maternal antibodies which (unlike influenza virus) cross the placenta readily and in quantity by means of Fc-receptor facilitated transport in order to protect the fetus and neonate against infectious disease (Osuga et al., 1992; Devi and Robbins, 1991).

Several of the antibody-mediated autoimmune diseases have counterparts in the fetus and neonate because antibodies of the IgG class are transported across the placenta to the fetus, irrespective of their antigen-specificity, where they attain higher concentrations than in the maternal circulation. For example, there are neonatal forms of Graves' disease and myasthenia gravis caused by antibodies against the thyrotrophin receptor and the skeletal muscle acetylcholine receptor, respectively (Munro et al., 1978; Papazian, 1992). Neonatal pemphigus vulgaris is a disease of cell-adhesion caused by maternal antibodies against a cadherin type cell-adhesion molecule of the skin which prevent adhesion of epidermal cells (Amagai et al., 1991). Given the abundance of cell-adhesion molecules and receptors in the developing brain, these examples suggest to us that antibodies of comparable specificity directed against brain antigens could impair brain development with neuroanatomical consequences similar to those seen in schizophrenic brains. Although the teratogenic properties of antibodies against cell-adhesion molecules have not been investigated in mammals, Fraser and Edelman found that antibodies against NCAM severely disrupted the development of the retino-tectal map in *Xenopus* embryos (Edelman, 1984). Indeed, several of the neuropathological phenomena of the schizophrenic brain may be due to disturbed neuronal migration in the late stages of cortical development (Conrad and Scheibel, 1987; Beckman and Jakob, 1991) - a process which is critically dependent on cell-adhesion molecules (Edelman, 1984). Thus, the observations of Fraser and Edelman could be very relevant to the developmental neurobiology of schizophrenia and suggest that NCAM and its relatives would be obvious candidate antigens for our putative teratogenic antibodies.

Although the transplacentally mediated autoimmune disorders mentioned above are transient in nature and subside naturally in postnatal life as maternal IgG is catabolised by the fetus, some such disorders result in permanent defects. For example, complete congenital heart block arising in the offspring of women with Sjogren's syndrome or SLE as a result of transplacentally transmitted anti-Ro and/or anti-La antibodies is a permanent neurophysiological defect caused by a failure of the ventricular conduction system of Purkinje fibres to develop properly (Harley et al., 1992). Similarly, kernicterus arising as a consequence of haemolytic disease of the newborn (caused by maternal erythrocyte Rhesus alloantibodies) results in permanent damage to the basal ganglia and hippocampus of the immature fetal brain (Stirrat, 1989). Also, although some of the disease-states mediated by transplacentally acquired antibodies are manifest as a corresponding disease state in the mother, quite frequently this is not the case. Thus, congenital heart block is often an indicator of subclinical disease (usually Sjogren's syndrome) in the mother. Also, haemolytic disease of the newborn is not associated with any maternal disease, although it may be precipitated accidentally by immunisation of the mother with tetanus toxoid in late pregnancy (Gupte and Bhatia, 1980).

The hypothesis that maternal antibodies are teratogenic agents responsible for perturbed brain development in schizophrenia is consistent with the timecourse of transfer of maternal IgG to the human fetus which commences at week 12 of gestation when Fc receptors first appear on placental cells, and is well-underway by mid gestation (Adinolfi, 1985). Also, the blood-brain barrier in man is not fully mature until after birth - as evident from the occurrence of kernicterus which is partly dependent on the permeability of the fetal/neonatal blood-brain barrier to bilirubin from lysed erythrocytes. It would therefore be anticipated that anti-brain antibodies derived from the maternal circulation would reach the fetal brain. Indeed, antibodies reach the fetal CSF in significant quantities as demonstrated by the presence of maternal IgG allotypes in the fetal CSF in man (Adinolphi et al., 1976; Adinolfi, 1985). Also, specific maternal anti-viral antibodies (against herpes simplex virus) have been demonstrated to reach the fetal CSF in man (Osuga et al., 1992).

In support of the teratogenic antibody hypothesis we have cited several examples of disease states of the fetus which are known to be caused by transplacentally transmitted maternal antibodies, and which involve various mechanisms such as disruption of cell-adhesion and perturbation of neurodevelopment. Also, we have established that influenza viruses are capable of eliciting anti-brain antibodies in rabbit (Laing et al., 1989) and mouse, and that influenza in man can give rise to autoimmune phenomena such as acute disseminated encephalomyelitis (Sulkava et al., 1981; Johnson, 1987), and various non-tissue-specific autoantibodies directed against specific cellular antigens (Loza-Tulimowska et al., 1976). Moreover, evidence from experiments in mammalian species suggests that maternal autoantibodies can perturb the development of the fetal brain.

Maternal Anti-Brain Antibodies Disrupt Fetal Brain Development. The concept of anti-brain antibodies as agents which would perturb neurodevelopment was first posulated independently by Kirman (1975) as a possible explanation for mental retardation. Given the evidence of retarded development in schizophrenia (see Chapter 3), and the foregoing arguments concerning influenza virus elicited autoimmunity to brain antigens, Kirman's suggestion is therefore also relevant to schizophrenia. The first evidence of the tissue-specific teratogenic properties of anti-brain antibodies was provided by experiments performed by Salome Gluecksohn-Waelsch (1957) who auto-immunised rats against brain homogenate and observed a dramatically increased incidence of gross anatomical brain abnormalities in the mid-gestation fetuses of immunised mothers (Gluecksohn-Waelsch, 1957). Interestingly, in view of the foregoing arguments about subclinical encephalitis and the occurrence of fetal/neonatal disease as a manifestation of subclinical disease in the mother, the dose of brain homogenate used for immunisation was not adequate to elicit an autoimmune encephalitis in the rat strain used (i.e. there was no clinically evident brain disease in the mother) although it did elicit anti-brain autoantibodies. The gross nature of the developmental brain abnormalities in the offpsring, which included anencephaly and neural tube defects, may have reflected the early timing of the immunisation (which was carried out prior to conception), and also the targeting of multiple brain antigens by the autoantibodies in question. These effects were also *specific* since no comparable elevation in the incidence of brain abnormalities was evident in controls where heart homogenate was the immunising antigen.

Several subsequent investigations by various authors using different immunisation protocols and different observational parameters confirm that anti-brain antibodies specifically perturb the development of the rat brain with lasting neuroanatomical and behavioural consequnces (Rick et al., 1981; Adinolphi et al., 1982). Unlike the study of Gluecksohn-Waelsch, most of these studies have employed passive immunisation of pregnant rats by maternal administration of antisera to brain antigens during pregnancy. Thus, Karpiak and Rapport (1975) used a rabbit antiserum raised against rat brain synaptosomal antigens which was administered late in the gestation of rats. The male offspring of treated mothers exhibited abnormally low scores in tests of avoidance conditioning, including increased response latencies and poor retention of behavioural tasks. Unfortunately, the many brain antigens targeted by such an antiserum preclude the implication of any specific antigenic molecule as being responsible for the observed effects. However, comparable adverse behavioural effects of anti-ganglioside antibodies were also observed when the fetus was exposed via administration of antiserum to pregnant rats, specifically implicating gangliosides as relevant antigens (Rick et al., 1981). In support of these findings Kasarskis et al. (1981) also found that postnatal administration of antibodies to G_{MI} ganglioside (by intracisternal injection) to five day old rats resulted in cytological abnormalities in brain tissue, even at this late stage of development, including disturbances of axodendritic arborization and synaptogenesis,.

Groups of ectopic neurones, reminiscent of the heterotopic nests of neurones in the pre-alpha cell layer of the entorhinal cortex of the schizophrenic brain (Jakob, and Beckmann, 1986), occur naturally in the cerebral cortex and hippocampus of two autoimmune strains of mice, the New Zealand Black (NZB) and BXSB strains (Sherman et al., 1990). Interestingly, these disturbances are most prominent in the marginal zone and subplate - cortical regions which are strongly positive for immunoglobulin-immunoreactive material in the developing rat brain (Fairen et al., 1992), and which have been implicated by the observations of Jones and colleagues of misplaced diaphorase-positive neurones in the schizophrenic brain (Akbarian et al., 1993a,b). Galaburda and colleagues, noting similarities between these developmental brain abnormalities in autoimmune mice and those of dyslexia, suggested that maternal autoantibodies reacting with fetal brain tissue may be responsible for the neuroanatomical concomitants of dyslexia (Sherman et al., 1985). The NZB and BXSB mouse strains also exhibit behavioural abnormalities which, as shown by ova-transfer experiments, are determined by development in an autoimmune uterine environment (Denenburg et al., 1991).

It is clear from the rat studies described above that maternal anti-brain antibodies can perturb fetal brain development with both anatomical as well as subsequent behavioural manifestations. However, the ova transfer experiments of Denenberg et al. (1991), which demonstrate the role of maternal antibodies in determining abnormal behaviour, also demonstrate that the neuronal ectopias of the autoimmune mouse strains are determined independently of maternal autoimmune influences on the fetal environment. This latter finding suggests a genetic determination for the neuronal ectopia of the autoimmune mice. Perhaps therefore genes which determine the abnormal autoimmune phenotypes of these mouse strains are also involved in the genetic determination of abnormal brain development (Nowakowski, 1988; Jones and Murray 1991)? For example, molecules of the immunoglobulin superfamily which are involved in brain development may also have immune functions: e.g. NCAM (synonyms CD56, Leu19) - which is a surface molecule of natural killer cells and certain T-lymphocytes. These findings urge caution in ascribing the neuroanatomical findings in schizophrenia to the effects of maternal antibodies on the fetal brain during development, since they could manifestly originate via other (genetic) mechanisms. However, the association of abnormal behaviour with fetal exposure to maternal autoantibodies emphasizes the importance of *behavioural* studies, which are more relevant to the bizarre behaviour that characterizes schizophrenia than are neuropathological studies. Also, since no causal relationship has yet been established between the neuropathological abnormalities of schizophrenia and the clinical syndrome of schizophrenia, it is possible that the neuropathological phenomena are only incidentally related to schizophrenia and can exist independently, as is the case with the neuronal ectopia and behavioural abnormalities of the mice. Thus, perhaps as many as one third of schizophrenic brains exhibit no evidence of neuropathological abnormalities at the macroscopic or microscopic level (Jakob and Beckman 1986).

Conrad and Scheibel have noted parallels between their observations of pyramidal cell disarray in the hippocampus of a subgroup of schizophrenics and abnormalities of neuronal migration in reeler and staggerer mice (Conrad and Scheibel 1987, 1993) which are thought to originate from defects in regulation of the adhesive properties of NCAM (reeler) and related molecules mediating adhesion of neurons and radial glia (staggerer) (Edelman, 1982; Pinto-Lord et al., 1982; Nowakowski, 1988). On the basis of these observations, Kovelman and Scheibel have postulated that fetal infection by influenza virus is responsible for the perturbed neurodevelopment of schizophrenia, and that removal of NCAM's polysialic acid by the influenza virus neuraminidase is the molecular mechanism of this perturbation (Conrad, and Scheibel, 1987). Although we concur with the view of Scheibel and colleagues that cell-adhesion molecues such as NCAM could well be involved in the developmental brain pathology of schizophrenia, we have argued above that infection of the fetus by influenza virus is an unlikely explanation. Also, the Kallmann's syndrome variant model of schizophrenia (Cowen and Green, 1993) argues that the analogous trait features of Kallman's syndrome (which is caused by deletion of an NCAM related gene 'KALIG1' on the X-chromosome, Bick et al., 1992) and schizophrenia indicate defective function (but not deletion) of this gene in the developing schizophrenic brain. It is clear that most cases of Kallman's syndrome and the characteristic abnormalities of reeler and staggerer mice have a genetic basis. Moreover, it is implied in the Kallmann's syndrome variant model of schizophrenia that the putative functional defect of KALIG1 is genetically determined. However, although the teratogenic antibody hypothesis also implicates molecules which are functionally related to NCAM, it implies no defect in the genes encoding them, since in general autoantigens do not exhibit pathologically significant allotypic variation. Rather, it invokes an interaction between maternal immune response genes and an environmental trigger (infectious agents including influenza virus) in the developmental origins of schizophrenia. However, it is eminently possible that both genetic mutations and autoantibodies could impair the function of the same cell-adhesion molecule in different individuals. For example, in angioedema (a disorder of complement regulation) there are congenital and acquired forms of the disease caused by germline mutations and autoantibodies (respectively) each of which impair the function of C1-inhibitor (Agostoni and Cicardi, 1992).

Fetal Antigens as Targets of Autoimmunity. One of the mechanisms that has been advanced to explain the the occurrence of autoimmunity during and following infection is the expression of embryonic antigens which become re-expressed from time to time during post-infectious tissue repair, which involves the re-enactment of certain developmental processes (Roitt, 1988). Thus, molecules involved in repair that are not expressed continuously have little opportunity to impose 'peripheral' immunological tolerance, which requires maintenance by continuous exposure to the immune system (Hammerling et al., 1993). Such molecules are therefore at increased risk of adventitious autoimmune reactions. Indeed, it has been suggested that a common origin in embryonic ectoderm may be a characteristic feature of tissue-specific autoantigens in autoimmune disorders such as multiple sclerosis, pemphigus vulgaris and vitiligo (Tadmor, 1992). The effects of maternal antibodies against a fetal antigen present in developing ectodermal tissues as well as brain could explain both the neuropathological abnormalties and also the minor physical anomalies of schizophrenia which involve predominantly structures of ectodermal origin (Guy et al., 1983; Green et al., 1988; Cannon et al., 1993). Moreover this view is supported by evidence that infection (and neoplasia) can give rise to antibodies against *fetal* antigens.

Infectious mononucleosis, which is caused by primary infection with Epstein Barr virus, is associated with the production of various autoantibodies including rheumatoid factor and autoantibodies recognising several cytoskeletal antigens. In some cases autoantibodies are also produced which recognise a fetal erythrocyte autoantigen 'i'and its adult counterpart 'I'which may result in cold-agglutinin haemolytic anaemia (Linde, 1992). The i antigen is expressed by various fetal tissues and by certain tumours and is therefore classed as an oncofetal antigen. It is thought that oncofetal antigens such as i are differentiation antigens with roles in embryogenesis (Feizi, 1985). Anti-i antibodies are not however specific to Epstein-Barr virus infection, since they may also be elicited by other infections such as *Mycoplasma pneumoniae* (Feizi, 1993). Also, an elevated incidence of anti-I antibodies has been reported in schizophrenia (Spivak et al., 1991), which we would interpret as suggestive evidence of a familial (i.e. maternal) tendency to produce these antibodies. The common capacity of EBV and *Mycoplasma pneumoniae* infections to elicit Guillain Barre' syndrome (Cook et al., 1987) may also indicate a shared capacity to initiate common autoimmune reactions against nervous tissue. Also, mycoplasma infections occasionally give rise to neuropsychiatric complications which are thought in most cases to be caused by autoimmunity to brain tissue (Koskiniemi, 1993). Interestingly, in the case of *Mycoplasma pneumoniae*, the anti-Ii antibodies are in fact anti-receptor antibodies - since the I carbohydrate functions as a receptor for the epithelial adherence of the mycoplasma (Feizi, 1993).

Epstein-Barr virus also brings about the re-expression of carcinoembryonic antigen in infected B-lymphocytes (Khan et al., 1993) - so called because it is also expressed by certain cancerous   and fetal tissues. Carcinoembryonic antigen is a prominent tumour antigen and, like NCAM, a (putative) cell-adhesion molecule of the immunoglobulin superfamily. In mammalian species several members of the immunoglobulin superfamily (e.g. CD4, ICAM1, carcinoembryonic antigen, poliovirus receptor) some of which are also cell-adhesion molecules, are subverted by viruses for use as virus receptors (White and Littman, 1989). The physical association of these molecules with viruses may render them prone to autoimmune reactions, in an analogous way to mycoplasma-induced anti-Ii antibodies. For example, CD4 (the HIV receptor) is targeted by autoantibodies produced by a subgroup of HIV-1 infected individuals (Kowalski et al., 1989). Also, influenza viruses use sialoconjugates including various glycoproteins and gangliosides as their cellular receptors (Bergelson et al.,1982) and may, according to the above reasoning, be capable of eliciting autoimmunity against these molecules. Thus, NCAM contains sialic-acid terminated oligosaccharide side chains which resemble those of glycophorin - the influenza virus· receptor of erythrocytes (Krog and Bock, 1992) which may mean that NCAM is capable of acting as a receptor for influenza virus.

Moreover, the capability to elicit autoantibodies to sialoconjugate antigens (such as NCAM) is not limited to viruses, since infection with group-B meningococci or antigenically cross-reactive microbes gives rise to antibodies against the polysialic acid moiety characteristic of the fetal form of NCAM (distinct from its N-linked *oligo*saccharides) (Nedelec, 1990). Since influenza is a risk factor for group-B meningococcal meningitis (Jones, 1994), it is possible that immune responses to encapsulated bacteria could underly the pro-schizophrenic effects of maternal influenza. Neoplasia too can provoke autoimmunity to fetal antigens of the nervous system. Thus, a recent report by Antoine et al. describes immune responses against multiple fetal antigens of brain and retina in a patient with simultaneous paraneoplastic posterior uveitis and cerebellar degeneration associated with small cell lung cancer (Antoine et al., 1993).

Alterations in gene expression caused by infection (e.g. by growth factors and cytokines) and by neoplasia may be involved in the re-expression of fetal antigens and autoantigens. For example, infection of hepatoma cells with influenza virus, or treatment of these cells with interferon alpha upregulates the expression of a hepatic autoantigen (Licinio et al., 1993). Also, influenza virus infection is known to be a potent inducer of interferon alpha in man (Murphy and Webster, 1990), and interferon alpha therapy can precipitate autoimmune thyroid disease (see above). Taken together, the above observations demonstrate that infectious agents can bring about the re-expression of fetal antigens, including molecules of the immunoglobulin superfamily, and can in some instances elicit autoimmune reactions against them.

Shared Oncofetal Antigens of Lung and Brain. Many infectious agents are capable of interacting with sialoconjugate receptors of the respiratory epithelium. We have emphasised the role of host factors in determining individual susceptibility to particular autoimmune diseases. From this we have developed the hypothesis that several infectious agents, including influenza-A, may be capable of eliciting a common autoimmune reaction against brain tissue involving fetal antigen(s) of ectodermal distribution, resulting in perturbed neuro/ectodermal development and subsequent schizophrenia. This hypothesis is based on observations that diverse infectious agents can bring about the same autoimmune reaction (e.g. mycoplasma and EBV induced autoantibodies and Guillain Barré syndrome), and that very few autoimmune disorders can be ascribed to infection with a single infectious agent. In fact, the only specified infectious agent other than inluenza-A so far implicated (tentatively) in the gestational origins of schizophrenia is varicella zoster (see Chapter 7), so the concept of several (but not many) infectious agents being involved is a prediction of the present hypothesis rather than a tenet upon which the hypothesis is based. However, there are indications that other infectious agents might be involved. Thus, the recent study of Adams et al. (1993) indicates that the season of birth effect in schizophrenia cannot be accounted for solely by influenza, since in three separate datasets it peaks too early to be explained by mid-trimester influenza. Perhaps therefore other seasonal respiratory infections are also involved.

In the light of the above observations on fetal antigens as targets of autoimmunity, it is pertinent to consider not only what common antigens are shared by respiratory epithelium and brain, but also those which are likely to be re-expressed during tissue repair in the context of an infection, and which may therefore be targeted by autoimmune reactions. The ciliated epithelium of the lung is interspersed with neuroepithelial cells which function as oxygen sensors and are essentially specialized neurones (Youngson et al., 1993). Analogous groups of cells responsible for olfaction exist in the olfactory epithelium. The neuroepithelial cells of lung epithelium express many neuronal markers such as neuron specific enolase and L-DOPA decarboxylase (Youngson et al., 1993) which could fuel post-infectious autoimmune reactions reacting with adult and fetal brain tissue. Also, NCAM is expressed in the fetal lung on ordinary ciliated epithelial cells (Bobrow et al., 1991), and is a prominent tumour antigen expressed by SCLC (Komminoth et al., 1991). SCLC cells are cells of the 'APUD' lineage (i.e. amine precursor uptake and decarboxylation) which are derived from the same stem cells as the respiratory epithelial cells (and neuroepithelial cells) and exhibit many of the functions and properties of aminergic neurones. Indeed small cell lung cancer cells are capable of uptake of the Parkinsonian toxin 1-methyl-4-phenyl pyridinium (MPP+) (Marini et al., 1992), which is one of the characteristic properties of the dopamine reuptake carrier (Gerlach et al., 1991). This indicates a latent capacity of lung respiratory epithelial cells (or rather their stem cells) to express NCAM and various other molecules characteristic of dopaminergic neurones, when induced to proliferate by neoplasia or reparative hyperplasia following infection.

Influenza-A virus infects and lyses the epithelial cells of the respiratory tract which must be replaced to prevent bacterial infection and to restore the function of the epithelium. We suggest that tissue repair during and following respiratory infections results in the hyperplasia of respiratory epithelial stem cells, and that hyperplasia - analogous to neoplasia - results in the reparative re-expression by these cells of sialoconjugate oncofetal antigens, including the fetal form of NCAM and certain enzymes and transporters of aminergic neurones. This process, being analogous to the inappropriate expression of nervous system antigens by tumours, and occurring in the context of a vigorous ongoing immune response against influenza virus, is liable to provoke autoimmune reactions against lung/brain oncofetal antigens. In a pregnant woman in mid gestation, the resulting autoantibodies would cross the placenta and react with fetal brain antigens thereby disrupting the latter stages of cortical development.

Changes in Maternal Immunity During Pregnancy. Pregnancy results in adaptive changes in the maternal immune system which are necessary to avoid the immune rejection of the fetus, which in some respects can be considered an allograft (Innes et al., 1989). Thus, the fetal part of the placenta, which interfaces with the maternal immune system, and fetal lymphocytes which reach the maternal blood during pregnancy, provoke antibody production against paternally derived fetal alloantigens, including HLA (Innes et al., 1989; Nelson et al., 1993). Also, immune responses during pregnancy appear to be biased towards antibody-mediated as opposed to cell-mediated immunity. These factors may serve to guard against the immunological rejection of the fetus, since allograft rejection is primarily a cell-mediated process. These observations have interesting parallels in the effects of pregnancy on autoimmune diseases. Thus, rheumatoid arthritis, which is caused predominantly by cell-mediated immune mechanisms, tends to be ameliorated by pregnacy (Da Silva and Spector, 1992), whereas systemic lupus erythematosus (an autoantibody-mediated disease) is liable to exacerbate during pregancy (Varner, 1991). Also, Sydenham's chorea may recur during pregnancy - manifesting as chorea gravidarum, apparently as a result of anti-phospholipid antibodies (Omdal and Roalso, 1992). Thus it is possible that changes in immunity associated with pregnancy may favour the development of maternal anti-brain antibodies which perturb fetal brain development.

Birth Order and Maternal Age During Pregnancy. Studies of birth order in schizophrenia have reached no definitive conclusions because of methodological difficulties, although a recent report by Sham and colleagues suggests that having siblings 3-4 years older may double one's risk of schizophrenia (Sham et al., 1993). Sham et al. interpret this data as evidence in support of the view that maternal virus infection during pregnancy is responsible for subsequent schizophrenia in the offspring: i.e. the infection being transmitted from siblings of kindergarten age to the pregnant mother. This interpretation accords with observations of the winter seasonality of sudden infant death syndrome which can be explained by spread of respiratory infection from children at kindergarten to family members at home (Guntheroth et al., 1992). Also, there are indications that maternal age during pregnancy may be associated with an increased risk of schizophrenia in the offspring, although uncertainty still exists because maternal age and season of birth are connected variables (Dalen, 1988). Maternal age is well known to be a risk factor for chromosomal abnormalities such as trisomy 21 (Down's syndrome), so this effect in schizophrenia could, in principle, derive from a (subtle) chromosomal abnormality. However, there is also a linear increase in the incidence of autoantibodies with age. Thus, the teratogenic antibody hypothesis can also explain the association of schizophrenia in the offspring with increased maternal age during pregnancy, since older mothers could be more liable to produce the offending antibodies.

Predictions and Tests of the Teratogenic Antibody Hypothesis

Schizophrenia research has been disadvantaged by the peculiarly human nature of the condition and the consequent lack of any experimental model system in a non-human species which would allow the testing of etiological hypotheses. The teratogenic antibody hypothesis differs from the autoimmune hypothesis of schizophrenia in a number of important respects, not least in its testability. For example, the teratogenic antibody hypothesis predicts that autoantibodies elicited by infectious agents will be neuroteratogenic. Thus, it should be possible, by administering antibodies against appropriate brain antigens to pregnant animals (rodents and non-human primates) to reproduce neuropathological and behavioural phenomena which are comparable to those which have been observed in schizophrenics. Thus, it has been demonstrated convincingly in rodents that anti-brain antibodies have neuroteratogenic properties and cause corresponding behavioural effects upon the offspring. These studies were not, of course, designed to assess how closely these phenomena approximate to the neuropathology and clinical syndrome of schizophrenia. This could be a fruitful area for future studies. Further research with transplacentally administered antibodies should concentrate upon the candidate antigens identified in this paper: namely the 37 kDa antigen implicated in influenza virus induced autoimmunity, NCAM and its relatives, and other oncofetal antigens shared between lung and brain. There is also a case for further studies with anti-ganglioside antibodies, since these have already been implicated as potential targets of the putative teratogenic antibodies.

According to the teratogenic antibody hypothesis, the mothers of schizophrenics should produce characteristic autoantibodies against brain antigen(s), and the offspring of these mothers should produce these antibodies, irrespective of whether they are schizophrenic, at a lower incidence than the mothers, but at a higher incidence than the general population. Although the hypothesis predicts that these antibodies need only be present transiently during pregnancy, it is nevertheless possible that they are produced continuously thereafter. It might therefore be possible to detect them decades after the event, when one or more offpring has become schizophrenic. We are currently investigating this possiblility.

Pregnant women infected by influenza who produce anti-brain antibodies may produce offspring who develop schizophrenia, and perhaps also mental retardation. We are currently identifying a large cohort of pregnant women who undergo intercurrent influenza during pregnancy (estimated to reach 200), using serological diagnosis (which is much more reliable than the clinical diagnosis of influenza). We will follow the offspring and seek evidence of retarded development, and determine how this relates to maternal autoantibody production.

The teratogenic antibody hypothesis also makes certain predictions about the genetics of schizophrenia. The hypothesis predicts a tendency towards maternal inheritance, at least in winter/spring born schizophrenics. Thus, the genetic predisposition to schizophrenia is postulated to be determined, in part, by the immune-response genes of the mother (e.g. HLA and T-cell receptor genes). The female offspring of that mother, whether or not they have schizophrenia, will themselves be at increased risk of giving rise to schizophrenic offspring, since they will be more likely than randomly selected individuals to have inherited the offending immune-response genes and to produce teratogenic antibodies during pregnancy. The male offspring of that mother however, even if they produce the offending antibody, will not pass it on (transplacentally) to their offspring, and will be less likely to give rise to schizophrenic offspring.

Whether the antigen recognised by the putative teratogenic antibodies is an autoantigen or an alloantigen will also have implications for the inheritance of schizophrenia. Thus, although an autoantigenic target would imply a tendency towards maternal inheritance, the immune response to a paternally derived alloantigen would, by definition, require a genetic input from the father - i.e. the gene encoding the alloantigen. This scenario would not therefore imply a tendency towards maternal inheritance.

CONCLUSIONS

We have considered the evidence for autoimmunity as a mechanism for the causation of schizophrenia in adult life. We conclude that this hypothesis, though capable of explaining many of the enigmatic epidemiological features of schizophrenia, has difficulties in terms of the lack of neuroanatomical evidence supporting postnatal changes in the schizophrenic brain, and in the relative impermeability of the adult blood-brain barrier to antibodies. Evidence of impairment of the blood-brain barrier in some schizophrenics and of ongoing immune responses in the schizophrenic brain do not, so far, provide a compelling argument for infection or autoimmunity as etiological factors in postnatal life. By contrast, the teratogenic antibody hypothesis, while consistent with all of the immunological data, can explain in addition: i) the pro-schizophrenic effects of matenal influenza; ii) the minor physical anomalies associated with schizophrenia; iii) the developmental nature of the neuropathology of schizophrenia; and iv) the absence of evidence of gross postnatal pathology in the schizophrenic brain. It is also supported by the existence of several disease states of the fetus and neonate which are known to be caused by maternal auto- and allo-antibodies, including two which affect neural systems (congenital heart block and kernicterus), and is consistent with the permeability of the placenta and fetal blood-brain barrier to maternal antibodies. Also, since the production of pathogenic antibodies is linked to defence against infectious disease, both phenomena being determined by immune response genes (such as HLA), the teratogenic antibody hypothesis can also explain the putative heterozygote advantage of the schizophrenia genes as superior immunity to infection, and the genetic predisposition to schizophrenia as being influenced by maternal immune response genes. Finally, the teratogenic antibody hypothesis is also supported by observations in rodents of the neuroteratogenic and behavioural effects of maternally administered anti-brain antibodies on the offspring. Maternal administration of antibodies against candidate antigens implicated by the present hypothesis in rodent and primate species may allow testing of the hypothesis in model systems.

ACKNOWLEDGEMENTS

We wish to thank Mandy Harris and Neil Smallheiser for comments on the manuscript, and Robin Murray and Seymour Kety for helpful discussion. Ongoing work referred to on influenza virus induced autoimmunity and on influenza in pregnancy is funded by grants from the Medical Research Council, the Stanley Foundation, The Royal Society and Action Research (PL, PL, PL/WLI and WLI/PL respectively).

REFERENCES

Abramsky, O., and Litvin, Y., 1978, Autoimmune response to dopamine receptor as a possible mechanism in the pathogenesis of Parkinson's disease and schizophrenia, *Perspect.Biol.Med.* 22:104.

Adams, D.D., 1980, Thyroid-stimulating autoantibodies, *Vitamins and Hormones*. 38:119.

Adams, D.D., 1987, Protection from autoimmune disease as the third function of the major histocompatiblity gene complex, *Lancet* ii:245.

Adinolphi, M., Beck, S.E., Haddad, S.A., and Seller, M.J., 1976, Permeability of the blood-csf barrier to plasma proteins during foetal and perinatal life, *Nature* 259:140.

Adinolphi, M., Rick, J.T., Liebowitz, S., and Gregerson, N., 1982, Effects of brain antibodies during development, and in mature animals, *Padiatrische Fortbildungskurse fur die Praxis* 53:178.

Adinolfi, M., 1985, The development of the human blood-CSF-brain barrier, *Dev. Med. and Child Neurol.* 27:532.

Agostoni, A., and Circardi, M., 1992, Hereditary and acquired C1-inhibitor deficiency: biological and clinical characteristics in 235 patients, *Medicine* 71:206.

Akbarian, S., Vinuela, A., Kim, J.J., Potkin, S.G., Bunney, W.E., and Jones, E.G., 1993a, Distorted distribution of nicotimnamide adenine dinucleotide phosphate diaphorase cells in temporal lobe of schizophrenics implies anomalous cortical development, *Arch. Gen. Psychiatry* 50:178.

Akbarian, S., Bunney, W.E., Potkin, S.G., et al., 1993b, Altered distribution of nicotinamide adenine dinucleotide phosphate diaphorase cells in frontal lobe of schizophrenics implies disturbances of cortical development, *Arch. Gen. Psychiatry* 50:169.

Aldrich, M.S., 1993, The neurobiology of narcolepsy cataplexy, *Progress in Neurobiol.* 41:533.

Alexander, R.C., Coggiano, M., Daniel, D.G., and Wyatt, R.J., 1990, HLA antigens in schizophrenia, *Psychiatric Res.* 31:221.

Amagai, M., KlausKovtun, V., and Stanley, J.R., 1991, Autoantibodies against a novel epithelial cadherin in Pemphigus vulgaris, a disease of cell-adhesion, *Cell* 67:869.

Amital Tephizla, H., Sela, B., and Schoenfeld, Y., 1992, Autoantibodies to brain and polynucleotides in patients with schizophrenia: a puzzle? *Immunol. Res.* 11:66.

Antoine, J.C., Honnorat, J., Vocanson, C., et al., 1993, Posterior uveitis, paraneoplastic encephalomyelitis and autoantibodies reacting with developmental proteins of brain and retina, *J.Neurol.Sci.* 117:215.

Arnold, S.E., Lee, V.M.Y., Gur, R.E., and Trojanowski, J.Q., 1991, Abnormal expression of two microtubule associated proteins (Map2 and Map5) in specific subfields of the hippocampal formation in schizophrenia, *Proc. Natl. Acad. Sci.* 88:1085.

Asaka, A., Okazaki, Y., Namura, I., Juji, T., Miyamoto, M. and Ishikawa, B.N., 1981, Study of HLA antigens among Japanese schizophrenics, *Brit. J. Psychiatr.*, 138:498.

Baekkeskov, S., Aansstoot, H.J., Christagu, S., et al., 1990, Identification of the 64K autoantigen in insulin-dependent diabetes as the GABA-synthesising enzyme glutamic acid decarboxylase, *Nature* 347:151.

Beckman, H., and Jakob, H., 1991, Prenatal disturbances of nerve cell migration in the entorhinal region: a common vulnerability factor in functional psychoses? *J. Neural Transm.* 84:155.

Bergelson, L.D., Bukrinskaya, A.G., Prokkazova, N.V., et al., 1982, Role of gangliosides in reception of influenza virus, *European Journal of Biochemistry* 128:467.

Bergquist, J., Bergquist, S., Axelsson, R., and Ekaman, R., 1993, Demonstration of immunoglobulin-G with affinity for dopamine in cerebrospinal fluid from psychotic patients, *Clinica Chimica Acta.* 217:129.

Bick, D., Franco, B., Sherine, R.J., Heye, B., Pike, L., and Crawford, J., et al., 1992, Intragenic deletion of the KALIG-1 gene in Kallmann's syndrome, *New Engl. J. Med.* 326:1752.

Bisno, A.L. Rheumatic fever, *in: "Textbook of Medicine,"* edited by Wyngaarden, J.B. and Smith, L.M. Philadephia: Saunders, 1985, p. 1527-1533.

Bloom, F.E., 1993, Advancing a neurodevelopmental origin for schizophrenia, *Arch. Gen. Psychiatr.* 50:224.

Bobrow, L.G., Happerfield, L., and Patel, K., 1991, The expression of small cell lung cancer related antigens in foetal lung and kidney, *Brit. J. Cancer.* 63:56.

Bocci, V., 1988, Central nervous system toxicity of interferons and other cytokines, *J. Biol. Regul. Homeost. Agents.* 2:107.

Bonfa, E., Golombek, S.J., Kaufman, L.D., and et al., 1987, Association between lupus psychosis and anti-ribosomal-P protein antibody, *New. Engl. J. Med.* 317:265.

Boos, J, and Esiri, M,M,. 1986. Viral Encephalitis, Blackwell Scientific, Oxford.

Boyle, M,. 1990. Schizophrenia: a scientific delusion?, Routledge, London.

Braun, W.E., 1992, HLA molecules in autoimmune diseases, *Clinical Biochemistry* 25:187.

Brimijoin, S., Balm, M., Hammond, P., and Lennon, V.A., 1990, Selective complexing of acetylcholinesterase in brain by intravenously administered monoclonal antibody, *J. Neurochem.* 54:236.

Cannon, M., Byrne, M., and Sham, P.C., 1992, Secondary creases in the palmprints of schizophrenic patients, *Schiz. Research* 6;105.

Carter, M., and Watts, C.A.H., 1971, Possible biological advantage among schizophrenics' relatives, *Brit. J. Psychiatr.* 118:453.

Chengappa, K.N.R., Carpenter, A.B., Yang, Z.W., Brar, J.S., Rabin, B.S., and Ganguli, R., 1992, Elevated IgG anti-histone antibodies in a subgroup of medicated schizophrenic patients, *Schizophrenia Res.* 7:49.

Chengappa, K.N.R., Yang, Z.W., Schurin, G., Farooqui, S.M., Rabin, B.S., and Ganguli, R., 1993, Antibodies to D-2 receptors in neuroleptic-naive schizophrenia patients, *Biol. Psychiatry* 33:97.

Chess, S, Korn, S,J, and Fernandez, P,B,. 1971. Psychiatric disorders of children with congenital rubella, Brunner/Mazel, New York: pp. 1-178.

Chiovato, L., Tonacherra, M., Lapi, P., Fiore, E., Vitti, P., and Pinchera, A., 1992, Thyroid autoimmunity and neuropsychological development, *Acta Medica Austriaca* 19:91.

Cohen, J.A. and Lisak, R.P. Acute disseminated encephalomyelitis. In: *Clinical Neuroimmunology,* edited by Aarli, J.A., Behan, W.M.H. and Behan, P.O. Oxford: Blackwell, 1987, p. 192-213.

Conover, P.T., and Roessmann, U., 1990, Malformational complex in an infant with intrauterine influenza viral infection, *Arch. Pathol. Lab. Med.* 114:535.

Conrad, A., and Scheibel, A.B., 1987, Schizophrenia and the hippocampus: the embryological hypothesis extended, *Schiz. Bulletin* 13:577.

Cook, S.D., Dowling, P.C. and Blumberg, B.M. Infection and autoimmunity in the Guillain-Barre syndrome. In: *Clinical Neuroimmunology,* edited by Aarli, J.A. and Behan, P.O. Oxford: Blackwell, 1987, p. 225-243.

Cowen, M.A., and Green, M., 1993, The Kallman's syndrome variant model of the schizophrenias, *Schiz. Res.* 9:1.

Dalen, P., 1988, Schizophrenia, season of birth and maternal age, *Brit. J. Psychiatr.* 153:727.

Da Silva, J.A.P., and Spector, T.D., 1992, The role of pregnancy in the course and aetiology of rheumatoid arthritis, *Clinical Rheumatology* 11:189.

Darnell, R.B., Furneaux, H.M., and Posner, J.B., 1991, Antiserum from a patient with cerebellar degeneration identifies a novel protein in Purkinje cells, cortical neurons and neuroectodermal tumours, *J. Neurosci.* 11:1224.

De Lisi, L.E., Boccio, A.M., and Riordan, H., 1991, Familial thyroid disease and delayed language development in first admission patients with schizophrenia, *Psychiatry Res.* 38:39.

De Lisi, L.E., Weber, R.J., and Pert, C.B., 1985, Are there antibodies against brain in sera from schizophrenic patients? review and prospectus, *Biol. Psychiatr.* 20:110.

Denenburg, V.H., Mobraaten, L.E., Sherman, G.F., et al., 1991, Effects of autoimmune uterine/maternal environment upon cortical ectopias, behavior and autoimmunity, *Brain Res.* 563:114.

Denman, A.M., 1991, Sex hormones, autoimmune diseases and immune responses, *Brit. Med. J.* 303:2.

Devi, S.J.N.,and Robbins, J.B., 1991, Antibodies to poly[(2-8)-alpha-N-acetylneuraminic acid] and poly[(2-9)-alpha-N-acetylneuraminic acid] are elicited by immunization of mice with Escherichia coli K92 conjugates: potential vaccines for groups B and C meningococci and E.coli K1, *Proc. Natl. Acad. Sci. (USA)* 88:7175.

de Vries, R.R.P., MeeraKhan, P., Bernini, L.F.,vanLoghem, E., and vanRood, J.J., 1979, Genetic control of survival in epidemics, *J. Immunogenet.* 6:271.

Doniach, D., Botazzo, G.F. and Drexhage, H.A. The autoimmune endocrinopathies. In: *Clinical Aspects of Immunology*, edited by Lachmann, P.J. and Peters, D.K. Oxford: Blackwell, 1982, p. 903-937.

Drlicek, M., Liszka, U., Jellinger, K., MohnStaudner, A., Lintner, F., and Grisold, W., 1992, Circulating antineuronal antibodies reach neurons in vivo: an autopsy study, *J. Neurol.* 239:407.

Eaton, W.W.,Hayward, C., and Ram, R., 1992, Schizophrenia and rheumatoid arthritis - a review, *Schizophrenia Research* 6:181.

Edelman, G., 1982, Embryonic to adult conversion of neural cell adhesion molecules in normal and staggerer mice, *Proc. Natl. Acad. Sci.*(USA) 79:7036.

Edelman, G., 1984, Cell-adhesion molecules: a molecular basis for animal form, *Scientific American* 250 (4):80.

Fairen, A., Smith-Fernandez, A., Marti, E., DeDiego, I., and de la Rosa, E.J., 1992, A transient immunoglobulin-like reactivity in the developing cerebral cortex of rodents, *Developmental Neuroscience* 3:881.

Fananas, L.,Moral, P., Panaders, M.A.,and Bertranpetit, J., 1992, Complement genetic markers in schizophrenia C3, BF and C6 polymorphisms, *Hum. Hered.* 42:162.

Feenstra A, Kirch DG, Bracha HS, and Wyatt RJ, 1989, Lack of evidence for a role of T-cell-associated retroviruses as an etiology of schizophrenia, *Biol. Psychiatry*.

Feizi, T., 1985, Demonstration by monoclonal antibodies that carbohydrate structures of glycoproteins and glycolipids are onco-developmental antigens, *Nature* 314:53.

Feizi, T., 1993, Carbohydrates and the pathogenesis of *Mycoplasma pneumoniae* infection and AIDS - some observations and speculations, *Clin. Infect. Dis.* 17(Suppl 1):S63.

Forrester, J.V. Immunological findings in diseases of the eye. In: *Clinical Neuroimmunology*, edited by Aarli, J.A. and Behan, P.O. Oxford: Blackwell, 1987, p. 291-312.

Gamboa, E.T.,Wolf, A., Yaho, M.D., Harter, D.H., and Duffy, P.E., 1974, Influenza virus antigen in post-encephalitic Parkinsonian brain, *Arch. Neurol.* 31:228.

Ganguli, R., Rabin, B.S.,Kelly, R.H., Lyte, M., and Ragu, U., 1987, Clinical and laboratory evidence of autoimmunity in acute schizophrenia, *Ann. N.Y. Acad. Sci.* 496:676.

Ganguli, R., Rabin, B.S.,and Brar, J.S., 1992, Antinuclear and gastric parietal cell antibodies in schizophrenic patients, *Biol. Psychiatr.* 32:35.

Ganguli, R., Rabin, B.S.,and McAllister, C.G., 1993a, CD5+ B-lymphocytes in schizophrenia: no alterations in numbers or percentages as compared with control subjects, *Psychiatry Res.* 48:69.

Ganguli, R., Brar, J.S.,Chengappa, K.N.R.,Yang, Z.W.,Nimgaonkar, V.L.,and Rabin, B.S.,1993b, Autoimmunity in schizophrenia: a review of recent findings, *Annals Med.* 25:489.

Gendelman, H.E., Wolinsky, J.S.,Johnson, R.T., Pressman, N.J.,Pezeshkpour, G.H., and Boisset, G.F., 1984, Measles encephalomyelitis: lack of evidence of viral invasion of the central nervous system and quantitative study of the nature of demyelination, *Ann. Neurol.* 15:353.

Gerlach, M., Riederer, P., Przuntek, H., and Youdin, M.B.H., 1991, MPTP: Mechanisms of neurotoxicity and their implications for Parkinson's disease, *Eur. J. Pharmacol.* 208:273.

Gibbs, C.J. and Gajdusek, D.C. Neurologic diseases of man with slow virus aetiology. In: *Membranes and Viruses in Immunopathology*, New York: Academic Press, 1972, p. 397-409.

Gluecksohn-Waelsch, S., 1957, The effect of maternal immunization against organ tissues on embryonic differentiation in the mouse, *J. Embryol. Exp. Morph.* 5:83.

Green, M.F.,Satz, P., Soper, H.V., and Kharibi, F., 1988, Relationship between physical anomalies and age at onset of schizophrenia, *Am. J. Psychiatr.* 144:666.

Gregersen, P.K., 1993, HLA associations with rheumatoid arthritis: A piece of the puzzle, *J. Rheumatol.* 19 Suppl 32:7.

Gregson, N.A.,Koblar, S., and Hughes, R.A.C., 1993, Antibodies to gangliosides in Guillain-Barre' syndrome: specificity and relationship to clinical features, *Quarterly J.Med.* 86:111.

Guntheroth, W.G., Lohmann, R., and Spiers, P.S., 1992, A seasonal association between SIDS deaths and kindergarten absences, *Public Health Reports* 107:319.

Gupte, S.C.,and Bhatia, H.M., 1980, Increased incidence of haemolytic disease of the new-born caused by ABO-incompatibility when tetanus toxoid is given during pregnancy, *Vox Sang.* 38:22.

Guldner, H.H., Szostecki, C., Grottzner, T., and Will, H., 1992, IFN enhance expression of Sp100, an autoantigen in primary biliary cirrhosis, *J. Immunol.* 149:4067.

Guy, J.D., Majorski, L.V., Wallace, C.J., and Guy, M.P., 1983, Peripheral tolerance as a multi-step mechanism, *Immunological Reviews* 133:93.

Hammerling, G.J., Schonrich, G., Ferber, I., and Arnold, B., 1993, Peripheral tolerance as a multi-step mechanism, *Immunological Reviews* 133:93.

Hancock, S.L., Cox, R.S., and McDougall, I.R., 1991, Thyroid disease after treatment of Hodgkin's disease, *New Engl. J. Med.* 325:599.

Harley, J.B., Scofield, R.H., Reichlin, M., 1992, Anti-Ro in Sjogren's syndrome and systemic lupus erythematosus, *Rheum. Dis. Clin. North America* 18:337.

Heath, R.G., McCarron, K.L., and O'Neil, C.E., 1990, Antiseptal brain antibody in IgG of schizophrenic patients, *Biol. Psychiatr.* 25:725.

Henneberg, A.E., Ruffert, S., Henneberg, H.J., and Kornhuber, H.H., 1993, Antibodies to brain tissue in sera of schizophrenic patients: preliminary findings, *Eur. Arch. Psyciatr. Clin. Neurosci.* 242:314.

Hill, A.V.S., Elvin, J., Willis, A.C., et al., 1993, Molecular analysis of the association of HLA-B53 and resistance to severe malaria, *Nature* 360:434.

Husmann, M., Roth, J., Kabat, E.A., Weisgerber, C., Frosch, M., and BitterSuermann, D., 1990, Immunohistochemical localization of polysialic acid in tissue sections: Differential binding to polynucleotides and DNA of a murine IgG and a human IgM monoclonal antibody, *J. Histochem. Cytochem.* 38:209.

Hussain, M., Wozniak, A.J., and Edelstein, M.B., 1993, Neurotoxicity of antineoplastic agents, *Critical Reviews in Oncology/Hematology* 14:61.

Huxley, J., Mayr, E., Osmond, H., and Hoffer, A., 1964, Schizophrenia as a genetic morphism, *Nature* 204, 4995:220.

Innes, A., Cunningham, C., Power, D.A., and Catto, G.R.D., 1989, Fetus as an allograft: Noncytotoxic maternal antibodies to HLA-linked paternal antigens, *American Journal of Reproductive Immunology* 19:146.

Jakob, H., and Beckman, H., 1986, Prenatal developmental disturbances in the limbic allocortex in schizophrenics, *J. Neural Transm.* 65:303.

Johnson, R.T., 1987, The pathogenesis of acute viral encephalitis and postinfectious encephalomyelitis, *J. Infect. Dis.* 155:359.

Jones, D.M., 1994, Influenza and meningococcal disease, *Lancet* 343:119.

Jones, P., and Murray, R.M., 1991, The genetics of schizophrenia is the genetics of neurodevelopment, *Brit. J. Psychiatry* 158:615.

Jonsson, S.A.T., 1991, Marriage rate and fertility in cycloid psychosis: Comparison with affective disorder, schizophrenia and the general population, *Eur. Arch. Psych. and Clin. Neurosci.* 241:119.

Kaldor, J., and Speed, R.B., 1984, Guillain-Barre syndrome and *Campylobacter jejuni*. *Brit. Med. J.* 288:1867.

Karpiak, S.E. and Rapport, M.M., 1975, Behavioral changes in 2-month old rats following prenatal exposure to antibodies against synaptic membranes, *Brain Res.* 92:405.

Kasarskis, E.J., Karpiak, S.E., Rapport, M.M., Yu, K., and Bass, N.H., 1981, Abnormal maturation of cerebral cortex and behavioral deficit in adult rats after neonatal administration of antibodies to ganglioside, *Dev. Brain Res.* 1:25.

Kaufmann, C.A., Weinberger, D.R., Stevens, J.R., et al., 1988, Intracerebral inoculation of experimental animals with brain tissue from patients with schizophrenia. Failure to observe consistent or specific behavioural and neuropathological effects, *Archives of General Psychiatry* 45:648.

Kemper, T.L., and Bauman, M.L., 1993, The contribution of neuropathologic studies to the understanding of autism, *Neurologic Clinics* 11:175.

Kendler, K.S. The genetics of schizophrenia: an overview. In: *Handbook of Schizophrenia*, edited by Tsuang, M.T. and Simpson, J.C. Amsterdam: Elsevier, 1988.

Kerwin, R., Patel, S., and Meldrum, B., 1990, Quantitative autoradiographic analysis of glutamate binding sites in the hippocampal formation in normal and schizophrenic brain post mortem, *Neuroscience* 39:25.

Khan, W.N., Hammarstrom, S., and Ramos, T., 1993, Expression of antigens of the carcinoembryonic antigen family on B cell lymphomas and Epstein-Barr virus immortalised B cell lines, *Int. Immunol.* 5:265.

Kilidireas, K., Latov, N., Strauss, D.H., et al., 1992, Antibodies to the human 60kDa heat-shock protein in patients with schizophrenia, *Lancet* 340:569.

King, D.J., and Cooper, S.J., 1989, Viruses, immunity and mental disorder, *Brit.J.Psychiatr.*154:1.

Kirch, D.G., Kaufmann, C.A., and Papadopoulos, N.M., 1985, Abnormal cerebrospinal fluid protein indices in schizophrenia, *Biol. Psychiatr.* 20:1039.

Kirch, D.G., Alexander, R.C., Suddath, R.L., et al., 1992, Blood-CSF barrier permeability and central nervous system immunoglobulin G in schizophrenia, *Journal of Neural Transmission* 89:219.

Kirch, D.G., 1993, Infection and autoimmunity as etiologic factors in schizophrenia: a review and reappraisal, *Schizophrenia. Bull.* 19:355.

Kirchlach, A.V., Fischer, E.G., and Kornhuber, H.H., 1987, Failure to detect dopamine receptor IgG autoantibodies in sera of schizophrenic patients, *J. Neural Transm.* 70:175.

Kirman, B.H. Immune reactions as a possible cause of hitherto unclassified encephalopathy and mental retardation In: *Proc. 3rd Congr. Int. Ass. Scientific Study of Mental Deficiency*, Warsaw: Polish Medical Publishers, 1975.

Kliks, S.C., Nisalak, A., Brandt, W.E., Wahl, L., and Burke, D.S., 1989, Antibody-dependent enhancement of dengue virus grown in human monocytes as a risk factor for dengue hemorrhagic fever, *Am. J. Trop. Med. Hyg.* 40:444.

Knight, A., Knight, J.G., Laing, P., and Adams, D.D., 1984, Co-existing thyroid and gastric autoimmune diseases are not due to crossreactive autoantibodies, *J. Clin Lab. Immunol.* 14:141.

Knight, J., Knight, A., and Pert, C.B., 1987, Is schizophrenia a virally triggered antireceptor autoimmune disease? *Biological Perspectives of Schizophrenia* (edited by H.Helmchen and F.A.Henn), 107.

Knight, J., Knight, A., and Ungvari, G., 1992, Can autoimmune mechanisms account for the genetic predisposition to schizophrenia? *Brit. J. Psych.* 160:533.

Knight, J.G., 1982a, Dopamine receptor stimulating autoantibodies: a possible cause of schizophrenia, *Lancet* ii:1073.

Knight, J.G. and Adams, D.D. The genetic basis of autoimmune disease. In: *Receptors, antibodies and disease*, edited by Evered, D. and Whelan, J. London: CIBA Foundation, 1982b, p. 35-56.

Knight, J.G., and Adams, D.D., 1978, Three genes for lupus nephritis in NZB x NZW mice, *J.Exp.Med.* 147:1653.

Knight, J.G., and Adams, D.D., 1982, The genetic basis of autoimmune disease, *Ciba Foundation Symposium* 90:35.

Knight, J.G., Knight, A. and Pert, C.B. Is schizophrenia a virally triggered antireceptor autoimmune disease?. In: *Biological Perspectives of Schizophrenia*, edited by Helmchen, H. and Henn, F.A.New York: Wiley, 1987, p. 107-127.

Knight, J.G., Knight, A., Menkes, D.B., and Mullen, P.E., 1990, Autoantibodies against brain septal region antigens specific to unmedicated schizophrenia, *Biological Psychiatry* 28:467.

Komminoth, P., Roth, J., Lackie, P.M., BittersSuermann, D., and Heitz, P.U., 1991, Polysialic acid of the neural cell adhesion molecule distinguishes small cell lung carcinoma from carcinoids, *Am. J. Pathol.* 139:297.

Koren, E., Reichlin, , M.W., Koscec, M., Fugate, R.D., and Reichlin, M., 1992, Autoantibodies to the ribosomal P proteins react with a plasma-membrane related target on human cells, *J.Clin.Invest.* 89:1236.

Koskiniemi, M., 1993, CNS manifestations associated with Mycoplasma pneumoniae infections: Summary of cases at the University of Helsinki and review, *Clinical Infectious Diseases* 17:S52.

Kowalski, M., Ardman, B., Basiripour, L., Blohm, D., Haseltine, W. and Sodroski, J., 1989, Antibodies to CD4 in individuals infected with human immunodeficiency virus type-1, *Proc.Natl.Acad.Sci.(USA)* 86:3346.

Krog, L., and Bock, E., 1992, Glycosylation of neural cell adhesion molecules of the immunoglobulin superfamily, *APMIS.* 100:53.

Laing, P., Knight, J.G., Hill, J.M., et al., 1989, Influenza viruses induce autoantibodies to a 37 kDa brain-specific protein in rabbit, *Proc. Natl. Acad. Sci. (USA)* 86:1998.

Licinio, J., Seibyl, J.P., Altemus, M., Charney, D.S., and Krystal, J.H., 1993, Elevated CSF levels of interleukin-2 in neuroleptic-free schizophrenia patients, *Am. J. Psychiatry* 150:1408.

Lieberman, J.A., Yunis, J., Egea, E., Canoso, R.T., Kane, J.M., and Yunis, E.J., 1990, HLA B38,DR4,DQw3 and clozapine induced agranulocytosis in Jewish patients with schizophrenia, *Arch. Gen. Psychiatr.* 47:945.

Linde, A., 1992, Diagnosis and pathogenesis of infectious mononucleosis and other EBV associated diseases, *Rev.in Med. Micro.* 3:43.

Lindstrom, J., Shelton, D., and Fujii, Y., 1988, Myasthenia gravis, *Adv. Immunol.* 42:233.

243

Linington, C., Berger, T., Perry, L., et al., 1993, T-cells specific for myelin oligodendrocyte glycoprotein mediate an unusual autoimmune inflammatory response in the central nervous system, *Eur. J. Immunol.* 230:1364.

Lock, C.B., Parkes, J.D. and Welsh, K.I. Narcolepsy and immunity. In: *Clinical Neuroimmunology*, edited by Aarli, J.A. and Behan, P.O. Oxford: Blackwell, 1987, p. 404-420.

Loza-Tulimowska, M., Semkow, R., Michalak, T., and Nowoslawski, A., 1976, Autoantibodies in sera of influenza patients, *Acta Virol.* 20:202.

Ludgate, M., Dong, Q., Dreyfus, P.A., et al., 1989, Definition, at the molecular level, of a thyroglobulin-acetylcholinesterase shared epitope: study of its pathophysiological significance in patients with Graves' opthalmopathy, *Autoimmunity* 3:167.

Marini, A.M., Fridman, R., Kanemoto, T., Martin, G.R., Guo, Y., and Passaniti, A., 1992, The neurotoxin 1-methyl-4-phenylpyridinium: A selective cytostatic agent in small-cell lung cancer cell lines with neuroendocrine properties, *J. Natl. Cancer Inst.* 84:1582.

Mason, D., 1991, Genetic variation in the stress response: susceptibility to experimental allergic encephalomyelitis and implications for human inflammatory disease, *Immunol. Today* 12:57.

McAllister, C.G., Rapaport, M.H., Pickar, D., et al., 1989, Increased numbers of CD5+ B-lymphocytes in schizophrenic patients, *Arch. Gen. Psychiatr.* 46:890.

McGregor, J.A., Burns, J.C., Levin, M.J., Burlington, B., and Meiklejohn, G., 1984, Transplacental passage of influenza A/Bangkok (H3N2) mimicking amniotic fluid infection syndrome, *Am. J. Obstet. Gynecol.* 149:856.

McGuffin, P. and Stuart, E., 1986, Genetic markers in schizophrenia. *Hum. Hered.* 36:65.

McMichael, A.J., Ting, A., Zweerink, H.J, and Askonas, B.A., 1977, HLA restriction of cell-mediated lysis of influenza virus-infected human cells, *Nature* 270:524.

McNeil, H.P., Chesterman, C.N., and Krilis, S.A., 1991, Immunology and clinical importance of antiphospholipid antibodies, *Adv. Immunol.* 49:193.

McNeil, T.F., 1991, Obstetric complications in schizophrenic patients, *Schiz. Res.* 5:89.

Mednick, S.A., Machon, R.A., Huttenen, M.O. and Bonnet, D., 1988, Adult schizophrenia following prenatal exposure to an influenza epidemic, *Arch. Gen. Psychiatr.* 45:189.

Menninger, K.A., 1928, The schizophrenic syndrome as a product of acute infectious disease, *Arch. Neurol. Psychiatr.* 20:464.

Milich, D.R., Jones, J., Hughs, J., and Maruyama, T., 1993, Role of T-cell tolerance in the persistence of hepatitis-B virus infection, *J. Immunotherapy* 14:226.

Miyanaga, K., Machiyama, Y., and Juji, T., 1984, Schizophrenic disorders and HLA-DR antigens, *Biol. Psychiatry* 19:121.

Montplaisir, J., and Poirier, G., 1987, Narcolepsy in monozygotic twins and non-genetic factors in narcolepsy, *5th Int. Congr. Sleep Res.* 401:1.

Mukherjee, S., and Schnur, D.B., 1989, Family history of type 2 diabetes in schizophrenic patients, *Lancet.* ii:495.

Mullis, K.B., and Faloona, F.A., 1987, Specific synthesis of DNA *in vitro* via a polymerase-catalysed chain reaction, *Meth. Enzymol.* 155:335.

Munro, D.S., Dirmikis, S.M., Humphries, H., Smith, T., and Broadhead, G.D., 1978, The role of thyroid stimulating immunoglobulins of Graves' disease in neonatal thyrotoxicosis, *Brit. J. Obst. and Gyn.* 85:849.

Murphy, B.R. and Webster, R.G. Orthomyxoviruses. In: *Virology*, edited by Fields, B.N., Knipe, D.M. and et al. New York: Raven Press, 1990, p. 1091-1152.

Nasrallah, H.A., McCalley-Whitters, M., Bigelow, L.B., and Rauscher, F.P., 1983, A histological study of the corpus callosum in chronic schizophrenia, *Psych. Res.* 8:251.

Nedelec, J., Boucraut, J., Garnier, J.M., Bernard, D., and Rougon, G., 1990, Evidence for autoimmune antibodies directed against neural cell adhesion molecules (N-CAM) in patients with group B meningitis. *J. Neuroimmunol.* 29:49.

Nelson, J.L., Hughes, K.A., Smith, A.G., Nisperos, B.B., Branchaud, A.M., and Hansen, J.A., 1993, Maternal-fetal disparity in HLA class II alloantigens and the pregnancy-induced amelioration of rheumatoid arthritis, *N. Engl. J. Med.* 329:466.

Nepom, G.T., 1988, Genetics and disease association of the major histocompatibility complex, *Curr. Op. Immunol.* 1:107.

Nimgaonkar, V.L., Ganguli, R., Rudert, W.A., Vavassori, C., Rabin, B.S., and Trucco, M., 1993, A negative association of schizophrenia with an allele of the HLA DQB1 gene among African Americans *Schizophrenia Res.* 8:199.

Nojima, Y., Minota, S., Yamada, A., Takaku, F., Aotsuka, S., and Yokahari, R., 1992, Correlation of antibodies to ribosomal P protein with psychosis in patients with systemic lupus erythematosus, *Ann. Rheum. Dis.* 51:1053.

Nowakowski, R.S., 1988, Development of the hippocampal formation in mutant mice, *Drug Dev. Res.* 15:315.

Ohno, S., 1991, Many peptide fragments of alien antigens are homologous with host proteins, thus canalizing T-cell responses, *Proc. Natl. Acad. Sci.* 88:3065.

Olerup, O., Schaffer, M., Hillest, J., and Sanders, C., 1990, The narcolepsy associated DR15, DQ6, DW2 haplotype has no unique HLA-DQalpha or DQbeta restriction fragments, and does not extend to the HLA-DP subregion, *Immunogenetics.* 32:41.

Omdal, R., and Roalso, S., 1992, Chorea gravidarum and chorea associated with oral contraceptives -diseases due to antiphospholipid antibodies, *Acta Neurologica Scand.* 86:219.

Oskenberg, J.R., Begovich, A.B., Erlich, H.A., and Steinman, L., 1993, Genetic factors in multiple sclerosis, *J. Amer. Med. Assn.* 270:2362.

Osuga, T., Murishima, T., Hanada, N., Nishikawa, K., Isobe, K., and Watanabe, K., 1992, Transfer of specific IgG and IgG subclasses to herpes simplex virus across the blood-brain barrier in preterm and term newborns, *Acta Paediatrica.* 81:792.

Papazian, O., 1992, Transient neonatal myasthenia gravis, *J. Child Neurol.* 7:135.

Parkes, J.D. Narcolepsy and the hypersomnias. In: *Sleep Disorders,* edited by Herne, J.A. and Page, M.L. Southampton: Duphar, 1989, p. 40-45.

Pert, C.B., Knight, J.G., Laing, P., and Markwell, M.A.K., 1988, Scenarios for a viral etiology of schizophrenia, *Schizophrenia Bull.* 14:243.

Pfister, G.M., Hanson, D.R., Roerig, J.L., Landbloom, R., and Popkin, M.K., 1992, Clozapine induced agranulocytosis in a native American: HLA typing and further support for an immune-mediated mechanism, *J. Clin. Psychiatr.* 53:242.

Pinto-Lord, M.C., Evrard, P., and Caviness, V.S., 1982, Obstructed neuronal migration along radial glial fibres in the neocortex of the Reeler mouse: a Golgi-EM analysis, *Dev. Brain Res.* 4:379.

Posner, J.B., 1992, Pathogenesis of central-nervous-system paraneoplastic syndromes, *Revue Neurologique.* 148:pp502.

Rabin, B.S., and Ganguli, R., 1991, Elevated IgG and IgM anticardiolipin antibodies in a subgroup of medicated and unmedicated schizophrenic patients, *Biol. Psychiatr.* 30:731.

Rakonczay, Z., Hammond, P., and Brimijoin, S., 1993, Lesion of central cholinergic systems by systemically administered acetylcholinesterase antibodies in newborn rats, *Neuroscience.* 54:225.

Ramphal, R., Donelly, W.H., and Small, P.A.Jr., 1980, Fatal influenzal pneumonia in pregnancy: failure to demonstrate transplacental transmission of influenza virus, *Am. J. Obstet. Gynecol.* 138:348.

Ravenholt, R.T., and Foege, V.H., 1982, Influenza, encephalitis lethargica and Parkinsonism, *Lancet.* ii:860. Rick, J.T., Gregson, A., Adinolphi, M., and Liebowitz, S., 1981, The behaviour of immature and mature rats exposed prenatally to anti-ganglioside antibodies, *J. Neuroimmunol.* 1:413.

Rick, J.T., Gregson, A., Adinolphi, M., and Liebowitz, S., 1981, The behaviour of immature and mature rats exposed prenatally to anti-ganglioside antibodies, *J. Neuroimmunol.* 1:413.

Riley, E., and Olerup, O., 1992, HLA polymorphisms and evolution, *Immunol. Today.* 13:333.

Ritsner, M., Sherina, O., and Ginath, Y., 1992, Genetic epidemiological study of schizophrenia: Reproduction behaviour, *Acta Psychiatrica Scandinavia.* 85:423.

Roberts, G.W., and Bruton, C.J., 1990, Notes from the graveyard: neuropathology and schizophrenia, *Neuropathol. Applied Neurobiol.* 16:3.

Roberts, G.W., 1990, Schizophrenia: the cellular biology of a functional psychosis, *Trends in Neuroscience.* 13:207.

Roitt, I.M. Autoimmune diseases. In: *Essential Immunology,* London: Blackwell, 1988, p. 254-273.

Rudduck, C., Beckman, L., Franzen, G., Jacobssen, L., and Lindstrom, L., 1985, Complement factor C4 in schizophrenia, *Hum. Heredity.* 35:223.

Rushton, D.I., Collie, M.H., Sweet, C., Husseini, R.H., and Smith, H., 1983, The effects of maternal influenza viraemia in late gestation on the conceptus of the pregnant ferret, *J. Pathol.* 140:181.

Safranek, T.J., Lawrence, D.N., Kurland, L.T., et al., 1991, Reassessment of the association between Guillain-Barre syndrome and receipt of swine influenza vaccine in 1976-1977: Results of a two-state study, *Am. J. Epidemiol.* 133:940.

Schneebaum, A.B., Singleton, J.D., West, S.G., and et al., 1991, Association of psychiatric manifestations with antibodies to ribosomal-P proteins in systemic lupus erythematosus, *Am. J. Med.* 90:54.

Sham, P.C., Maclean, C.J., and Kendler, K.S., 1993, Risk of schizophrenia and age difference with older siblings: evidence for a maternal viral infection hypothesis, *Brit. J. Psychiatr.* 163:627.

Shaw, S.Y., Larusen, R.A., and Lees, M.B., 1986, Analogous amino acid sequences in myelin proteolipid and viral proteins, *FEBS Lett.* 207:266.

Sherman, G.F., Galaburda, A.M., and Geschwind, N., 1985, Cortical anomalies in brains of New-Zealand mice - a neuropathologic model of dyslexia, *Proc. Natl. Acad. Sci. (USA).* 82:8072.

Sherman, G.F., Morrison, L., Rosen, G.D., Behan, P.O., and Galaburda, A.M., 1990, Brain abnormalities in immune defective mice, *Brain Res.* 532:25.

Shima, S., Yano, K., Sugiura, M., and Tokunaga, Y., 1991, Anticerebral antibodies in functional psychoses, *Biol. Psychiatr.* 29:322.

Silver, M.L., Guo, H.C., Strominger, J.L., and Wiley, D.C., 1992, Atomic structure of a human MHC molecule presenting an influenza virus peptide, *Nature.* 360:367.

Sirota, P., Firer, M.A., Schild, K., et al., 1993a, Autoantibodies to DNA in multicase families with schizophrenia, *Biol. Psychiatr.* 33:450.

Sirota, P., Firer, M., Schild, K., et al., 1993b, Increased anti-Sm antibodies in schizophrenic patients and their families, *Prog. in Neuro-Psychopharmacol. and Biol. Psychiatr.* 17:792.

Spillane, J.D., and Wells, C.E.C., 1964, The neurology of Jennerian vaccination, *Brain.* 87:1.

Spivak, B., Radwan, M., Brandon, J., et al., 1991, Cold agglutinin autoantibodies in psychiatric patients: their relation to diagnosis and pharmacological treatment, *Am. J. Psychiatry.* 148:244.

Steinman, L., 1993, Autoimmune disease, *Scientific American.* Sept.:74.

Stevens, J.R., 1982, Neuropathology of schizophrenia, *Archives of General Psychiatry.* 39:1131.

Stevens, J.R., 1988, Schizophrenia and multiple sclerosis, *Schizophreia Bulletin.* 14:231.

Stevens, J.R., Papadopoulos, N.M., and Resnick, M., 1990, Oligoclonal bands in acute schizophrenia: a negative search, *Acta Psychiatrica Scandinavia.* 81:262.

Stirrat, G.M. The immunology of diseases of pregnancy. In: *Immunology of Pregnancy and its Disorders*, edited by Stern, C.S. Kluwer: Dodrecht, 1989, p. 143-164.

Sugiura, M., Tokunaga, Y., Maruyama, S., Ishido, S., Yokoi, Y., and Sasaki, K., 1989, Detection of anti-cerebral autoantibodies in schizophrenia and Alzheimer's disease *J. Clin. Lab. Immunol.* 28:1.

Sulkava, R., Rissanen, A., and Pyhala, R., 1981, Post-influenzal encephalitis during the influenza A outbreak in 1979/80, *J. Neurol. Neurosurg. Psychiatr.* 44:161.

Tadmor, B., Putterman, C., and Naparstek, Y., 1992, Embryonal germ layer antigens: Target for autoimmunity, *Lancet* 339:975.

Tiwari, J.L. and Terasaki, P.I., 1985. HLA and Disease Associations, Springer-Verlag, New York:

Todd, I. and Bottazzo, G.F. HLA Expression and Autoimmunity. In: *Molecular Bases of Human Diseases*, edited by Polli, E.E.: Elsevier Science Publishers, 1993, p. 51-58.

Todd, J.A., 1990, Genetic control of autoimmunity in type 1 diabetes, *Immunol. Today.* 11:122.

Torrey, E.F., 1973, Slow and latent viruses in schizophrenia, *Lancet.* 2:22.

Torrey, E.F., 1988, Stalking the schizovirus, *Schizophrenia Bulletin.* 14:223.

Varner, M.W., 1991, Autoimmune disorders and pregnancy, *Seminars in Perinatology.* 15:238.

Villemain, F., Magnin, M., Feuillet Fieux, M.N., and Bach, J.F., 1988, Anti-histone antibodies in schizophrenia and affective disorders, *Psychiatr. Res.* 24:53.

Vincent, A., Lang, B., and Newsom-Davis, J., 1989, Autoimmunity to the voltage-gated calcium channel underlies the Lambert-Eaton myasthenic syndrome, *Trends in Neurosciences.* 12:496.

Vogel, F. and Motulsky, A.G. Natural selection. In: *Human Genetics*, Berlin: Springer Verlag, 1986, p. 433-511.

Warren, R.P., Singh, V.K., Cole, P., et al., 1991, Increased frequency of the null allele at the complement C4B locus in autism, *Clinical and Experimental Immunology.* 83:438.

White, J.M., and Littman, D.R., 1989, Viral receptors of the immunoglobulin superfamily, *Cell.* 56:725.

Wilcox, J.A., and Nasrallah, H.A., 1987, Childhood head trauma and psychosis, *Psychiatric Res.* 21:303.

Wright, P., Murray, R.M., Ronaldson, P.T., and Underhill, J.A., 1993, Do maternal HLA antigens predispose to schizophrenia? *Lancet.* 342:117.

Wright, P., Murray, R.M., Ronaldson, P.T., and Underhill, J.A., 1993, Do maternal HLA antigens predispose to schizophrenia? *Lancet* 342:117.

Yawn, D.H., Pyeatte, J.C., Joseph, J.M., Eichler, S.L., and Garcie-Bunuel, R., 1971, Transplacental transfer of influenza virus, *J. American Med. Assoc.* 216:1022.

Yoss, R.E., and Daly, D.D., 1960, Hereditary aspects of narcolepsy, *Trans. Am. Neurol. Assoc.* 85:239.

Youngson, C., Nurse, C., Yeger, H., and Cutz, E., 1993, Oxygen sensing airway chemoreceptors, *Nature.* 365:153.

PARTICIPANTS

Dr. Christopher Barr
Social Science Research Institute
University of Southern California
Los Angeles, California 90089-1111
USA

Dr. Helmut Beckmann
Department of Psychiatry
University of Wuertzburg
15 Fuechslienstrasse
8700 Wuertzburg, Germany

Robert M. Bilder
Hillside Hospital, Long Island Jewish
        Medical Center
Albert Einstein College of Medicine
Glen Oaks, New York 11004, USA

Dr. Anna Bonfanti
Psychiatric Branch
Department of Biomedical and
        Technological Sciences
DSNP-H.S. Raffaele
Via Prinetti 29
10127 Milano, Italy

Dr. N.J. Brandt
Rigshospitalet, Section of Clinical
        Genetics, 4062
Blegdamsvej 9, DK-2100
Copenhagen, Denmark

Dr. Patricia Brennan
Social Science Research Institute
University of Southern California
Los Angeles, California 90089-1111
USA

Dr. Giovanna Calabrese
Psychiatric Branch
Department of Biomedical and
        Technological Sciences
Instituto Scientifico
DSNP-HS Raffaele
Via Prinetti 29
20127 Milano, Italy

Dr. Robert Cancro
Department of Psychiatry
New York University Medical Center
550 First Avenue
New York, New York 10016, USA

Dr. Tyrone Cannon
University of Pennsylvania
Department of Psychology
3815 Walnut Street
Philadelphia, Pennsylvania 19104
USA

Dr. Jimsie Cutbush
Prince Charles Hospital
Rode Road
Brisbane, Queensland
Australia

Dr. Rudolf Cohen
Universitat Konstanz
Sozialwissenschaftliche
    Fakultat
Postfach 5560-D-7750
Konstanz 1, Germany

Cristina B. Colombo, M.D.
Psychiatric Branch, Department of
Biomedical and Technological Sciences
Instituto Scientifico
HS Raffaele, Via Prinetti 29
20127 Milano, Italy

Dr. David Cotter
Saint John of God Hospital
Cluain Mhuire Family Centre
Newtownpark Avenue
Blackrock, County Dublin
Ireland

Karen Dykes
Social Science Research Institute
University of Southern California
Los Angeles, California 90089-1111
USA

Dr. Jonas Eberhard
Department of Neurology
Roskiloe AMP
Sygehus 4000
Rioskilde, Denmark

Gabriel A. de Erausquin, M.D., Ph.D.
Department of Veterans Affairs
        Medical Center
950 Campbell Avenue
West Haven, Connecticut 06516
USA

Mr. Savas Erdogan
Psychiatry Specialist
Anicara Numune State Hospital
Iller Sokak No. 3 1/2
Mebusevleri
Tandogan, Turkey

Dr. F. Sibel Ertan
Department of Neurology
Cerrahpasa Medical School
University of Istanbul
Istanbul, Turkey

Mr. Turan Ertan, M.D.
Department of Psychiatry
Cerrahpasa Medical Faculty
University Istanbul
Istanbul, Turkey

Julie Evans
London Guild Hall University
Calcutta House
Old Castle Street
London E17 NT, United Kingdom

Lisa Eyler-Zorrilla
University of Pennsylvania
Department of Psychiatry
3815 Walnut Street
Philadelphia, Pennsylvania 19104-6196
USA

Karen Finello, Ph.D.
High Risk Infant Project
Los Angeles County/USC
        Medical Center
5828 Temple City Blvd., Suite 2
Temple City, California 91780

Dr. Anders Fink-Jensen
Pharmaceuticals Division
Novo Nordisk A/s
Novo Nordisk Park
DK 2760 Malov, Denmark

Kirsten Fleming, Ph.D.
National Institute of Mental Health
2700 Martin Luther King, S.E.
Washington, DC 20032, USA

Dr. Orsola Gambini
H.S. Raffaele
Instituto Di Ricovero E Cura
A Carattere, Scientifico
Via Prinetti 29
20127 Milano, Italy

Dr. Joseph Gogos, M.D., Ph.D.
Department of Cellular and
    Developmental Biology
Harvard University
16 Divinity Avenue
Cambridge, Massachusetts 02128
USA

Dr. Gamyanka Guetova
Institute of Physiology
Dept. Exp. Pharmacology
Bontchev str. bl. 23
1113 Sofia, Bulgaria

Ms. Meggin Hollister
Social Science Research Institute
University of Southern California
Los Angeles, California 90089-1111
USA

Dr. Istvan Horvath
KICLM Organizing Committee
Institute for Psychology
Budapest, Pf. 398
Hungary 1394

Dr. Matti Huttunen
Department of Psychiatry
University of Helsinki
Lapinlahdentie, SF 00180
Helsinki 18
Finland

Dr. Edward Jones
Department of Anatomy and
    Neurobiology
University of California, Irvine
317 Med. Surg. II
Irvine, California 92717 USA

Peter B. Jones
Genetics Section
Institute of Psychiatry
De Crespigny Park
Denmark Hill
London SE5 8AF
United Kingdom

Dr. Sven Jonsson
University of Lund
Department of Psychiatry and
    Neurochemistry
PO Box 638
S-220 09 Lund, Sweden

Dr. Guilla Jonsson
University of Lund
Department of Psychiatry and
    Neurochemistry
PO Box 638
S-220 09 Lund, Sweden

Ms. Maria Karayiorgou
Center for Cancer Research
Massachusetts Institute of Technology
77 Massachusetts Avenue
Cambridge, Massachusetts 02139-4307
USA

Dr. Britt af Klinteberg
Department of Psychology
University of Stockholm
S-106-91 Stockholm, Sweden

Mr. Ersin Koylu, M.D.
Ege University, School of Medicine
Dept. of Physiology
35100 Bornova
Izmir, Turkey

Dr. Peter Laing
University Hospital
Queens Medical Center
Nottingham NG7 2UH
United Kingdom

Dr. Bengt Lögdberg
University of Lund
Department of Neuropathology
Solvegatan 25
S-223 62 Lund
Sweden

Dr. Melvin Lyon
Department of Psychiatry and
      Behavioral Sciences
University of Arkansas for Medical
      Sciences
4301 West Marham, Mail Slot 554
Little Rock, Arkansas 72205-7199
USA

Dr. William McClure
Biological Sciences
LAS - Natural Sciences & Math
University of Southern California
Los Angeles, California 90089-2520
USA

Mr. John McGrath
Clinical Studies Unit
Wolston Park Hospital
WACOL Q 4076
Australia

Dr. Ricardo Machón
Social Science Research Institute
University of Southern California
Los Angeles, California 90089-1111
USA

Dr. Athanasios Maras
Central Institute of Mental Health
PO Box 122120
68072 Mannheim, Germany

Dr. Sarnoff A. Mednick
Social Science Research Institute
University of Southern California
Los Angeles, California 90089-1111
USA

Prof. Herbert Y. Meltzer
Case Western Reserve University
2040 Abington Road
Cleveland, Ohio 44109 USA

Dr. Robin Murray
Professor of Psychological Medicine
King's College Hospital and the
      Institute of Psychiatry
De Crespigny Park
London SE5 8AF, United Kingdom

William T. O'Connor
Department of Pharmacology
Karolinska Institute, Box 60-400
Stockholm, S104-01, Sweden

Stephen C. Olson, M.D.
Department of Psychiatry
The Ohio State University College of
      Medicine
473 West 12th Avenue
Columbus, Ohio 43210-1228 USA

Dr. Adrian Raine
Department of Psychology
University of Southern California
Los Angeles, California 90089-1061
USA

Dr. Birgitte Reinholdt
Institute for Preventive Medicine
Psykiatrisk Afdeling
1399 Copenhagen K, Denmark

Dr. Fred Rist
Central Institute of Mental Health
Box 122120
68072 Mannheim, Germany

Dr. A. Rossi
Cattedra de Clinica Psichiatrica
      dell' Universita de L'Aquila
c/o Ospedale S. Maria di Collemaggio
67100 L'Aquila, Italy

Dr. Ratna Sircar
Dept. of Psychiatry - F109
Albert Einstein College of Medicine
1300 Morris Park Avenue
Bronx, New York 10461
USA

Neil R. Smalheiser, M.D., Ph.D.
Joseph P. Kennedy, Jr. Mental
        Retardation Research Center
University of Chicago
Department of Pediatrics
5841 South Maryland Avenue, Box 413
Chicago, Illinois 60637 USA

Ms. Susan Stack
Social Science Research Institute
University of Southern California
Los Angeles, California 90089-1111
USA

Dr. Paolo Stratta
Cattedra de Clinica Psichiatrica
        dell' Universita de L'Aquila
c/o Ospedale S. Maria di Collemaggio
67100 L'Aquila
Italy

Dr. Kay Thomas
Faculty of Law
Queensland University of Technology
Locked Bag 2, Post Office, Red Hill
Queensland 4059, Australia

Dr. P. Tienari
Department of Psychiatry
University of Oulu
Kajaanintie 43
SF-90220 Oulu, Finland

Dr. Harry Uylings
Netherlands Institute for Brain Research
Meibergdreef 33
1105 AZ Amsterdam ZO
The Netherlands

Dr. Francis Varghese
University of Queensland
Department of Psychiatry
Princess Alescandra Hospital
Ipswich Road
Brisbane, Queensland, Australia

Dr. Peter Venables
University of York
C/o Derwent Cottage
Newton-on-Derwent
York YO4 5DA, United Kingdom

Dr. John Waddington
Royal College of Surgeons in Ireland
Department of Clinical Pharmacology
123, St. Stephen's Green
Dublin 2, Ireland

Dr. Edgar Williams
University of Southern California
Department of Educational Psychology
Los Angeles, California 90089-0031

Dr. Mary L. Williams
Long Beach City College
520-103 Chelsea Court
Long Beach, California 90803 USA

INDEX

Environment 13, 14, 27, 101, 121, 171
  abnormal 17
  autoimmune uterine 231
  environmental confounders 120
  environmental determinants 170
  environmental factors 7, 33, 44, 61, 62,
    117-120, 124, 128, 132, 170
  environmental injury 147
  environmental insult 4, 23, 62
  environmental medicine 117
  environmental stressors 61, 62
  fetal 231
  gene/environment interaction 186
  in utero 7
  maternal 21
  rearing 167
Erlenmeyer-Kimling, L. 152
Ernhart, C.B. 121, 128
Eyler-Zorrilla, M.A. 4, 57, 66
Fahy, T.A. 204
Falkai, P. 2, 3, 29, 32, 73, 74, 85, 89, 131,
    145
Fananas, L. 218
Feenstra, A. 223
Feighner, J.P.
  Feighner Criteria 181, 183
Feinberg, I. 41
Feizi, V. 233
Ferm, T.H. 123
Fine, P.E.M. 151
Fish, B. 5, 28, 45, 145, 152, 167
Fisman, M. 131
Flechsig, P. 40
Flor-Henry, P. 71, 73, 74
Foerster, A. 166, 209
Fohrman, E.B. 144
Forrester, J.V. 219, 224
Fraser, F.C. 15, 16, 22, 229
Friauf, E. 34, 41
Frith, C.D. 106, 111
Frost, D.O. 39
Gaffney, G.R. 132
Galaburda, A.M. 33, 34, 71, 86, 88, 231
Gamboa, E.T. 225
Ganguli, R. 217, 219, 220
García, I. 147
Garcia-Rill, E. 109
Gendelman, H.E. 223
Gender 159, 162
  differences in effect of teratologic
    insult 19
  effect and prevalence of SBAs 59
  effect of hormones 22
  in results of holeboard testing 100
Genetic 14, 18-24, 33, 45, 47, 48, 59,
    61-63, 88, 182-184, 196, 199
  basis 232
  determinants 190
  determination 170, 180, 216, 217, 231,
    232

  effects in teratogenicity 15
  factors 118, 132, 167, 170, 185, 187,
    216
  heterogeneity 186
  high risk children 152
  linkage 187
  mechanisms 232
  mutations 232
  ontogenetic 28, 44, 45, 47, 48
  pathogenetic mechanisms involving
    primary lesions 146
  phylo-ontogenetic 122, 123
  predisposition 7, 13, 169, 191, 196,
    214-217, 219, 228, 237
  protective effects 178
  risk 6, 64, 65, 68, 85, 96, 184, 185, 191
  risk factors in an etiological model 4
  studies 219
  versus sporadic cases 185
  vulnerability 196
Genetics 17, 215, 237
  in teratology and neurodevelopment 2
Gerber, B.B. 122
Gerlach, M. 98-100, 103, 106, 111, 235
Geschwind, N. 71, 73, 86, 88
Ghafour, S.Y. 121, 126
Gibbs, C.J. 223
Gibson, J.L. 123
Giguere, M. 34
Gilani, S.H. 121
Gilles, F.H. 95, 96, 107
Girault, J.A. 139, 140
Gittleman-Klein, R. 152
Glick, S.D. 106
Gliosis 29, 131
  absence of as a form of disturbance 3
  and dysplasia 2
  cytoarchitectural disturbances 3
Gluecksohn-Waelsch, S. 230
Godfrey, K.M. 151
Goldman-Rakic, P.S. 38, 41, 43, 44
Goldstein, G.W. 122, 126
Goldstein, L. 15
Goodman, R. 75
Gosh, A. 46
Gottesman, I.I. 7, 61, 62, 177
Gould, E. 109
Graham, J.M. 44
Grant, L.D. 126
Green, M.F. 6, 232, 233
Greenamyre, J.T. 140
Gregersen, P.K. 217
Gregg, N. 15, 22, 119
Gregson, N.A. 223
Griesinger, W. 177
Grinker, R.R. 183
Grüsser, O.J. 28
Gualtieri, C.T. 6
Gunther, W. 40
Guntheroth, W.G. 236